SPECIAL TOPICS IN CARDIAC SURGERY

Edited by **Cuneyt Narin**

INTECHWEB.ORG

Special Topics in Cardiac Surgery
Edited by Cuneyt Narin

Published by InTech
Janeza Trdine 9, 51000 Rijeka, Croatia

Publishing Process Manager Molly Kaliman
Technical Editor Teodora Smiljanic
Cover Designer InTech Design Team

First published February, 2012
Printed in Croatia

A free online edition of this book is available at www.intechopen.com
Additional hard copies can be obtained from orders@intechweb.org

Special Topics in Cardiac Surgery, Edited by Cuneyt Narin
p. cm.
ISBN 978-953-51-0148-2

Contents

Preface

The perioperative period is vitally important in outcomes of patients undergoing cardiac surgery. The proper evaluation of preoperative period, as well as improvement in standards of perioperative care of these patients have been helping to reduce mortality and morbidity rates following the cardiac surgery. Accordingly, the content of present textbook mainly covers various topics related to perioperative period in cardiac surgery. In order to organize the content, two books have been created. The first book focuses on topics both in preoperative and early postoperative periods of cardiac surgery. The book covers not only classical chapters such as anesthesia for pediatric heart surgery and management of pulmonary hypertension in intensive care unit, but also currently "hot" topics consisting of strategies of blood conversation and heparin induced thrombocytopenia. The second book covers miscellaneous issues such as fungal endocarditis after cardiac surgery, off pump versus on pump coronary artery bypass surgery and arrhythmia after cardiac surgery.

This book should prove to be a useful reference for trainees, senior surgeons and nurses in cardiac surgery, as well as anesthesiologists, perfusionists, and all the related health care workers who are involved in taking care of patients with heart disease which require surgical therapy.

This book aims to improve the knowledge and understanding of readers with regard to the background of perioperative period in cardiac surgery.

I hope these internationally cumulative and diligent efforts will provide patients undergoing cardiac surgery with meticulous perioperative care methods.

Numerous international authors have participated in the creation of this book. I have compiled their valuable experiences and contributions about critical issues in the field of cardiac surgery.

I greatly acknowledge the precious assistance of Ms. Molly Kaliman of InTech Publisher. I also would like to thank Ilker Kiris, MD, for his productive ideas in the course of preparing this book.

Finally, upcoming decades should see even greater advances in the field of care of patients undergoing cardiac surgery. I assure that improvements in technologies and surgical skills will help to accomplish this goal.

To my wife, Gokce and to our children, Kaya and Kayra.

Assoc. Prof. Cuneyt Narin, MD
Department of Cardiovascular Surgery,
Selcuk University Meram Medical School, Konya,
Turkey

1

Intensive Care Management of Patients in the First 24 Hours After Cardiac Surgery

Villalobos J. A. Silva, Aguirre J. Sanchez, Martinez J. Sanchez,
Franco J. Granillo and Garcia T. Zenón
Universidad Nacional Autónoma de México (UNAM), Tamaulipas
México

1. Introduction

The cardiac surgery continues having a fundamental roll in the therapeutic arsenal of many heart deseases in spite of the spectacular advances that determined drugs or different forms of interventionist cardiology have experimented during the past few years. The present impact of the heart surgery is due to the constant increase of the cardiovascular risk factors, related to the increase in the life expectancy in last the three decades, the clinical approach of the ischemic cardiopathy towards the repair has taken to the creation and development of techniques and methods at the moment used in the miocardic revascularization surgery; the roll of the coronary surgery initiated by Sabiston in 1962 and popularized by Favaloro in 1967 has had an exponential development with the purpose of to exclude the ill part from the artery by placing a bypass to improve the perfusion of the ischemic area. Nevertheless the other side of the balance is the pharmacological treatment whose objective is to look for the balance between the supply and demands in the ischemic scope at the expense of a smaller consumption of oxygen (VO2), diminution of the inflammatory local metabolism, control of trombotics phenomena, etc. Now on the basis of the knowledge and acquired experience we establish a margin of durability of 90% to 10years in grafts of internal mammary (AMI) and 50-60% of venous grafts (HV), depending on the vascularized area and the type of vein, in relation to the arterial grafts the average life is of 90% to 5 years with sufficient information of early stenosis problems. Most of the post-operated patients recover in a fast and complete form, which depends on the quality of the performed surgery and an opportune and suitable handling as all the symptoms of the organism recover of the effects of: anesthesia, cardiopulmonary derivation (CEC) and surgical stress. Nevertheless some patients who present combinations of indicators of preoperative risk like: age outpost, antecedents of miocardic revascularization, recent and acute miocardic heart attack (IAM), ejection fraction (EF) low or diabetes, have a much greater surgical risk to the one of the habitual patient. At the moment there are certain characteristics that have determined a fast recovery as they are the early extubation, to avoid major sedation, the disconnection of the support devices and the suspension of drugs as rapidly as possible. A fast treatment before a: Low cardiac cost, alteration of the pulmonary function, hemorrhages, coagulopathy and fever is essential to be able to obtain a fast recovery of the patients; at the moment the surgical indications of the miocardiac revascularization (RVM) have been based in relation to the number and degree of affectation of the coronary arteries, decreased ventricular function and more and more by the increase of percutaneous interventions there are patients with greater risk and worse diagnosis which has modified the results in the last years, as well as a reduction in the number of surgeries per year. Mortality in Europe and the United States is lower than 2,5% with a survival that oscillates respectively between 97-80% of 1 to15 years. Its reduction increased as of the eighth year, is in relation to the average life of the grafts, its occlusion, progression of the disease and development of its comorbidities. [1,2,3.]

2. Preoperative surgical risk

From the antiquity, man has tried to anticipate or predict the facts to come, that is to say the prediction of the results in cardiovascular surgery has been and continues being a goal. The stratification of the patients in different risk levels, previous to the accomplishment of a cardiovascular surgery has diverse intentions, among them the clinical decision making with respect to the accomplishment or not of the surgical procedure or the derivation of the patient for another type of treatment. It is necessary to establish preoperative conducts that can reduce the risk to cost-effectiveness, to establish the stratification of the risk sometimes is difficult, being implicit some factors of individual risk that can be interpreted of different way and has like objectives:

1. Identification of patients of high risk with critical allocation, to adapt the perioperatory problems.
2. To diminish the morbidity and mortality, establishing strategies of preoperative, intraoperating and post-operative treatment.
3. It is indispensable to know the heart disease suitably. (Physiopathology, diagnosis, treatment, and perioperatory complications).
4. A suitable evaluation and treatment of the cardiopathy surgical patient, requires a team work and communication between: patient-surgeon, cardiologist and **intensivist**.
5. Several factors are known that modify the individual risk as they are the age, the sort, previous the cardiovascular function, the renal diseases and you will tilt, respiratory function and other related factors.

John and collaborators established 7 fundamental criteria like and 13 important criteria which are an influence in the morbi-mortality of the post operated patient. (CHART 1)

Age

Every time it is more frequent than patients with age greater to 60 years, are admitted. The cardiovascular risk is increased by above of 65 years by the presence of his comorbidities, age outpost with cardiac symptoms and a key point is the selection of this type of patients, since with this secondary mortality to the surgery is determined. In these patients it is frequent the existence of important complications as they are the low cardiac cost, acute myocardial infarct of the perioperatory, surgical re-intervention by bleeding, acute renal insufficiency, pneumonia, prolonged ventilation, all these increase to the percentage of complications and mortality.

Gender

Many studies exist that have determined that the woman has a greater risk of mortality after the coronary revascularization; because they have minor corporal surface and the size of the coronary glasses is smaller. As far as the sort it does not seem to be predictive of mortality in valvular procedures, mitral and aortic.

Predictors of post-CABG mortality	
Age Sex Urgency of operation Prior heart surgery LVEF Percent stenosis of LM coronary artery Number of major coronary arteries with >70% stenosis	Height Weight PCI during current admission Date of most recent MI History of angina Ventricular arrhythmia CHF Mitral regurgitation DM CVD PVD COPD Creatinine level

Chart 1.

Cardiovascular state

Is the most important aspect of perioperative mortality, the important factors are: severe valvular disease, reoperation, left ventricular function, infarct to the myocardium previous, cardiac insufficiency, emergency surgery and upheavals of the rate.

Respiratory function

The pulmonary disease chronicle is a risk factor to prolong the mechanical ventilation, to have a more difficult weaning, and associated to the pulmonary arterial hypertension, its extubation requires major care.

Mortality

The explanation of the diminution in mortality has been the present methods of myocardic protection with retrograde cardioplegia, hypothermia since the ischemia diminishes triphosphate of adenosine (ATP), altered sanguineous flow, calcium overload, reduction of intracellular calcium sensitivity, sarcoplasmatic dysfunction and the presence of free oxygen radicals. The morbidity and mortality fall significantly in spite of being increased the risk factors, the tendency of the secondary complications of comorbid sufferings have increased until in 30-40%.

The preoperative cardiovascular evaluation provides recommendations for stratification with risk and handling of proposals by the American College of Physicians: Medical history, clinical exploration, ECG, X-ray of thorax, laboratories, tests ECG to the exercise, ambulatory monitoring (Holter), ventriculography to radio nuclear, heart ultrasound, coronary angiography, thallium scintiscanning. [4,5,6,7,8,9] (CHART 2)

In resistance to indices of multi-factor risk, the functional classification New York Heart Association (NYHA) and the American Society of Anesthesiology (HANDLE) are used of routine by the anesthesiologist. Nevertheless, these classifications do not designate a predicting result after the surgery reason why its predictive ability in operating room is limited.

ASA

Healthy patient, with a process located without systemic affection.

PREOPERATIVE EVALUATION OF CARDIAC SURGERY
History
1. History of bleeding: Use of antiplatelet and anticoagulant medication.
2. Smoking (COPD, bronchospasm).
3. Alcoholism (cirrhosis)
4. Diabetes (reactions to protamine, prior infection)
5. Neurological symptoms.
6. Venous insufficiency.
7. Distal vascular reconstruction.
8. Urologic symptoms.
9. Gastric ulcer or gastrointestinal bleeding.
10. Infections (Urol)
11. Allergies
Physical Examination.
1. Skin infection / rash.
2. Dental Caries (dental)
3. Vascular examination (carotid, abdominal aneurysm and peripheral pulses)
4. Heart / Lung (congestive heart failure, new murmur).
5. Varicose veins.
Laboratories
1. Hematologic: PT, PTT, platelets, Hb, Time Ivy.
2. Chemistry: Electrolytes, BUN, QS, PFHS.
3. Urinalysis.
4. Chest X-ray AP and lateral.
5. Electrocradiogram.

Chart 2.

Patient with slight systemic disease.
Patient with serious, but non incapacitated systemic disease.
Patient with serious and incapacitated systemic disease, that constitutes a constant threat for the life.
Dying patient, whose life expectancy does not exceed the 24 hours, is realized or not it to his surgery.

NYHA

Patient with heart disease, without limitations of physical activity.
Patient with disease, with slight limitation ofordinary physical activity, fatigue, palpitations, designs or angina pain.
Patient with heart disease, with noticeable limitation of physical activity, less than the ordinary physical activity, cause tires, palpitations design or pain angina.
Patient with heart disease, incapacity to walk and physical activity, symptoms of cardiac insufficiency, angina.
There are over 100 studies of perioperatory risk-prognosis stratification that have tried to identify adverse predictive factors, the greater limitation of these studies is that they were realized in a single institution, small groups, or the cardiac experience of the anesthesiologistwas the one taken into account. Between the preoperative risk-prognosis

classifying stratification, transoperatory and post-operative factor risks are the following scales: Parsonnet, Tumman, Higgins, Tu, Hannan, Connor, Cleveland Clinic, EuroSCORE, Ontario Provincial Risk (OPR) among others, which vary in predicting correlation of risk of morbidity and mortality in relation to distribution of patients by risk, the average one hoped, and the averageobservada.[10, 11.12.13] (Chart 3)

3. Stratification of risk using data base

The basic information of data is used to improve the clinical practice producing reports with validity and application, evaluating the results, optimizing and improving the cares of the patient, the high mortality is identified in a small and specific sub-group classified like of high risk. The obtained results are used to change institutional programs diminishing mortality in patients of high risk like of smaller risk, mainly in patient put under coronary revascularization diminishing the mortality from 4,5% to 1,5%.

The European for System Cardiac Operative Risk Evaluation (EuroSCORE) is a predicting logistic model of hospitable mortality in patients submissive cardiac intervention, starting off of 18 variables of risk and with a coefficient beta associated to each of them, it provides the probability of dying of each individual, this model was created and validated initially in across-sectional study of 19,030 European patients in 1999, and it has become, since then, in the used model more in the world in this type of patients. Most of the authors agree in raising that the Euroscore is a system simple additive that it provides to facultative a tool of easy handling to consider the death risk. A variant of the much more simple logistic model, denominated Euroscore additive, that awards a weight determined to each factor of risk that presents the patient, the sum of these weights exists provides the approximated probability to die.

The interesting exercise to compare logistic Euroscore with additive already has been realized, but in fact it contributes certain confusion, and the conclusions that are obtained are understood easily observing.

The preoperative surgical risk models are made on the basis of cardiac surgery using cardiopulmonary bypass (CPB). However, it can be applied to off-pump cardiac surgery, as evidenced by Vazquez Roque, in a study in 208 patients undergoing bypass surgery without cardiopulmonary bypass and found that the mean EuroSCORE was significantly higher in patients who died. When comparing patients with and without major complications can see that the mean EuroSCORE was also significantly higher in patients with major complications.

Without fatal perioperative morbidity results in an increase of stay in postoperative care unit and overall hospital stay, this increases resource consumption and costs per patient. The EuroSCORE proved to have a discriminating power and acceptable calibration in predicting these events, we can say that Euroscore, despite being designed a risk score based on patients who underwent cardiac surgery using CPB may be used to predict the risk of death and major complications in patients who are going to be revascularized without the use of cardiopulmonary bypass. This is a novel technique that still suffers from risk scores based on the preoperative characteristics of their own patients. The study uses databases Euroscore retrospective studies, to provide predictive models of morbidity, mortality and prolonged stay in the postoperative intensive care unit, which can be used to improve the quality of postoperative care in different institutions is a tool to categorize patients for cardiac surgery in several subgroups.

Risk factors	Punctuation
Female sex	1
Morbid obesity	3
Hypertension (p. s.> 140 mmHg)	3
EJECTION FRACTION	
Good> 50%	0
Moderate 30-49%	2
Poor <30%	4
age years	
70-74	7
75-79	12
>80	20
Reoperation	
Primary	5
Secundary	10
Preoperative BIAC	2
Left Ventricular Aneurysm	5
Emergency surgery and angioplasty	10
Dialysis	10
Catastrophic States	10-50
Mitral valve surgery	5
PAP > 60mmHg	8
Aórtic	5
Gradient > 120 mmHg	7
Revascularization + Valve Surgery	2

Chart 3.

Due to differences in adult cardiac surgery in the countries of Europe the EuroSCORE is responsible for assessing the quality of surgical care, the analysis is performed for each individual to individual and predicting mortality among the countries of the study is were: Germany, England, Spain, Finland, France and Italy. The EuroSCORE model was satisfactory in all countries with a p <0.05, despite epidemiological differences between European countries the discriminative power of EuroSCORE was good in Spain and in other countries excellent. [14, 15,16,17, 18,19,20.]

4. Cardiac risk evaluation of anesthetic (CARE)

The scale used most recently is called Cardiac Anesthesia Risk Evaluation Score (CARE), prospective studies in cardiac surgery demonstrated a significant number of prognostic information was obtained from only a few clinical variables or clinical trial, were validated and compared with 3.548 patients with Parsonet, Tuman, and Tu, the CARE is a simple risk classification predicts morbidity and mortality on a scale which means ordinary CARE1 low risk, high risk means CARE5 and Care 2-4 as intermediate risk, based on clinical trial recognized three variables: [21.22]

Scale of anesthetic Cardiac Risk Assessment (CARE).

- Heart disease stable without other medical problems, surgery scheduled for a low surgical risk.
- stable heart disease with one or more controlled medical problems, set to a low-risk surgery.
- uncontrolled medical problem, or patient scheduled for surgery high risk.
- uncontrolled medical problem, scheduled for surgery high risk.
- advanced or chronic heart disease, scheduled for cardiac surgery that delayed it can complicate or improve their lives.

Cardiopulmonary bypass (CBP)

On-pump bypass also known as cardiopulmonary bypass is a method used in coronary bypass surgery, this device has been used in cardiac surgery since 1960, due to the high incidence of perioperative mortality due to low spending, it is increasingly used in the last decade, increasing its survival up to 60%. Cardiac surgery and cardiopulmonary bypass activate the inflammatory response, characterized by cardiovascular and pulmonary disorders, this inflammatory response that occurs during cardiac surgery is presented by three processes:

- Contact of blood with the cardiopulmonary bypass machine.
- Development of ischemia and reperfusion injury.
- Release of endotoxins.

The extent and duration of the inflammatory response depend on many factors including the composition of the solution pump, the presence of pulsatile perfusion, pharmacological agents used to reduce the response, the use of mechanical filtration, the type of extracorporeal circuit and temperature during cardiopulmonary bypass. During CPB flow decreased splenic occurs, which induces the crossing of endotoxins by the lumen, activating the inflammatory response, endotoxins are potent initiators of the inflammatory cascade, which in turn causes production of cytokines and complement activation.

A frequent complication of systemic inflammatory response is the evolution to multiple organ failure (MOF) including respiratory failure, shock and renal failure, development of FOM is the most important determinant for the postoperative increases those patients who have risk factors such as prolonged mechanical ventilation (intubation ≥ 48 hours), increased volumes of lower urinary nitrogenous and persistence of vasopressors, resulting in an increase in mortality to 41%. The inflammatory response and also condition FOM phenomena of hemolysis, thrombocytopenia and leukopenia, in the first 24 hours of the end of cardiopulmonary bypass can be seen that the total count of leukocytes undergoes an increase with significant changes in the differential count, the leukocytosis persisted in 72 hours, in the differential count reports a significant increase in neutrophils and monocytes and decreased lymphocyte counts during the first days. Postoperative fever in the second and third day in patients undergoing cardiac surgery is accompanied by an increase in neutrophils, two times the initial value during cardiopulmonary bypass activation of neutrophils is manifested by leukocyte sequestration in the pulmonary circulation at the time of reperfusion of the vascular bed can lead to endothelial and parenchymal injury, in immunocompromised patients and prolonged intubation favors the development of infections. Neutrophils represent the most significant source of oxygen free radicals, which is associated with myocardial dysfunction and pulmonar.[23, 24,25,26,27.]

The CBP decreased flow causes splenic bacterial translocation which conditions, these cross the intestinal lumen and activate the inflammatory response have different degrees of hemodynamic compromise, noting in addition sequential elevations of endotoxin followed by elevations in levels of cytokines and these correlate the degree of myocardial dysfunction. Endotoxins are potent initiators of the inflammatory cascade causing cytokine production, production and complement activation, their presence is associated with the development of lactic acidosis, decreased peripheral vascular resistance and left ventricular dysfunction. The cardiovascular effects of cytokines are mediated by nitric oxide which involves interaction between leukocytes and endothelium and the mechanisms that cause these effects are the presence of circulating endotoxin, lipopolysaccharide (LPS) of gram-negative bacterial cell wall that interact with host cells to promote the release of mediators, lipopolysaccharide increases because the immune response by binding to protein carriers of LPS forms a complex that is a thousand times more potent to induce the release of tumor necrosis factor (TNF) and the union lipopolysaccharide occurs between the CD14 receptor of macrophages is that the activation of kinases and TNF. The inflammatory response can be maintained by several factors including the production of cytokines such as TNF-alpha (α), interleukin 1 (IL-1), IL-1 (beta), interleukin 2 (IL-2), interleukin 6 (IL-6), interleukin 8 (IL-8), interleukin 10 (IL-10), interferon and colony stimulating factors, which may be related to postoperative complications. The release of cytokines produce clinical manifestations in patients with cardiopulmonary bypass, such as fever, altered level of consciousness that occurs microembolisms due to encephalopathy. The crystalloid solutions used to prime the pump bypass hemodilution while causing turbulence and osmotic pressure during cardiopulmonary bypass cause lesions in the cell membrane of erythrocytes and hemolysis eventually causing mainly postoperative bleeding and coagulopathy platelet dysfunction. It is possible that renal failure during cardiopulmonary bypass is due to changes in renal perfusion during periods of hypotension or, for low blood flow, vasoconstriction and microembolism, likewise, hemoglobinuria may also cause significant renal dysfunction as a result of hemolysis during CPB, cardiopulmonary bypass can also cause susceptibility to infections, Sabick et al found that deep sternal infection occurs in 2% in patients undergoing extracorporeal pump versus 0.2% in off-pump patients ($p < 0.04$).[28]

Intra aortic balloon counterpulsation (BIAC)

The intra-aortic balloon counterpulsation is the method used in the treatment of severe cardiac dysfunction and potentially reversible in the perioperative and postoperative cardiac surgery is indicated in the shock associated with myocardial infarction or other complications intractable cardiac ischemia, with or without infarction, ventricular failure post CPB, and so on.

There are two main effects of this device, the first is to increase coronary blood flow improved myocardial oxygen availability by increasing diastolic perfusion pressure and the second is the blood moves during balloon inflation reduces ventricular work by reducing afterload with rapid deflation in systole and thus decreasing myocardial oxygen demand, this increases the heart rate up to 20%, thus the signs associated with BIAC surgical procedure are:

Low cardiac output syndrome, perioperative
As a bridge to cardiac transplantation
Acute mitral insufficiency
Perioperative arrhythmias are difficult to control

Christeson, showed that the use of preoperative IABP reduced hospital costs and length of stay in revascularized and reoperation, Dietl, also reported a stay of 10 days vs. 12 days in those with BIAC those who did not have it at a cost average hospital stay of $ 4000 per paciente. Although minor complications associated with IABP placement has been estimated at 6.5% and higher (vascular surgery and requiring transfusion) of 2.1% is greater than the benefit conferred on all preoperative placement to reduce mortality significantly vs to who are placed in the postoperative period (mortality 8.8% vs 28.2%, $p < 0.0001$) in conclusion, the use of BIAC has increased over the past 10 years, significantly as evidenced by the record made in 29, 961 patients England and Canada, where the increase in aortic counterpulsation in cardiac surgery in the last 6 years is 47%. [29.30.]

Initial assessment and aost-aurgical therapy (TiPQ)

There should be a systematic evaluation of the patient immediately on arrival to postoperative intensive care unit (TiPQ), communication with the surgical team and anesthesia should provide an overview of the intervention performed and the response of the cardiovascular system and perioperative hemodynamic treatment and handling of medication. Although initially it may focus attention on an aspect of patient status (eg, existing arrhythmia on arrival), it is essential to develop a systematic approach to evaluation. The patient is fully independent and dysfunction of the elements of support systems can be fatal quickly. Surgical dressings must be kept intact during the first 24 hours in order to control the infection. If handling is necessary for diagnostic purposes must follow a strict technique. Upon transfer, the patient should continue with the pharmacological management started in the operating room and continued monitoring that includes at least fan movement, Electrocardiography digital, non-invasive blood pressure (PBIN) and pulse oximetry (SO2). Upon arrival to the ICU should be corroborated electrocardiographic tracing displayed on the monitor and make an immediate transfer line 12-lead ECG or chest circle when necessary. Capnography (PECO2) and central venous pressure (CVP) are measures that must be reactivated immediately, it also calibrates the transducer invasive blood pressure monitor confirms his bed and his blood pressure is checked immediately after the pacemaker (MCP) epicardial and functionality, if the patient arrives with pulmonary catheter also must be calibrated immediately and make a hemodynamic profile to assess their cardiovascular status at the time and determine current therapeutic recommendations behaviors common pulmonary catheter placement are EF <40%, patients with combined valve implantation (aortic-mitral) or severe acute heart failure diagnostic doubt its hemodynamic profile. It is important to immediately verify the patency of chest tubes and immediately upon arrival quantify pleural drainage at 15, 45 minutes and hourly for the first 24 hours, and assess their macroscopic features and clot formation. The ventilatory parameters must be set in the next 5 minutes upon arrival and assess the degree of de-recruitment and the need for alveolar opening Pa02/Fi02 if their relation ship is less than 200 mm Hg and if their hemodynamic status is not compromised, the monitoring hypothermia and its management is immediate. During the first 15 minutes should be evaluated central venous saturation (SvO 2), arterial blood gases, acid-base status, serum electrolytes (ABG) and serum examinations required, such as hemoglobin, platelets, hematocrit, serum electrolytes, coagulation, time Ivy, myocardial enzymes, prealbumin, liver function tests (LFT), nitrogenous, Cystatin C, urine sediment and start of urine collection for urinary urea nitrogen (NUU), subsequent tests are given in the next 6 hours or before be necesario.[31, 32,33,34,35]

5. Postoperatively not complicated

At present, the cardiovascular monitoring is noninvasive and invasive integral part of the intensive care critically ill cardiac patient.

Cardiovascular monitoring

The proper outcome after cardiac surgery depends on preoperative and postoperative status of the myocardium rather than coronary anatomy in the postoperative period is uniformly diminished contractility compared to the preoperative magnitude and duration of this depression depends on the severity of chronic dysfunction, the presence of recent ischemic events, efficacy and complications of operative procedures and the intraoperative course. All intraoperative events play a significant role in recovery processes are the most important anesthetic management, cardioplegia and cardiopulmonary bypass duration. Events and preoperative and intraoperative interventions vary in magnitude and duration but in characteristic result in reduced myocardial contractility and compliance, which affects the postoperative management and eventual evolution. Ejection fraction in the preoperative less than 35%, the presence of ischemia or infarction in the immediate preoperative have substantial postoperative management, patients with outflow tract obstruction by a disease associated with hypertrophic chronic hypertension or stenosis aortic present particular difficulties postoperatively. It is always important to optimize left ventricular preload in TiPQ evaluated through filling pressures but not always filling pressures adequately reflect preload, defined as ventricular end-diastolic volume, so that ideally should be monitored with end-diastolic volume index and cardiac index continued, ie in real time. Patients with chronic volume overload, as in those with mitral regurgitation are dependent on adequate volume resuscitation in these patients the response of blood pressure and heart rate are usually a better guide to the proper preload because pulmonary occlusion pressure and pulmonary artery pressure are insensitive, except at the ends of hypovolemia and fluid overload in this situation, blood pressure and cardiac index can significantly change before filling pressures. [36.37]

Ventricular work is a crucial element in the postoperative management of heart surgery, the hypertrophic ventricular pressure overload or are intolerant to significant changes in heart rate when the heart rate is high, the filling time can be shortened enough to compromise the volume of end-diastolic volume and thus cardiac output, in contrast, when heart rate is below the time needed to develop the maximum end-diastole, cardiac output may decline relative to the low frequency. Assuming that the preload is adequate, a heart rate between 90 and 100 beats per minute is optimal for a hypertrophic myocardium, where compliance is significantly diminished synchronized atrioventricular contraction plays a significant role in ensuring optimal preload, so these patients require sinus rhythm or a dual-chamber pacemaker. The ventricle with volume overload in contrast, is more tolerant of tachycardia and loss of atrioventricular synchrony. When ventricular compliance at the end of diastole decrease as a result of increased heart rate, systolic emptying may be better in these patients, sinus rhythm below 75 beats per minute tends to be more deleterious to an abnormal rhythm frequencies above 90 per minute, with low heart rates, prolonging the diastolic filling time committed ventricular ejection fraction because the ventricle is more dilated. Ultimately in ventricles with volume overload tachycardia and loss of atrioventricular synchrony can be better tolerated than sinus bradycardia. Determining the degree of reduction in contractility admission to TiPQ is problematic, the main contributors to the decrease in postoperative contractility including ejection fraction before surgery less than 35%, CPB time, especially if the duration exceeds 120 minutes. In patients undergoing valve procedures, it is advisable to perform intraoperative transesophageal echocardiography at the end of CPB as this is useful to assess valve function and ventricular dynamics. If the preoperative ejection fraction is greater than 35% and the operative course was satisfactory, decrease myocardial compliance in the first 4-6 hours in the unit and then quickly returns TiPQ values similar to or better than the preoperative values. Patients with an ejection fraction before surgery less than 35%, presence of perioperative ischemia or complicated operative course may require a longer time to recover or make permanent dysfunction, myocardial depression may persist for an extended period of time. These factors may affect the withdrawal of ventilatory support and necessitate the use of oxygen in prolonged, the tachypnea may be a reflection of compromised perfusion rather than primary respiratory failure.

Maintaining normal blood pressure is critical in the early hours of postoperative necessarily invasive measurement must be continued for at least 24 hours for analysis beat to beat but if it is non-invasive measurement must be measured regularly every 5 minutes but the objectivity of plethysmographic measurements are reliable non-invasive automatic in the absence of intense vasoconstriction and a very high frequency. Class I recommendation, level of evidence C. The optimal MAP in the first 6 postoperative hours especially in revascularized patients should be 65 to 80mmHg, maintaining adequate tissue perfusion to all organs and prevent bleeding at the sites of anastomosis of the bypass. The goal of hemodynamic monitoring of critically ill patients is to assess the adequate perfusion and tissue oxygenation, using intermittent or continuous measurement of oxygen saturation both considered acceptable, although the measurement of lactate may be useful lacks precision as a measure of status tissue metabolism in patients with mechanical ventilation is recommended central venous pressure of 12-14 mm Hg to offset the increase in intrathoracic pressure especially those with PEEP> 5mmHg. A similar consideration is the elevation of intra-abdominal pressure (IAP is approximately normal. 5-7 mmHg in critically ill patients) as it is inversely proportional to tissue perfusion pressure (PPP) and dependent on the mean arterial pressure (MAP) ie: PPA = MAP - IAP.

The good use in the immediate postoperative period of Swan-Ganz implies a broad knowledge of hemodynamics by the doctor for a proper training and constant use of the device, much of the value of this catheter for monitoring the hemodynamic status is based on their ability adequate to measure pulmonary capillary pressure which we take as a measure of left ventricular preload. The subsequent interpretation of a good wedge pressure curve are not simple things, implies among other things, the tip of the catheter has been placed in a part of the lung that the condition of zone 3, the ball was not over-inflated or default, the catheter is floating in the right place and has not migrated back, there is no strong auto-PEEP and various other things. However there are many more and more data, which indicate that the use of postoperative pulmonary catheter in heart depends on many factors that have little to do with their true indications or the severity of the patient also has serious complications observed in studies presented to the placement of a Swan-Ganz pulmonary artery in this group of patients where metabolic changes, hypothermia, cardioplegia, ischemia or myocardial stunning favor residual arrhythmias, thromboembolic events, infections, pulmonary infarction or to knotting of the catheter, not to mention does not improve cardiovascular survival in critically ill patients.

You must have a central venous line and periodically monitor the central venous saturation (SvO2) and good availability in the administration of appropriate fluids for resuscitation in the first six hours following the early goals of Rivers and colleagues, as therapy guided by objectives has been shown to improve survival in critically ill patients susceptible to revival under the supervision of personnel in these areas.

During the first hours must meet the physiological parameters already discussed, however those who do not meet these criteria should be reassessed therapeutic conduct, analyze ECG, diuresis, PVC, the need to correct up to 30% hematocrit and evaluate the need for inotropic or increase in dosage especially if the central venous saturation is <70%, or GC-invasive measurements have decreased their acceptable ranges. The SvO 2 is a determinant and with greater sensitivity in the postoperative monitoring of oxygenation, perfusion, oxygen consumption and microcirculatory level, now has shown that goal-directed resuscitation, in which this has been a decisive objectives in the first six hours significantly decreased cardiopulmonary morbidity and mortality in patients to assess critical to tissue oxygenation indirectly: this is defined as adequate oxygen supply to demand, the supply is always greater than consumption (VO2), in cases of circulatory shock and severe hypoxemia there is a significant fall in DO2 but the VO2 is maintained by the compensation determined by the EO2%, which explains a security mechanism that ensures the proper use until it descends DO2 a critical point where consumption becomes dependent on the contribution anaeróbico initiating cellular metabolism. [38,39]

The use of PiCCO (press contour cardiac output) can continuously monitor cardiac output, the variability of pulse pressure and stroke volume. Likewise, estimates of the severity of intermittent pulmonary edema, intravascular volume and intrathoracic cardiac chambers, two measures related to ventricular preload.

Electrocardiographic monitoring or driving is important in the first six hours after a stroke thoroughly evaluated on admission electrocardiogram to TiPQ, you need continuous monitoring of electrical activity and identify arrhythmias or morphological changes that warrant immediate management. You also have to periodically assess the proper functioning of epicardial pacemaker generator. Management should be initiated when the ventricular rate is above 110lat/min.

Respiratory monitoring

First of all clinical assessment remains the mainstay in respiratory monitoring, inspection of the chest is important from the patient's arrival to TiPQ is important to assess that there is synchrony in movements of both amplexación amplexión and thorax as well as observation of permeability each of chest drains and their exact position placed by the surgical team must verify proper endotracheal tube position, surely the next step is auscultation of lung regions in search of clinical syndromes or abnormal sounds that suggest some clinical suspicion is necessary to assess respiratory mechanics measurements in our patient by the ventilator as well as scheduling parameters. Sets the following startup parameters:

Mode: Assist-control (volume or pressure)
Respiratory rate = 10-15 L / min;
Tidal volume = 6-8 ml / kg;
FiO2 = to maintain SaO2> 90%.

Over 90% of postoperative patients reach TiPQ Units with mechanical assistance in breathing, so the generally invasive respiratory monitoring, however, is always important clinical evaluation since joining our service to have an initial assessment and observe its evolution in the first 24 hours. Not established the need for routine use of PEEP in patients without complications due to decreased functional residual capacity (FRC) in these patients and atelectasis appear 5 minutes after the onset of anesthesia are not important and no impact on arterial oxygenation postoperatively. However, in the first hour is important to evaluate the relationship and consider PaO2/FiO2 lung history to give an appropriate value, it is also important to rule out existence of residual pleural effusion or pneumothorax because both entities are also involved in lowering the ratio PaO2/FiO 2, and evaluated these considerations and having a stable hemodynamic status can be performed alveolar recruitment maneuver (ARM) is a technique that uses a sustained increase in airway pressure with the aim of recruiting collapsed alveolar units, increasing lung area available for gas exchange and consequently arterial oxygenation. Recent studies concern the use of MRA after cardiac surgery, during which the authors believe that lung function and oxygenation are decreased> 20% with the use of cardiopulmonary bypass and the inflammatory response with the exponential growth atelectasis. Cardiac surgery with cardiopulmonary bypass includes the complete collapse of the lungs, thus, the move will improve oxygenation by opening collapsed lung regions. The results of current work suggest that alveolar recruitment maneuvers are safe procedure in patients with cardiovascular surgery and reduces the frequency of postoperative atelectasis.

The decline of ventilatory support should generally be within 24 hours, ideally Fast-track implementation of the ventilation is the goal in most patients (Fast-track cardiac anesthesia-FTCA-). The importance of predicting the timing of weaning is that both the early weaning as the unnecessary prolongation of mechanical ventilation is deleterious to the patient. In addition only with the clinical trial is difficult to predict how successful disconnection accurate (50% positive predictive value and 67% negative predictive value) because these results justify the implementation of objectives and accurate methods to identify patients who are able to adequately of extubated successfully.

Early extubation is associated with a significant reduction in costs associated with mechanical ventilation, there is now several modalities to a quick and safe extubation, spontaneous ventilation with pressure support (VPS) with 2 dual ventilation PEEP levels (BiLevel) or that pressure release ventilation (APRV).

Patients extubated within 24 hrs it has decreased PaO2/FiO2 ratio <200 is recommended the use of noninvasive mechanical ventilation for 24 hrs demonstrated by Yoshiyuki Takami et al, as it must be part of primary treatment strategy in patients with acute pulmonary edema in this group of patients and reduces the need for endotracheal reintubation and lower mortality when compared against conventional treatment with oxygen therapy in postoperative heart patient.

Pulse oximetry has been used to transfer the patient to the operating room TiPQ unit and required at all times to monitor the state of oxygenation does not replace the determination of arterial blood gases, however the devices currently are more sensitive and less margin for error, which has gained considerable ground in noninvasive respiratory monitoring. The most common cause of inaccurate readings of SpO_2 is movement, affects the ability of light to travel from the light-emitting diodes (LED) to the photodetector, parkinsonism, seizures, tremors, cause problems with detecting saturation with falsely high measurements in low perfusion states, such as low cardiac output, vasoconstriction, hypothermia, hypovolemia, severe hypotension, particularly in cardiac surgery, the oximeter reading is difficult, however, this noninvasive method provides reliable early the decrease in oxygen saturation before they show clinical signs of hypoxemia.

Capnometry capnography and monitoring is a noninvasive method useful in the postoperative cardiovascular since it is constantly evaluating the level of carbon dioxide (CO_2) exhaled and its graphical representation is undoubtedly an important tool in the management of mechanical ventilation in the first hours after surgery. Carbon dioxide the patient is transported from the cells into the lungs through the venous blood, mostly in the form of bicarbonate (HCO_3) and dissolved in small amounts in plasma and bound to hemoglobin, the amount of CO_2 that comes the alveoli is determined by its production and flow of venous blood that is, its perfusion (Q), on the other hand, their removal is an almost direct function of alveolar ventilation (V). Therefore, the $PaCO_2$ is the result of the relationship between ventilation and perfusion: the ratio = V / Q

1. In the case where the alveolar ventilation equals pulmonary blood perfusion, $PaCO_2$ is very similar to $PaCO_2$ in these cases changes in the $PaCO_2$ almost exactly reflect those observed in $PaCO_2$.
2. In cases where ventilation is inappropriately high with respect to the infusion, ie there is a high degree of "dead space" (VD), $PaCO_2$ is considerably lower than $PaCO_2$.
3. In cases where the ventilation is decreased in relation to infusion, $PaCO_2$ is close to the values of PCO_2 in venous blood, ie the $PvCO_2$, and results in a V / Q low. This occurs in those clinical situations in which the airways or alveolar sick or increased pulmonary blood perfusion.

As evaluated in the above three points the lungs are not physiologically homogeneous and therefore carbon dioxide at the end of expiration ($ETCO_2$) is the average of the mixture of all different types $PaCO_2$ alveoli. It's called $PaCO_2$-$ETCO_2$ gradient to the difference between arterial CO_2 pressure and the pressure of CO_2 in the alveoli ($ETCO_2$), which normally is 1-5 mmHg. This small difference is due to the small dead space that exists in normal conditions. But knowing the physiological concepts, translation in the immediate postoperative clinic may be:

- A $ETCO_2$ of 0 usually means the patient is not breathing, however, can also be the result of a malfunctioning fan or a disconnect from it.
- The decrease in $ETCO_2$ suggests a decreased production of CO_2, hypothermia or a fall in transport, low cardiac output, excessive alveolar ventilation, hyperventilation or a malfunctioning fan. fig 6
- Increased $ETCO_2$ may be the result of excessive production of CO_2, hyperthermia or sepsis or a decrease in alveolar ventilation

Arterial blood gases are essential to making the postoperative management of blood gases were performed on all patients from their initial arrival and subsequent to any adjustment or correction fan electrolyte and acid-base status, interpretation of blood gases is sometimes difficult; laboratory results must always be studied in light of the clinical picture, by the systematic approach to each of the values. In the critically ill patient post-operative heart surgery is also necessary to know the values of venous blood gases. The determination of arterial and venous blood gases provides three basic values through direct measurement of the respective electrodes:

1. Partial pressure of oxygen dissolved in plasma, PaO2.
2. Partial pressure of carbon dioxide dissolved in the plasma, PaCO2.
3. The degree of acidity or alkalinity of the plasma pH.

The PaO2 is the rate of oxygenation of the blood an indicator of the intensity of the presence of molecular oxygen dissolved in plasma, is the expression of the efficiency of alveolar ventilation-perfusion and alveolar capillary diffusion normal to achieve the transfer oxygen from inside the alveolus to pulmonary capillary blood. The PaCO2 is a ventilation parameter also reflects the respiratory component of acid-base and is a highly reliable method that reflects without confusion or error, unless you have a fan failure or bad programming environment with respect to individual clinical Patient postoperados.[40, 41,42,43]

Renal monitoring

The clinical value in the immediate postoperative period is important because the simple quantification of urine schedule can objectively evaluate renal function, however there are several circumstances where the patient usually attends with minimal deterioration and time indicated by decreased urine output, factors are multi-age, prior renal impairment, intravascular volume cash cytokines by CBP, controlled hypotension, bleeding, and so on. The incidence of acute renal failure (ARF) in cardiac surgery with cardiopulmonary bypass, between 1% and 45%, and in most schools in a 1% to 15%. The incidence of severe ARF that required renal replacement therapy techniques, the work varies between 1% and 11.1%, thanks to a study by Charujas and colleagues demonstrate and validate a "ARF score" in patients undergoing heart surgery and determine the risk of postoperative renal failure in taking a score: 1 to 17 than to predict the risk of acute renal failure expressed in percentage.

The CBP has also been involved for many years in the genesis of renal damage associated with cardiac surgery, initially manifested by microscopic or gross hematuria depending on the severity, though studies of the last fifteen years, using sensitive techniques to identify kidney damage have suggested greater importance of perioperative generator impairment and acute renal failure, as opposed to possible damage of CPB. Most of these studies have been performed in elective postoperative patients with normal preoperative renal function, recent studies comparing off-pump coronary surgery versus conventional coronary surgery, show no differences in postoperative renal damage, however the valve patients have been considered within the group at high risk of kidney damage. So today in the early hours 24 hours urine volume remains the most reliable parameter of renal impairment and prayers whatever their origin (hypovolemia, nephrotoxicity, ischemia, contrast, etc). [44,45,46,47]

Metabolic monitoring

Hyperglycemia in the perioperative period is associated with increased morbidity, decreased survival and increased costs. A number of observational studies have shown that improved control of glucose levels in diabetic patients undergoing coronary revascularization improves the outcome. Van den Berghe et al demonstrated in surgical ICU patients, 63% of whom were postoperative cardiac surgery, the control of glucose concentrations of 80-100 mg / dl was associated with a relative decrease in mortality over

40% when compared with controls. This study has been criticized for lack of blind control, administration of high doses of glucose control and high incidence of hypoglycemia. The current recommendation is to try to keep blood glucose below 150 mg / dl, this was secondary to a study called normoglycemia in Intensive Care Evaluation Survival Using Glucose Algorithm-Regulation (NICE-SUGAR) used to test the hypothesis that intensive of blood sugar reduces mortality 90 days in this study showed higher mortality from severe hypoglycemia. Because polyuria in the early hours, the release of antidiuretic hormone and hyperaldosteronism that characterizes the patient operated on with CPB, it is common the presence of hypokalaemia which must be corrected for values greater than 4.0 mEq / L, just as occurs hypomagnesemia should be corrected usually there is usually no changes in serum calcium or other ions that require correction.

The dilutional hyponatremia type being increased total body sodium, the use of mannitol and / or furosemide during CPB produces a polyuria in the first two to three hours postoperatively INSTANT that can reach 1000 ml / hour, with a tendency to normalize within hours, the usual consequence is the need to infuse fluids resulting hypovolemia. [48.49]

Neurological monitoring

It is essential in the first 24 hours because it is not uncommon to find deficits in different degrees and which are generally grouped into cognitive dysfunction, which is the most common disorder and unnoticed, and that their identification will be necessary to carry out mini-mental and demonstrate an early deficit and time of their higher mental functions. All patients coming to the unit with residual sedation TiPQ so within the next 6 hours there is a 95% elimination of sedatives, since coming patients should be evaluated clinically to assess the integrity of the stem bark and well-get a first impression to rule out diagnoses and cerebral ischemic event or bleeding. In patients who quickly integrates a focus fasciocorporal study should be completed image and a more detailed review to have an early management and prevent secondary damage. [50.51]

Moreover, patients with prolonged CPB tend to have greater involvement of cardiorespiratory function and hemodynamic instability preoperatively intraoperative surgery more complicated, hence the increased incidence of neurological disorders may be related to these factors rather than the CPB time, now happens with hypotension and cerebral hypoperfusion which is another postulated mechanism of neurological damage. The CBP is under hypothermia and anesthesia, both of which lower the cerebral metabolism and thus cerebral blood flow as there is less demand on the other hand, hemodilution decreases blood viscosity by decreasing its resistance to move, so lower blood pressure can keep the same cerebral blood flow. Thus, it alters the autoregulation curve of cerebral blood flow may keep it even with blood pressures of 50 to 60 mm Hg, studies measuring regional cerebral blood flow in patients during CPB have shown that blood pressure can reach 50 mm Hg without altered cerebral blood flow. Moreover, the flow can reach 19 cm 3 per 100 grams of tissue per minute without psychometric alterations detected between pre and post operative. Glasgow is interpreted evaluation at baseline and 6 hours by issuing a neurological assessment, monitoring with bispectral index (BIS) in patients who have to initiate a secondary sedation is necessary to identify a level of sedation adecuado.[52, 53, 54]

Hematologic monitoring

Hematologic monitoring after surgery is associated with anemia hemodilution and blood loss, the minimum necessary use of blood products has shown improvement in morbidity and mortality in recent years. This consideration has resulted from recent meta-analysis and evidence-based medicine, evidence shows the association of adverse effects such as increased costs, morbidity and mortality especially in the group <65 years so even 7.5gr hemoglobin can be well tolerated and no increased risk increase in elderly patients without ischemic but the minimum allowed is 8.5 grams, although a large number of scientific publications are those who prefer to have an algorithm in relation to individual patient characteristics as shown in the table below . The indications for transfusion in patients with coronary disease are valid when hypovolemia has been corrected, optimized hemodynamics and oxygenation after correction tachycardia. [55,56,57]

It is common in the postoperative cardiac surgery hours uncomplicated run smoothly. At approximately 36 hours the patient can be transferred to a general room with telemetric control.

6. Complicated postoperative

Cardiovascular

Hypotension and hypoperfusion injury may condition not directly related to the surgical procedure and include cardiac tamponade, a new myocardial ischemia, tension pneumothorax, hemothorax or significant bleeding related to arterial cannulation. Rarely produce acute thrombosis of a graft or coronary embolization. The electrocardiogram (ECG) may be of diagnostic aid because it is expected that the initial postoperative ECG changes does not show or reveal abnormalities preoperatively limited ST-T. If there are significant changes in ECG repeated, should be thought of an occlusive lesion of one of the grafts.

In the presence of suspected acute ischemia should indicate intravenous nitroglycerin, the risk of a perioperative myocardial infarction is present from the preoperative to the hospital and even after the diagnosis of acute myocardial infarction (AMI) presents difficulties in the perioperative You must have a combination of ECG, cardiac enzymes and echocardiography can occasionally make the diagnosis. Frequently observed nonspecific ECG changes a large percentage of patients have an increased enzyme and troponin I (TnI) generally exceeds the levels observed in AMI unrelated to cardiac surgery. The loss of graft thrombosis has been reported in up to 10% of grafts in the first week in the hours following the surgery, aspirin and possibly clopidogrel appears to reduce the prevalence of AMI diagnosis although postoperative postoperative AMI is difficult itself has a significant effect on morbidity and mortality in the long term.

Arrhythmias

Low cardiac output syndrome

The low cardiac output syndrome (LCOS), is characterized by decreased performance of cardiac function where the cause may damage myocardial and cardiogenic shock condition corresponds to a failure in the balance between central cardiac pump and control components peripherals, including: a) the tone of the peripheral circulation and b) neurohumoral regulators of vascular tone, with the arrival insufficient oxygenated blood to peripheral tissues to meet metabolic needs, their presence is associated with high mortality at that requires immediate diagnosis and treatment. The multiple causes can produce or aggravate this syndrome can be grouped, for descriptive purposes, the following pathogenic mechanisms:

1. Reduced preload. The major cause is the leakage of fluid into the interstitial space, excessive bleeding, polyuria, the use of high levels of positive end-expiratory warming excessive vasodilator drug use, cardiac tamponade, and so on.
2. Increase in afterload. It can affect both the left and right ventricle. in the cause of increased afterload are systemic hypertension, pulmonary hypertension, the replacement of the mitral valve in mitral regurgitation, etc..
3. Reduced contractility. The main causes of decreased contractility are perioperative AMI, drugs with negative inotropic effect, the phenomena exaggerated ischemia-reperfusion during aortic clamping, and so on. In relation to the phenomenon of ischemia reperfusion is important to note contractile deterioration often not immediately apparent to the patient's admission to the ICU. In these cases, there is a period of normo-or hyper ventricular early after reperfusion. This period is short (hours) and is followed by a gradual depression of systolic function, leading in many cases to a false sense of security in the early postoperative hours, when this phenomenon is unknown.
4. Changes in heart rate and heart rate. Are due to extreme bradycardia, supraventricular or ventricular tachyarrhythmias and impaired high-risk condition.
5. Metabolic and electrolyte. Acidosis, hypoxemia, hypo-or hypercapnia, hyperkalemia, hypocalcemia and may contribute to the development of this syndrome.
6. Inadequate surgical management. Sometimes not achieved the expected result from the technical point of view and this can generate a low output syndrome, such as poor condition can bridge aortocoronary junction in myocardial revascularization surgery, prolonged pump time with poor poor systemic perfusion and hypothermia induced, the presence of a residual stenosis in mitral commissurotomy, miss-match of prosthetic valve replacement or plasty, and so on.

The diagnosis of low cardiac output syndrome after surgery can be established through the clinic or by hemodynamic monitoring. Hypotension is the warning sign and used more widely, however, patients with moderate decrease in cardiac index may retain acceptable levels of low systemic blood pressure which minute volume is high or normal. Oliguria is the most common signs of urinary volume monitoring is time and calculate the minute volume through the renal plasma flow and rhythm of diuresis, but lacks specificity. No doubt the hypothermia of the extremities and the temperature difference between central and extremity: these signs are not very useful in the immediate postoperative period because patients usually come to body temperature, cardiovascular recovery with low and sometimes remain so for several hour, despite attempts to overheat. In the first hours after surgery are patients with marked vasomotor instability (vasoconstriction - vasodilation) for which no specific capillary filling. On the other hand in the first hours after surgery can be found lactic acidosis, which in many cases does not reflect the present situation, but situations of decreased perfusion in the operating room occurred body, markedly decreasing the diagnostic and prognostic value with other medical and Finally, the decrease in mixed venous saturation, this parameter depends on cardiac output and oxygen consumption level of the tissue, so in the first 60 minutes is more specific cardiac output. Due to the low sensitivity and specificity of symptoms from the first sign of consensus definitions in cardiovascular recovery, recently published, is required to make the clinical diagnosis of low cardiac output syndrome, patients present simultaneously at least 2 of the following criteria:

Hypotension (systolic blood pressure below 90 mmHg).

Oliguria (urine output less than 0.5 ml / kg / hr).

The hemodynamic evaluation allows continuous monitoring of cardiac function postoperatively, being indispensable implementation in this particular group of patients. This is done by direct measurement of cardiac output by thermodilution technique. Authors such as J. Kirklin consider being in the presence of low cardiac output when cardiac index less than 2.2 L/min/m2 in the early hours after surgery and less than 2.4 L/min/m2 in the first postoperative day, other authors consider the value 2.0 L/min/m2 index of heart as the limit for the diagnosis of low cardiac output syndrome, with values between 2 and 2.5 L/min/m2 cardiac index usually require therapeutic intervention, whatever its value must be accompanied by systemic vascular resistance values normal or elevated, for differentiation vasoplegic syndrome that presents with decreased systemic vascular resistance. The radionuclide ventriculography with Technetium 99 is an excellent diagnostic tool, with it you can obtain the ejection fraction as much of the left ventricle of the right ventricle, and allows cardiac tamponade diagnosed by the presence of pericardial blood or clots in relation to Echocardiography its main drawback is to obtain an acceptable acoustic window in this group of patients, however these problems have been solved with transesophageal echocardiography. LCOS mortality is very high, the study CONAREC III mortality of patients suffering from low cardiac output syndrome was 44.7%, compared to those patients who did not suffered and whose mortality was only 4.9% in the same study when considering all the excuses of death, this syndrome was the most frequent (28.9%) in patients undergoing coronary bypass surgery. Another study observed the ESMUCICA un12% mortality in CABG and valve surgery in 25-45%) and ESMUCICA II (26% mortality in valvular).

The therapeutic management should follow a similar pattern of the pathogenesis stating:

a. Optimize preload
b. Optimizing afterload
c. Optimizing the pace and heart rate.
d. Increase inotropy.

The optimal preload for each patient is different and depends on the heart for each patient and how they estimated. When you need to optimize the preload is used intravascular volume expansion with either colloids, crystalloids or both, while, as if what is required is a decrease in preload is done with diuretics, vasodilators, with predominant effect in the venous bed as nitroglycerin, mechanical ventilation with PEEP or hemofiltration if the patient is oliguric renal failure.

Afterload also depends on heart disease for each patient and if you have any other special situation. The most commonly used drugs to reduce vascular resistance and therefore afterload are vasodilators with predominant effect on the arterioles, such as sodium nitroprusside. Another important therapeutic elements are warming persist in hypothermic patients, sedation and analgesia in patients who have pain or anxiety they generate strong isometric muscle contraction, and oxygen in varying concentrations in those with hypoxemia and pulmonary vasoconstriction bed with increased pulmonary vascular resistance and consequently the right ventricular afterload. To get the rhythm and heart rate can be used atrial pacing in case of a sub-optimal heart rate in sinus rhythm and normal atrioventricular conduction, ventricular pacing in cases of atrial fibrillation with low ventricular response, and sequential pacing, atrioventricular case of complete atrioventricular block. The presence of tachyarrhythmias can be managed with drug therapy, over-stimulation or cardioversion shock as appropriate.

Commonly used catecholamines such as dopamine, dobutamine, isoproterenol, epinephrine, norepinephrine and inotropic catecholamines not milrinone and levosimendan, being necessary in many cases the combination of more than one. Catecholamines, particularly dopamine are the drugs most often used and indiscriminately without taking into account many times the preload. The most important are the catecholamines and phosphodiesterase inhibitors, there are few data concerning the use of levosimendan. these agents have proven effective in improving myocardial contractility or heart rate or both catecholamines are more potent chronotropic and inotropic agents determine side effects such as increased myocardial oxygen consumption of the myocardium, tachycardia, arrhythmias, and increased in afterload can make your job difficult. B-adrenergic receptors may also be downregulated in patients with previous heart failure. This has increased the interest in the use of inhibitors of phosphodiesterase III and more recently, the calcium sensitizer levosimendan. In a study by Labriola et al. Nijhawan et al.) Drug compared to placebo in patients with low cardiac output syndrome after surgery, in which documented an increase in cardiac output and ejection fraction and a decrease systemic vascular resistance in patients treated with levosimendan. Gillies et al. Conducted a systematic review of the literature on the use of inotropic agents in patients with cardiac surgery, in which certain recommendations were documented, each with a particular level of evidence.

Respiratory

Respiratory dysfunction in postoperative heart surgery patients is a common problem that results in a significant increase to 25% mortality and significant morbidity with impact on cost and hospital stay, atelectasis is a frequent occurrence in the immediate postoperative period The incidence of atelectasis in the postoperative period of 40 to cardiac 70%, the term is derived from Greek: Atel and ektasis mean incomplete expansion of a segment or lobe is characterized by volume loss and collapse of alveolar region manifested radiographically as an area opacified. The severity of atelectasis increases with more time to pump, more bridges and prolonged ischemia, the opening of the pleura, phrenic nerve injury, intraoperative and very low temperatures. Thoracotomy alters lung function by shallow breathing (restrictive functional pattern), and vital capacity may be reduced by up to 45 to 70%, the pain diminishes deep breath and a cough can lead to ineffective with the consequences in lung mechanics and bronchial hygiene. Another important factor is the presence of atelectasis, diaphragmatic paralysis caused possibly by phrenic nerve injury caused by surgery or by the use of topical agents or cold cardioplegia. Decubitus position maintained, leads to changes in regional distribution of ventilation and perfusion of the lung, lung inflation decreases along a vertical axis from ventral to dorsal supine and when spontaneous breathing begins immediately after surgery and in the supine position ventilation is distributed mainly dependent areas of the lung. In contrast, during mechanical ventilation, this pattern changes and the distribution of ventilation is primarily aimed at non-dependent areas in both positions, therefore, the subsidiaries tend to collapse. Studies have shown that prone position ventilation becomes more homogeneous. Mechanical restraint of ventilation is produced by several factors explain such as bronchial secretions accumulating in dependent areas, pleural effusion or dysfunction of chest drains in the first hours after surgery. Alveolar recruitment maneuver is a technique that uses a sustained increase in airway pressure with the aim of reducing atelectasis by recruiting collapsed alveolar units, increasing the lung area available for gas exchange and consequently arterial oxygenation. Different methods are used alveolar recruitment in the postoperative patient, it is important to know that before the maneuver is to have an adequate intravascular volume and residual sedation after surgery. Ventilatory strategies proposed to achieve alveolar recruitment in surgical patients are based on the use of pressure (PEEP or CPAP) ranging between 20 and 40 cm H2O for varying periods of time. The effects of positive end-expiratory should be monitored continuously, as some of the side effects include decreased venous return by increasing the average pressure of the airways, impaired lung perfusion overdistended areas (increase dead space), increased pulmonary vascular resistance and right heart dysfunction, barotrauma and impaired renal blood flow, which are frequent causes of hemodynamic compromise in critically ill patients with cardiovascular disease and those with intravascular volume deficit. Pleural effusion is frequently observed in the immediate postoperative period, but a considerable percentage persist for more than 30 days, the incidence is 41-87% in postoperative patients, although most are not significant pleural effusions, a study of 602 heart postoperative patients showed pleural effusion in 63%, more than 30 days but less than 5% need thoracentesis for resolution in those patients who had more than 5 days chest drains pleural related to infections associated with atelectasis and ipsilateral lung infection, said box by fever, productive cough and an alveolar infiltrate on chest radiograph. It is important to differentiate whether it is indeed a spill transudate or if there is a pulmonary complication due to an infection with a pleural early. To make this distinction using the criteria of Light, which are more sensitive at identifying exudates, they meet at least one of the following criteria: (transudates none)

1. Relationship between pleural fluid protein and serum 0.5,
2. Relationship between pleural fluid LDH and serum 0.6,
3. In pleural fluid LDH greater than the 2 / 3 parts of the upper limit of normal for serum LDH.

Other proposed criteria for an exudative pleural effusion are:

4. Cholesterol> 43 mg / dl,
5. Gradient-pleural serum albumin less than 1.2 g / dl.

The thoracic duct that enters the thorax through the right diaphragm and flows into the left subclavian vein, has collateral lymphatic sometimes can be injured during surgery and result in a chylothorax. This pleural fluid milky-white at times and some colored (yellow or red) in other, has high content of lymph (chylomicrons), with a triglyceride level above 100 mg / dl and cholesterol below 200 mg / dl , treatment includes not remove the chest tubes because the fistula may close spontaneously in the thoracic duct short time, starting with parenteral nutrition for 10 to 14 days to reduce the production of intestinal lymph and thereby reduce the flow through the thoracic duct. If despite these measures fail to control the chylothorax, pleurodesis can be performed. Injury or acute progressive respiratory insufficiency (ALI / ARDS) is a multifactorial process of respiratory damage from pulmonary or extrapulmonary origin and is defined by the European-American consensus.

In patients with postoperative heart surgery the incidence is 5 to 20% depending on the type of surgery, severity, time in surgery, bleeding, age, EuroSCORE, comorbidities, and so on.

In elderly patients shows the highest incidence due to low physiological reserve and are more likely to have postoperative complications, the impact of gender remains controversial, although female gender was not shown to be an independent predictor of LPA in a large study recent cohort, two small studies identified a strong association between female gender and the incidence of ALI after cardiac surgery. Vascular risk factors are independent predictors of LPA include diabetes, kidney failure, hypertension. These markers of systemic atherosclerotic disease are associated with an increased risk of major complications. Preexisting renal insufficiency is a strong predictor of ALI (OR, 2.3), which confirms the findings of several studies, increased atherosclerotic burden associated with renal failure. Chronic obstructive pulmonary disease (COPD) identified preoperative was also an independent risk factor, confirming that patients with COPD who are undergoing valve surgery or surgery RVM have two or three times the chance of LPA in severe COPD has been associated with excess postoperative mortality in patients with MVR. Pathophysiological observed that lung damage is mixed but the most important finding in the lungs during the early stages of ALI / ARDS is the presence of severe pulmonary edema secondary to increased permeability of capillary endothelium and alveolar epithelial barrier of . Simultaneously, increased pulmonary vascular resistance as a result of thromboembolic events and reflex vasoconstriction, these morphological characteristics are a complex reaction of the lung to different nosological agents and processes and not related to the nature of the causal process. During mechanical ventilation in the immediate postoperative behavior is rest to follow by pulmonary alveolar protection strategy as ALI / ARDS is a syndrome characterized by loss of functional residual capacity, increased lung and short circuits refractory hypoxemia FiO2. The standard or optimal tidal volume is difficult to determine, because in the inflamed lung or ALI / ARDS alveolar pressures each area has specific and requires its own level of PEEP to keep open during expiration. The alveolar pressures and volumes that can reach areas not dependent overdistended lung, are often insufficient to ensure the recruitment of regions dependent edema and atelectasis by maintaining recruitable lung areas open, there is distension of the healthy areas of the lung, it is explained that the regional compliance of the lung are different as well as mentioned Gattinoni.

Postoperative bleeding

One of the most frequent complications encountered in the management of patients, approximately 20% of patients present with significant bleeding and only 5% required reintervention. Predictive factors for bleeding include age, renal failure, cardiopulmonary bypass time, liver failure, hypothermia, secondary fibrinolysis, NSAIDs, etc; bleeding contributes to more days of ventilation hospital stay and mortality.

The definition of excessive bleeding in postoperative patients occurs in 5% -10% approximately and only 3% required reoperation, bleeding, and reoperation are 2 independent predictors of poor prognosis. In those patients with postoperative bleeding can be divided into two categories: surgical bleeding (bleeding venous layer anastomosis, sternum, anywhere stitches), non-surgical bleeding (caused by coagulopathy).

Risk factors for bleeding are preoperative such as pharmacologic agents (thrombolytic PTCA, antiplatelet drugs, anticoagulation) in the case of ASA should be discontinued 5-7 days before surgery and anticoagulation is recommended to have INR <1.5, five days prior to surgery, vitamin K malabsorption, liver disease due to decreased synthesis of clotting factors, SLE, amyloidosis, prior chemotherapy, and so on.

Intraoperative risk factors are: pump bypass, hypothermia, use of heparin during cardiopulmonary bypass generation of fibrinolytic activity and postoperative risk factors known are octogenarians, non-elective surgery, low BMI, CPB> 150 min, grafts ≥ 5, surgical reintervention.

During the first 6 hrs of PO should immediately obtained objective results of platelet count and coagulation, for early medical or surgical management, clinical criteria is in relation to the following table.

In the management of patients with heavy bleeding PO should commence administration of blood products such as red cell concentrates without doubt the goal is to maintain the optimum level in arterial blood content [CaO2 = CaO2 = Hb (g/100ml) x 1.34 (ml O2 / g) x% SaO2 + (PaO2 x 0.0031) = ml blood O2/100ml)]. They are prepared with 300 ml volume with low WBC (<5x106 cells) to reduce alloimmunization and avoid possible TRALI or lung damage. Cell salvage, the process by which collects a patient's own blood during surgery for later transfusion in the same patient is a reliable alternative to donor blood transfusion when needed. We found 23 studies investigating the effectiveness of cell salvage in cardiac surgery, conclude that apparently there is insufficient evidence to support the use of cell salvage in cardiac surgery but the methodology in the studies were flawed and may be biased.

Alterations in the number or function of platelets may have effects ranging from a clinically insignificant prolongation of bleeding time to large defects of hemostasis, platelet transfusion is usually required when it decreases the count: <50,000, is individualized 50-100 the case and over 100,000 were transfused if the time of Ivy is more than 10 minutes with continued bleeding. Can be obtained by platelet concentrates (40-70ml) or platelet apheresis (200-300ml).

The use of fresh frozen plasma in postoperative patients offers all the clotting factors and plasma proteins needed to improve the prothrombin time and clotting better ensure hemodilution coagulopathy, caution should be exercised in bleeding secondary to heparin, as a source ATIII natural and should not be used prophylactically. To replace clotting factors to be used a dose of 10 to 20 mL / kg, which could increase the concentration factor by 20% immediately after infusion. [58,59,60]

The cryoprecipitate is a concentrate of plasma proteins of high molecular weight cold rush its volume is approximately 15 to 20 mL after removing the supernatant plasma containing concentrations of factor VIII: C (procoagulant activity), 80 to 120 U; factor VIII: vWF (von Willebrand factor), 40 to 70%, fibrinogen, 100 to 250 mg, and Factor XIII, 20 to 30%.

Most of the work with hemostatic agents were designed to assess the therapeutic efficacy and to assess potential toxic effects, so that there are still definite data on the safety of hemostatic agents. Many studies on these agents have used perioperative blood loss and other parameters with endpoints of little clinical importance, whereas other studies did not have enough power to evaluate the clinical outcome of importance, such as mortality or need for reoperation.

Pharmacological agents that decrease postoperative bleeding are desmopressin is a synthetic analogue of natural vasopressin, with the advantage of having less vasoconstriction, is recommended for use in the immediate postoperative hemostatic, unlike aprotinin has fewer side effects such as anaphylaxis, thrombosis and renal failure. Aprotinin has been used in recent times but because it is a bovine protein, there is an increased risk of anaphylaxis, especially if you already had previous exposure, and its cost is higher. When used at low doses acts as antidiuretic hormone and is 10-20 times the dose that increases hemostatic function and plasma levels of factor VIII, von Willebrand factor (vWF) and tissue plasminogen activator (tPA), releasing these factors endothelium and liver. Also observed increased platelet aggregation, the result is the shortening of bleeding time. Administered

IV (0.3ug/Kg), SC (0.3ug/Kg) but for obvious reasons dministration IV is recommended in postoperative patients. The best response is expected between 30-60min after parenteral administration.

Inside are antifibrinolytic drugs: aprotinin (a direct inhibitor of the fibrinolytic enzyme plasmin) is the only drug approved by published and the Food and Drug Administration (FDA) to minimize transfusion requirements in coronary bypass surgery, directly inhibits the fibrinolytic enzyme plasmin, plasma kallikrein, tissue trypsin and activated coagulation factor XII, the highest recommended dose is> 700mg.

Are also used tranexamic acid and aminocaproic acid, but have not been approved by the FDA for this indication, their mechanisms of action are the first to inhibit the binding of plasmin to fibrin occupying the binding sites of lysine of the proenzyme plasminogen and the second is the same mechanism of action, but 10 times more potent. Doses are 10-30g and maintenance 1-3gr/hr and the second 3-10gr with 20-250mg/hr maintenance.

There are reviews of meta-analysis on the effectiveness of antifibrinolytic agents compared with placebo, aprotinin or tranexamic acid, but not aminocaproic acid, reduced the need for blood transfusion by 30% and saved about 1 unit of blood per operation. There was no difference in efficacy between regimens with high or low doses of aprotinin, while varying doses of tranexamic acid and aminocaproic's not possible to assess the relationship between dose and efficacy. As for the most relevant clinical events, the relative risk of reoperation for excessive bleeding was significantly reduced in patients receiving aprotinin, compared with those receiving placebo, although the mortality rate remained unchanged. Both tranexamic acid and aminocaproic acid significantly decreased these events. Therefore, the results of the work checked and reviews indicate that antifibrinolytic drugs are effective hemostatic agents in cardiac surgery. Reductions in transfusion requirements and reoperation for bleeding seem to be confirmed by the narrow confidence intervals of likelihood ratios, indicators of relative risks. There were no sufficient data on the effectiveness that allow definitive conclusions regarding the use of antifibrinolytic agents in other situations. [61,62,63,64,65,66,67]

While other review reports that aminocaproic acid and tranexamic acid are safe, it is noteworthy that the works included were smaller than the jobs studied aprotinin. Therefore, the authors say, the safety data are not reliable, especially with regard to thrombosis. Currently, the Blood Conservation using Antifibrinolytics: a randomized work in a population submitted to cardiac surgery (Randomized Trial in a Cardiac Surgery Population) or BART, which is still enrolling patients, is designed to enroll 2970 patients with indications for cardiac surgery high risk, to determine whether aprotinin is superior to tranexamic acid or aminocaproic acid to reduce the risk of massive postoperative bleeding. Secondary endpoints were overall mortality and adverse effects such as cardiovascular disease and kidney failure. For all available data, the authors argue that the evidence that aprotinin reduces perioperative bleeding and immediate postoperative transfusion requirement is sound. However, note that despite the large number of clinical trials that have addressed the drug, its effectiveness in reducing the need for reoperation has just emerged from reviews and lack of evidence about its effect on mortality. [68,69,70]

Recombinant activated factor VII (rFVIIa) acts locally at the site of tissue injury and alterations of the vascular wall by binding to exposed tissue factor, generating small amounts of thrombin sufficient to activate platelets. The activated platelet surface can then form a template on which rFVIIa half the direct or indirect activation of coagulation to generate thrombin in the end much more and convert fibrinogen to fibrin. The clot is stabilized by inhibition of fibrinolysis, secondary to activation of the inhibitor of thrombin-activatable fibrinolysis mediated by rFVIIa. The availability of rFVIIa has expanded treatment options for acute bleeding in hemophilia patients. This drug is not a panacea, but it has efficacy in patients with trauma and excessive bleeding resistant to other treatments. However, the encouraging results obtained so far must be confirmed by other studies, are also necessary cost-effectiveness studies, as it is an expensive drug. The authors recommend to take with caution the results of studies recognized even before considering the evidence as a guideline. We have tried to increase the power and efficacy of rFVIIa by molecular engineering acting on DNA, but no studies. [71,72,73,74,75]

Perioperative myocardial

Although virtually all patients have some degree of increase in cardiac enzymes after surgery. The perioperative myocardial infarction is one of the most serious complications after CABG (RVM), an incidence of 5-20%, and is associated with significant morbidity and mortality in the post-surgical high. The pathogenesis of IPO vasa in the various mechanisms by which the placement of coronary artery bypass bridges leading to myocardial necrosis: The most common is acute occlusion of the hemoducto, twist it, subtotal graft stenosis or spasm, saying recent articles The presence of collateral arterioles protects perioperative stroke patients.

The perioperative myocardial infarction (IPO) type 5 belongs to heart and is defined according to the latest consensus established in 2007 by the AHA / ACC as an increase of at least 5 times the baseline or reference biomarkers, along with the emergence of new q waves left bundle branch block on electrocardiogram, or coronary angiography showing acute occlusion of hemoductos and imaging evidence of recent loss of viable myocardial tissue.

According to Thielmann, the increase in markers of myocardial damage, can be used to discriminate between perioperative stroke related to the placement of coronary artery bypass bridge, or another cause. So analyzing 3308 patients with MVR, I conclude that the 94 who underwent coronary angiography, 56 had stroke related to the placement of coronary artery bypass bridges, 38 was not related to the procedure. Levels of troponin I, rather than CK / CK-MB rose significantly in the first group with respect to the second, considering the troponin I as the best marker to discriminate between IM surgery associated with those who are not associate the procedure with a cutoff of 10.5 ng / ml, and those in which MI was directly associated with the placement of non-hemoductos with a cutoff of 35.5 ng / ml.

In peri-operative myocardial infarction not associated with coronary bypass grafts, is due to mechanisms such as inadequate cardioplegic perfusion, incomplete revascularization, distal coronary microembolization caused by surgical manipulation, recent unstable angina, poor left ventricular function. This early detection of perioperative myocardial infarction plays an important role in treating either early coronary angiography and angioplasty, trying to preserve left ventricular function as a predictor of long-term survival. Obviously the presence of perioperative myocardial infarction is associated with a high rate of heart failure and long-term mediately, as evidenced by Steuer, analyzing patients with MVR 7.493 assessing the number of readmissions for heart failure. Found that 7.7% (576) were readmitted for heart failure. Of these, 20% (114) had perioperative myocardial infarction. [76,77,78,79,80,81]

Tamponade

It is characterized by symptoms and signs of hemodynamic instability due to the restrictive effect on cardiac contraction, usually observed within the first 6hrs associated with poor permeability of their drains. The prevalence of this complication varies between different publications, ranging from 0.8% -8.5%, there are reports in which said one of the most frequent causes, to the use of internal mammary artery for coronary artery bypass bridge, on the other hand, the use of a single anterior mediastinal tube, instead of 2 tubes (front and back) has been associated with a high rate of pericardial fluid and as a result of these patients tamponade.La course evaluation should be carried out by echocardiography, and not just those with a radiological image suggestive of this entity (heart carafe), since by this method because of cardiac surgery postoperative patients identified only 50% of patients. This is important because several studies have shown that those patients who develop pericardial effusion, even without hemodynamic compromise, increased risk of supraventricular arrhythmias, sternal dehiscence, prolonged hospital stay and a significant reduction in exercise tolerance. [82,83,84]

Finally, the treatment will be those with hemodynamic compromise, is permeated drains, by performing emergency echocardiography and reoperation. [85,86,87,88,89]

Vasoplegic Syndrome

Vasoplegic syndrome (SV) is a severe form of systemic inflammatory response syndrome (SIRS), which ranks its expression on the cardiovascular system. A number of reports considered the vasoplegia as a recognized complication of cardiac surgery, the main clinical manifestation is the presence of hypotension, usually severe, which features the distinctive clinical feature of responding with little or no input from volume.

In cardiac surgery, the reported incidence is 8 to 10%, even up to 40%, these differences often depend on characteristics of the study population (ventricular function), the type of intervention assessed (use or not of CPB, type cardioplegia) and mainly from the diagnostic criteria used. As mentioned previously, the key point is the presence of hypotension, usually with a systolic blood pressure (SBP) <85 mm Hg, and / or mean arterial pressure (MAP) <50 mm Hg.Un clinical data necessary to consider the diagnosis of Vasoplegia is the lack of response to volume expansion. A hypotensive patient in the postoperative period of cardiac surgery, central venous pressure (CVP) reduced elevation of the same after the infusion of 500 or 1000 ml of solutions (even at higher volumes) should lead to the posing of vasoplegia. [90,91,92,93]

Strict diagnostic confirmation will require the use of hemodynamic monitoring, the presence of Swan Ganz catheter will allow a broader determination descended filling pressures, by providing values of pulmonary capillary pressure (PCP) reduced.

Diagnostic criteria

1. Clinical (only allow them to suspicion)
   Low blood pressure response with little or no volume expansion aapropiada
2. Hemodynamic
   Hypotension (SBP <85 mm Hg / TAM <50 mm Hg)
   Reduced filling pressures (CVP <5 mm Hg / Wedge <10 mm Hg)
   Minute volume and normal or elevated cardiac index (CI equal to or greater than 2.5 L/min/m2)
   Reduced systemic vascular resistance (SVR <800 dinas/seg/cm-5)

Vasopressor requirement (> 0.5 mcg / kg / min noradrenaline or> 10 mcg / kg / min dopamine)

3. Other
   a. In operating room, with open chest
      PVC hypotension with low (<5 mm Hg) refractory avolumen associated with excellent observation of left ventricular contractility.
   b. postoperative
      PVC hypotension with low (<5 mm Hg) refractory avolumen associated with echocardiography (bidimensionalcon good window or transesophageal) with apreciaciónde good left ventricular contractility.

The main therapeutic goal is sustain perfusion to vital organs like the kidney, brain, liver and heart. This also implies the initial use of volume, the use of two types of drugs, drugs with pressor effect, linked to its exclusive or non-selective action on alpha adrenergic receptors, such as metaraminol or phenylephrine among the first, and epinephrine, norepinephrine or dopamine among the latter. The use of drugs associated with beta-adrenergic effect, will result in some measure, an increase of myocardial oxygen consumption in the same direction, their association with postoperative arrhythmias, has also been reported. The second drawback associated with, and probably the most important clinical refractoriness to vasopressors is that certain forms of vasoplegia postoperative manifest. This refractoriness drugs raises the utility of antagonists or inhibitors of NO and the enzyme guanylate cyclase, we consider a rational therapeutic approach more physiological. Two drugs are the most studied, methylene blue, and vasopressin [94,95,96,97,98]

Methylene Blue (AM): its therapeutic action is based on the inhibitory effect of NO or blocking of the enzyme guanylate cyclase. This drug has been considered in several isolated reports in a series without a control group and essentially in a randomized control group. Leyh et al. reported 54 patients with refractory postoperative vasoplegia the use of norepinephrine, treated with 2 mg / kg AM. Fifty-one patients showed favorable hemodynamic changes in the course of one hour post-treatment. Three patients died in the hospital course of the picture (5.6%). The study lacked a control group. Another key finding is the shorter of the table between those treated with AM. In these, vasoplegia resolved completely within two hours after the start of infusion, whereas in those managed conventionally, the box is extended in time, such extension of time associating with a higher incidence of complications and late onset sepsis and multiorgan dysfunction . Several authors have agreed with this finding, giving unfavorable prognostic value of the persistence over time of the SV, accepting that a breakpoint located between 36 and 48 hours is a marker of poor prognosis.

Vasopressin: Vasopressin (antidiuretic hormone arginine vasopressin), Argenziano et al. described the association between the shock with vasodilatation after bypass surgery and deficiency of vasopressin. Which is secreted by the neurohypophysis regulates tubular permeability to water, typically having limited participation in the control of BP. Under conditions of hypotension, such as bleeding or vasoplegia itself is a rapid depletion of endogenous. It allows a rapid reversal of hypotension, especially in patients refractory to vasopressors. In addition, the hormone increases vascular sensitivity to catecholamines and increases urine output, based on its direct action on glomerular efferent arteriole, unlike catecholamines, whose site is located on the therapeutic afferent arteriole. The proposed dose is 0.05 to 0.1 unit / minute.

The use of off-pump surgery was associated with less inflammatory response, with lower incidence of postoperative SV. However, the picture is commonly seen and may present a favorable course. Vasoplegic syndrome is associated with a poor prognosis, when it is resistant norepinerina poorer prognosis with increased morbidity and mortality. The reported mortality after cardiac surgery is 24% in series reported by Levin and colleagues, and 25% in series reported by Gómez et al, in which case the syndrome persisted for up to 48hr vasoplegic. [99,100,101,102,103]

7. Drug therapy

The support with vasopressor, vasodilator and inotropic therapeutic behavior is common in the first 24 hours secondary to hemodynamic effects induced hypothermia, myocardial stunning, extracorporeal circulation, hypovolemia, sedation, and so on. Despite the frequency of use of catecholamines are well known adverse effects such as increased myocardial consumption, arrhythmogenic, favor delirium, and so on. [104,105,106]

Dobutamine

Amine as the structure similar to dopamine is primarily a beta-adrenergic agonist relatively selective beta-1. Is much more effective and positive inotropic and positive chronotropic capacity less arrhythmogenic than dopamine, has no affinity to dopamine receptors and therefore lacks the renal effect. A standard dose (2-15µg/kg/min) positive inotropic responses observed with a slight increase in heart rate and decreased peripheral resistance. [107,108]

In the perioperative setting is used primarily as inotropic, often combined with vasopressor either to maintain adequate cardiac output and blood pressure and to achieve a combined effect of cardiac output and perfusion. On the other hand as shown by Susana Lobo et. al; randomizing 50 patients over 65 high-risk cardiac surgery, receiving IV fluids liquid + vs Dobutamine, the largest number of perioperative complications observed was present in those who do not use vs those who had dobutamine infusion: 52 % vs 16%, and mortality at 60 days was 28% vs 8% in the dobutamine group. [109,110,111,112,113,114]

The drug's half life is 3-5 min, one of several effects is the progressive decrease in blood pressure and pulmonary wedge has an advantage over the effect of dopamine beta for a smaller effect observed tachycardic and arrhythmogenic action and dilation in the pulmonary circulation has been confirmed in the peripheral circulation. As observed Romson et al; administered dobutamine in varying doses and patients undergoing cardiopulmonary bypass the heart rate changes depending on the dose and this is lower in individuals over 65 years, there were minimal changes in blood pressure, instead a decrease in pulmonary capillary wedge pressure and central venous pressure increased systemic vascular resistance remained in a mild and constant left ventricular performance also increase due to increased heart rate [115,116]

Phosphodiesterase inhibitors

They are a family of enzymes involved in cellular physiology by regulating the concentration of intracellular second messengers are known at present eight of these isoforms of phosphodiesterases, which interests us is the number III. Cyclic AMP, produced from the stimulation of beta-adrenergic receptors may have two destinations: the culminating with an increase in cardiac contractility, and the other consisting of the degradation of cAMP to 5-AMP, produced by phosphodiesterase III . Inhibition of this enzyme protects cAMP, promoting their destination to the increase in contractility. It now has a group of inotropic drugs whose mechanism of action is precisely in the inhibition of phosphodiesterase-III. Of this group stand amrinone and milrinone for the extensive clinical experience has accumulated with its use. These substances belong to the bipyridines, this is a positive inotropic effect supplemented by a peripheral vasodilator, which contributes to a better ability to emptying of the heart. The hemodynamic effects of milrinone, administered as a loading dose of 50 micrograms / kg followed by continuous infusion of 0.35 to 0.75 micrograms / kg / min is significant reductions in diastolic pressure in the aorta, the mean aortic pressure and systemic vascular resistance by about 11% ejection fraction of left ventricle is increased by about 14%, these effects are closely related to plasma concentrations. [117,118,119,120]

In the postoperative period especially in patients receiving milrinone pump has several effects on pulmonary circulation and inotropism as evidenced Mitsunori et al, which randomized 30 patients undergoing cardiac surgery treated with milrinone was reported, reduced the mean pressure of right atrial pressure in the pulmonary artery wedge, mean pulmonary pressure and systemic vascular resistance without making a significant change in mean arterial pressure or heart rate.

On the other hand the use of Milrinone has been shown to be beneficial in patients undergoing CSRC bomb and right ventricular dysfunction prior. Jong H. et al analyzed the effect of infusion of milrinone in patients undergoing CSRC and right ventricular dysfunction (VD) found no increase in cardiac index, heart rate, and decreased systemic vascular resistance. Changes in right ventricular ejection fraction were not significant, whereas in cardiac output and RV afterload if they were, finally improves graft flow in the breast and in the middle cerebral artery during surgery of the CSRC.

Dopamine

Dopamine (D) precursor of norepinephrine in the biological synthesis, there are specific receptors for this substance, especially in the renal circulation, where it produces a vasodilatory effect which favors renal tubular function (Hiberman et.al 1984). At the heart there are dopamine receptors, but its function on contractility is weak and little known, this effect is not accompanied by an increase in resistance as pronounced as with peripheral epinephrine and norepinephrine under in vessels predominantly to dopamine receptor stimulation.

The mechanism of action is dose dependent at relatively low doses (1-5µg/kg/min) stimulates dopamine receptors predominantly with subsequent renal and mesenteric vasodilation (Szerlip, et. Al 1991). A moderate dose of 5-10 mg / kg / min stimulates beta adrenergic receptors leading to positive inotropic effects and high-dose alpha-adrenergic stimulation 10-15µg/kg/min carries peripheral vasoconstriction.

By perioperative is used for its effects on the renal circulation as well as its positive inotropic effect can be used in improving the ICC states inotropism significantly, the clinical effect is seen immediately as the drug's half life is 3 -4 min. Among its side effects can cause or exacerbate tachyarrhythmias, because its effect is mediated by increased levels of norepinephrine. At present medical evidence did not show benefit of using low doses of dopamine effect of splanchnic vasodilatation and renal function, however, this drug increases oxygen consumption at promoting tubular tubular ischemia, in addition there is poor correlation between blood levels with dose infused.

Norepinephrine

Its structure is similar to that of epinerfrina is the endogenous neurotransmitter for postganglionic sympathetic nervous system, its basic function is to stimulate alpha-1 receptors and less beta-1 receptors and beta-2. Intravenous administration of norepinephrine increases blood pressure by increasing peripheral vascular resistance due to this increase, heart rate tends to decrease due to a vagal reflex which overrides the stimulation of myocardial beta-1 receptors, their After stimulation of these receptors causes a recent positive inotropic effect especially at low doses.

Under normal conditions this amine decreases renal blood flow (with minimal changes in glomerular filtration rate) and mesenteric, splanchnic and liver. The administration of norepinephrine should be through a central line to avoid tissue necrosis. Is much more convenient administration via infusion and the usual dose is 0.01 to 0.1 mg / kg / min or 2-15 mcg / min. So perioperative norepinephrine may be used at low doses for its chronotropic effect and vasoconstrictive properties (intermediate dose). Especially for its effect on the peripheral circulation is indicated in cases where failure is demonstrated in the ability of vasoregulation, because it increases blood flow by increasing systemic blood pressure especially in shock. It should be used so cautious in patients with MAO inhibitors. The tx hypovolemic shock with norepinephrine leads to severe multiorgan hypoperfusion.

The use of norepinephrine in patients undergoing cardiac surgery is controversial because of fear that has regard to the commitment in the function mediated renal vasoconstriction. Hiroshi Morimatsu, et. randomized 100 patients to post-operative heart to norepinephrine infusion in line and this study was carried out monitoring of renal function with infusion of norepinephrine in postsurgical hypotension TAM <70 mmHg. The results was an increase in central venous pressure, decreased systemic vascular resistance index with increased heart rate will eventually change in serum creatinine of treaties. Kwak Y, showed that one of the applications of norepinephrine after surgery is the treatment of hypotension in patients with chronic pulmonary hypertension as they are benefiting from the control of blood pressure without increasing the PSAP but rather decreases many of them.

Nitroglycerin

Its mechanism of action is through biotransformation in vascular smooth muscle by activating guanylyl cyclase thereby resulting in an increase of cyclic GMP and thus vasodilation. The effectiveness of nitroglycerin decreases after 18-24 hr by a phenomenon of tolerance due to decreased formation of nitric oxide in this way. The NTG has the ability to vasodilate both beds (arterial and venous) at low doses, dominated by its vasodilatory effect and increases venous capacitance and thus decreasing venous pressure and diastolic filling. However high doses of nitroglycerin significantly increases venous capacitance and systemic arteriolar resistance, thereby decreasing the systolic blood pressure and cardiac output. As a mechanism the body responds by reflex sympathetic tachycardia and peripheral arteriolar vasoconstriction, despite this effect on the coronary circulation is vasodilation of both healthy and affected artery atherosclerosis, and also increase collateral circulation areas although its main effect is on the arteries coronary larger caliber and low on resistance of lesser caliber. On myocardial oxygen requirements, mainly affects the ventricular wall tension by increasing venous capacitance, which in turn decreases venous return to the heart leading to a decrease in ventricular wall tension and myocardial oxygen consumption. Another beneficial effect is that the decrease in pre-produced increase in LV perfusion and favoring the subendocardium.

Their metabolism is primarily via hepatic glutathione by organic nitrate reductase. Its effect is dissipated in 30-60 min intravenous Its effect is achieved after 90 seconds and is dose dependent. The usual dose of 0.5-3 mg is / kg / min infusion or 5-200 g / min and 0.5 mg bolus. In post-qx therapy use in peri-and post-qx:

- Myocardial ischemia associated with ventricular arrhythmias, especially when this is caused by halogenated anesthetics.
- Myocardial ischemia with an increase in pulmonary capillary pressure associated with a persistence in the inhalation anesthetics.
- Coronary Spasm
- Intravenous administration has been proposed as prophylactic coronary bypass surgery to prevent episodes of ischemia by vasospasm
- Useful for the treatment of hypertension during surgery RVM.

Sodium nitroprusside

One of the most commonly used vasodilators in the perioperative period, penetrating the endothelium acts to form nitric oxide, this results in the production of guanine monophosphate to guanine triphosphate. Thus cyclic GMP is the second messenger that triggers calcium binding. Its effect occurs seconds after the start of infusion. The commonly used dose is 1-40 mcg / min.

At low doses predominantly dilated arteries and arterioles, and how the dose increases also becomes a venodilators. As with nitroglycerin may occur reflexively tachycardia. And increased venous capacitance and thereby reducing cardiac output. On the other hand it is important to consider that as an important arteriodilatador can produce the phenomenon of coronary steal, mostly because it does not vasodilation in arteries affected by atherosclerosis, reducing the flow in the latter.

Among other effects has the ability to produce dilation of the pulmonary vascular bed arriving to produce hypoxia. Another effect is less desirable thiocyanate intoxication, which prevent tissue oxygen delivery by blocking the final stages of the respiratory chain.

Its administration should be in glucose solution covering both the drug and the line connecting the infusion pump. The usual dose is 40 - 300 micrograms / min. Going to be titrated according to a patient's response.

Vasopressin

Vasopressin also known as antidiuretic hormone is a peptide product of the hypothalamus and stored in the posterior lobe of the pituitary. Feedback effects in several organs including the brain where it acts as a neurotransmitter regulating body temperature, nociception and adenocorticotropica hormone release. In the pulmonary vasculature, moderate dose of vasopressin causes vasodilatation while high doses produce vasoconstriction. Vasopressin also has other effects on thrombosis and hemostasis, including platelet aggregation and release of factor VIII and von Willebrand.

Plasma levels of vasopressin in patients after undergoing bypass surgery ranges from 100 -200 pg / ml, while the hemorrhagic shock promotes the release of plasma concentrations of 1000 pg / ml. Several publications indicate that the usual dose of this drug is between 0.01 to 0.1 U / min, and is effective in patients with shock vasodilation without adverse effects.

Hypotension refractory to high doses of alpha-adrenergic agonists after cardiac surgery, after the use of cardiopulmonary bypass, has been referred to as Sx vasoplegic. This vasopressin has been used for this treatment with encouraging results. Masseti and colleagues studied 16 patients with intravenous vasopressin (0.1-1 IU / min) for the treatment of hypotension refractory to maximum dose of norepinephrine (> 30 mg / kg / min). Preoperative ejection fraction was 40.5% and NYHA functional class 3.5. Getting an increase in blood pressure of 89 mmHg baseline to 116, increase in SVR from 688 to 1043, decreased cardiac index from 2.6 to 2.9 L/min/m2, urine volume increased from 36.8 to 72.8 ml / h.

Whereas high doses of vasopressin and effective in the treatment of Sx vasoplegic after cardiac surgery with cardiopulmonary bypass.

In a recent study, Argenziano et al found that about 10% of patients undergoing cardiac surgery experienced hypotension by vasodilation after bypass surgery, which not necessarily is associated with cardiogenic or septic shock. Interestingly, in situations in which hypotension persists after surgery RVM, smooth muscle cells become less sensitive to circulating catecholamines. This phenomenon is due to decreased function of adrenergic receptors, the study of 50 patients conducted at Columbia Presbyterian Medical Center undergoing cardiac surgery were treated with vasopressin in the operating room or intensive therapy in the first 24 hr surgery (6). All patients had less than 60 mmHg TAM and decreased systemic resistance, despite support with catecholamines. This administration of vasopressin infusion of 0.09 U / min increased the TAM from 58 to 75 mmHg, the SVR increased from 920 to 1200 dyne s cm and achieving a reduction in the administration of norepinephrine in 32%.

Nesiritide

Brain natriuretic peptide also known as BNP is a neurohormone secreted by the left ventricle in response to increased stress (both pressure and volume in the varga) in the ventricular wall. Physiological actions of BNP include natriuresis, vasodilation and neurohormonal modulation. So the tx with BNP has emerged as a viable option in the tx of acute CHF. Moreover, its determination of serum is currently used to differentiate cardiac dyspnea pulmonary dela type. In general, levels of BNP 100pg/ml excludes minors 1 decompensated CHF, whereas values greater than 500pg/ml indicates decompensation.

Neseritide is the recombinant form of endogenous human BNP. Has been shown to decrease filling pressures, increase cardiac output and improve the clinical condition of patients with decompensated CHF. In August 2001 was approved by the FDA for tx of CHF in those with decompensated dyspnea at rest or with minimal effort. The recommended dose is 2μg/kg initial bolus followed by infusion of 0.01μg/kg/min extended to a maximum of 48 hr.

Several studies have examined the possible application of perioperative neseritide so, in patients with left ventricular dysfunction who will undergo heart surgery. In a study prospectivco, open, randomized controlled, Brackbill et al examined the use of perioperative infusion of neriritide and showed improvement compared with milrinone. We included 40 hemodynamically stable patients with LVEF 35% or less that were undergoing bypass surgery. And they were randomized to a bolus of nesiritide or milrinone intraoperatively followed by an infusion of any of them for 24 hr. The time spent in post-qx therapy was the primary outcome measure. The incidence of post-qx ICC, the rate of readmission within 30 days, mortality and other clinical parameters were compared. Patients receiving nesiritide had a hospital stay of 50.6 + / - 46.8 hours compared with 44.1 + / - 23.5 hours of receiving milrinone (p = 0.57). The incidence of post-qx ICC also showed no significant results in both groups (p = 0.25). On the third day of follow up, no significant differences in SBP readmission between the two drugs and there was no impact on mortality, the authors concluded that nesiritide does not reduce hospital stay post-qx like not modify other parameters of disease compared with nesiritide in MVR and stable ventricular function.

In a prospective double-blind (NAPA) Mentzer et al; consider the role nesiritide might play in patients with left ventricular dysfunction with MVR with cardiopulmonary bypass. Patients with ejection fraction less than or equal to 40% who underwent MVR and DCP were randomized to receive nesiritide or placebo for 24-96 hr after induction of anesthesia. The post-qx renal function, hemodynamic parameters and drug use (primary endpoints) were evaluated in patients with MVR with DCP, mortality and safety (secondary endpoints) were evaluated in all patients who received the drug, 303 patients randomized, 279 received the drug and 272 underwent MVR with DCP. Compared with placebo, nesiritide was associated with a slight increase in serum creatinine (0.15 + / - 0.29 mg / dl versus. 0.34 + / - 0.48 mg / dl, p <0.001) and a fall in glomerular filtration rate (- 10.8 + / - 19.3 mL/min/1.73 m (2) versus -17.2 + / - 21.9 mL/min/1.73 m (2), P = 0.001) during hospital stay or stay on 14. On the other hand, patients treated with nesiritide had a shorter hospital stay (p = 0.043) and lower mortality at 180 days. (P = 0.046). The authors concluded that nesiritide in the context of RVM with CPB is associated with improved renal function post-qx and possibly increased survival.

8. Medical treatment

Aspirin

There are currently a total of 8 studies with more than 2500 patients using aspirin CSRC. The doses used 325-1200 mg daily. Two of these studies showed significant benefit of aspirin a day after heart surgery. In contrast to the other 6 that saw no difference vs placebo with regard to occlusion of the bridges managed belatedly. In conclusion, the evidence so far suggests that the use of aspirin to reduce occlusion of coronary artery bypass bridges to 12 months after CSRC when given the 1st day after surgery, on the other hand is a medicine economic which is associated with few adverse effects and is of great benefit for patients with coronary artery disease peripheral with that aspirin should be given the most quickly as possible after cardiac surgery and continued indefinitely.

Hlipolipemiantes

There are three studies involving 1900 patients to evaluate the use of these agents on the occlusion of coronary artery bypass grafts and the risk of cardiovascular events): The Post-CABG trial, LOCATE (Lopid Coronary Angiography Trial) and Cholesterol Lowering Atherosclerotic Study (CLAS). All three showed a significant reduction in the progression of atherosclerosis in coronary artery bypass bridges. Thus the long-term use of lipid-lowering drugs prevent the progression of atherosclerosis in both native arteries and in coronary bridges and reduces cardiovascular events, it was shown that the use of these agents reduces the progression of atherosclerosis after 2 years RVM.

Pan et al, found that after adjusting the demographic and clinical differences, the preoperative use of statins was associated with a 50% reduction in mortality, but showed no benefit in the occurrence of AF or IM. Dotan et al, found that statins were associated with a significant decrease in cardiac mortality, unstable angina and arrhythmias 60 days to 1 year.

Beta blocker

Its use has been assessed by many studies, but in a perioperative cardiac surgery, Sjölander et.al, conducted a controlled double-blind study of 967 patients with MVR. Patients were randomized 4 to 21 days after RVM receiving 50 mg of metoprolol 2 times per day x 2 weeks and 100 mg of metoprolol per day vs placebo 2 x 2 years. There was no significant difference between the 2 study arms with respect to exercise capacity, however cn patients placebo had a higher rate of chest pain compared with the metoprolol group. On the other hand no significant difference in both groups with regard to revascularization, unstable angina, nonfatal MI or death at 2 years of follow-up.

Finally, Ferguson et al, in a cohort study investigated the use of preoperative B-blocker in 629 877 patients undergoing CSRC and showed a reduction to 30 days of drug-related mortality (OR 0.90, 95% CI0.87-0.93). This decrease was consistent with all groups of patients except those with LVEF <30% where there was no demonstrated benefit.

Calcium antagonist

Only one study has examined the effect of calcium antagonists initiated after surgery RVM, Gaudino et al; evaluating the benefits of calcium antagonists after the first year of revascularization. A total of 120 patients with normal perfusion function were randomized after 1 year of tx with 120 mg diatiazem to continue with or stop. No significant differences after 4 years of follow-up among the group of calcium antagonists and those who discontinued tx with respect to recurrence of angina (10% vs 12%), residual ischemia, 17% vs 18%) and cardiac death 2% vs 0%). In short there is little evidence to support the routine use of calcium antagonists or nitrates after cardiac surgery.

ACEI

Despite the known benefits of ACE inhibitors, only 4 studies examined perioperative prophylactic use of ACE inhibitors in patients with MVR. QUO VADIS In the study 149 patients were randomized to quinapril 40mg/día or placebo for 4 weeks before elective surgery RVM, treatment was continued for 1 year. The researchers found that quinapril significantly reduced 1-year clinical events, such as death from cardiovascular causes.

9. Anticoagulants and antithrombotics management

Thromboembolism and bleeding associated with anticoagulation comprise about 75% of the complications associated with prosthetic valves. antithrombotic therapy can reduce but not eliminate the possibility of this catrastofe. It is reported that the incidence of perioperative arterial thromboembolism is approximately 0.4 to 1.5% and the annual risk of stroke in high risk patients without anticoagulation is> 5.6% and <2.0% of major bleeding.

The risk for thrombus formation with prosthetic heart valves is seven times higher in the first month after valve replacement during the following months, years intracardiac position independent. The underlying pathophysiology of activation are factors in the systems of intrinsic and extrinsic coagulation of synthetic surface extracorporeal circulation of blood or from contact with surfaces or tissue devoid of collagen, a significant number of surgeons in favor of delaying the anticoagulant because the risk of bleeding, the incidence of pericardial tamponade and reoperation is eight times higher in

patients treated with high doses of heparin than in those treated with low-dose heparin for prevention of venous thrombosis.
Anticoagulation is recommended in the following cases:

- Lifetime on all patients with mechanical valves
- Lifetime in patients with biological valves who have other indications for anticoagulation Vgr: atrial fibrillation, heart failure, ventricular ejection fraction less than 30% left.
- For the first three months in patients with bioprostheses after insertion, with a target INR of 2.5. No emabrgo strategy with aspirin (low dose-100 mg DE75) is an alternative, but there have been no randomized studies supporting the safety of this strategy.

There is no consensus at the time of initiation of anticoagulation after surgery, but should begin during the first days postoperatively. (5 + -2)

10. References

[1] Lyons AS, Petruccelli RJ II. Medicine and illustrated history. New York: HN Abrams Inc, 1978.
[2] Vesalius A. De humani corporis fabrica. Budapest: Corvina / Magyar Helikon, 1972.
[3] Rutkow IM. Surgery. An illustrated history. St. Louis, Baltimore, Boston, Chicago, London, Madrid, Philadelphia, Sydney, Toronto: Mosby, 1993.
[4] Casey LC. Roles of cytokines in the pathogenesis of multisystem organ failure induced cardiopulmonary. Ann Thorac Surg 1993; S6: S92-S96.
[5] Huddy SP, Joyce WP. Pepper JR. Gastrointestinal Complications in Patients Who underwent cardiopulmonary 4.473 bypass surgery. Br J Surg 1991; 78:293-296.
[6] CHV Thakar, Jared JP, Worley S, Cotman K, Paganini EP. Renal dysfunction and Serious Infections After open-heart surgery. Kidney Int 2003; 64:239-246.
[7] Laffey J, Boylan J, Cheng D. The systemic inflammatory response to cardiac surgery. Anesthesiology 2002; 97:215-252.
[8] Kollef MH, Wragge T, Pasque Ch Determinants of Mortality and multiorgan dysfunction in cardiac surgery Patients Requiring Prolonged mechanical ventilation. Chest 1995; 107 (5) :1395-1401.
[9] Kalfin RE, Engelmann RM, Rousseau JA, Flack JE III, Deaton DW, Kreutzer DL, DK Dash. Induction of interleukin-8 expression cardiopulmonary bypass DURING. Circulation 1993; 88 [Part 2]: 401 - 406.
[10] Ascione R, Lloyd CT, Underwood MJ, Lotto A, Pitsis AA, Angelini GD. After coronary revascularization Inflammatory response With or Without cardiopulmonary bypass prospective randomized study. Ann Thorac Surg 2000; 69: 1198-1204.
[11] Nilsson L, Kulander L, Sven-Olov N, Eriksson O. Endotoxins in cardiopulmonary bypass. J Thorac Cardiovasc Surg 1990; 100:777-780.
[12] Pizzo PA. Empirical therapy and prevention of infections in the immunocompromised host. In: Mandell GL, Bennett JE. Dolin R, editors. Principles and practice of infectious diseases. 5th edition. New York: Churchill-Livingstone, 2000. pp. 3102-3112.
[13] Rossi F. The O2-forming NADPH oxidase of the phagocyte: nature, Mechanisms of activating and function. Biochim Biophysics Acta 1984, 853:65-71.

[14] Clermont G, Vergely C, Girard C, Rochette L. Cellular injury associated with extracorporeal circulation (in French) Ann Cardiol Angiol 2002; 51 (1) :38-43.
[15] Richard H, Marc S, Graeme R. The systemic inflammatory response to cardiopulmonary bypass: Pathological, Therapeutic, and pharmacological considerations. Anesth Analg 1997; 85, 766-782.
[16] Sabik JF, Gillinov AM, Blackstone EH, Vacha C, Houghtaling PL, Navia J. Does off pump coronary surgery reduce morbility and Mortality? J Thorac Cardiovasc Surg 2002; 124 (4) :698-706.
[17] Butler J, Rocker GM, Westaby S. Inflammatory response to cardiopulmonary bypass. Ann Thorac Surg 1993; 55:552-559. Nashef SA, Roques F, Hammill BG et al. Validation of European
[18] System for Cardiac Operative Risk Evaluation (EuroSCORE) in North American cardiac surgery. Eur J Cardiothorac Surg 2002; 22 (1) :101-5. Bridgewater B. Mortality data in adult cardiac surgery for named surgeons: retrospective Examination of Collected data prospectively on coronary artery surgery and aortic valve replacement. BMJ. 2005; 330:506-10.
[19] Nilsson J, Algotsson L, Hoglund P, Luhrs C, Brandt J. Comparison of 19 pre-operative Risk stratification models in open-heart surgery. Eur Heart J. 2006; 27:867-74.
[20] Nashef SA. Editorial comment EuroSCORE and the Japanese aorta. Eur J Cardiothorac Surg. 2006; 30:528-3.
[21] Pitkanen O: Intra-institutional predictor of outcome after-cardiac surgery: comparison entre a locally derived model and the EuroSCORE. Eur J Cardiothorac Surg 2000; 18: 703 - 710.
[22] Geissler HJ: Risk stratification in heart surgery: comparison of six score systems. Eur J Cardiothorac Surg 2000; 17: 400-406.
[23] Van Dijk D, Nierich AP, Jansen EW, Nathoo MH Suyker WJ, Diephuis JC, van Boven WJ, Borst C, Buskens E, Grobbee DE, Robles De Medina EO, of Jaegere PP. Early outcome after-versus off-pump coronary bypass on-pump surgery: results from a randomized study. Circulation. 2001, 104:1761-1766.
[24] Ranucci M, Soro G, Frigiola A, Menicanti L, Ditta A, Candido G, et al. Normothermic perfusion lung function and cardiopulmonary bypass After: effects in pulmonary Risk Patients. Perfusion 1997; 12:309-15.
[25] Diegel A, Doll N, Rauch T, Haberer D, Walther T, Falk V, et al. Humoral immune response coronary artery bypass grafting DURING: a comparison of limited approach, "off-pump" technique, cardiopulmonary bypass and Conventional. Circulation 2000; 102 (Suppl III) :95-100. Wan S, Izzat MB, Lee TW, Wan IY, Tang NL, Yim AP.
[26] Avoiding cardiopulmonary bypass in multivessel CABG you reduce myocardial injury and cytokine response. Ann Thorac Surg 1999; 68:52-7.
[27] Ascione R, Lloyd CT, Underwood MJ, Lotto AA, Pitsis AA, Angelini GD. After coronary revascularization Inflammatory response With or Without cardiopulmonary bypass. Ann Thorac Surg 2000; 69:1198-204.
[28] C. Weissman Pulmonary Complications After Cardiac Surgery. Semin Cardiothorac Vasc Anesth 2004, 8:185-213.

[29] Michaux I, Filipovic M, Skarven K, Schneiter S, Schumann R, Zerkowski HR, Bernet F, Seeberger MD. Effects of on-pump versus off-pump coronary artery bypass graft surgery on right ventricular function. J Thorac Cardiovasc Surg. 2006, 131:1281-1288.

[30] Pegg TJ, Selvanayagam JB, Karamitsos TD, Arnold RJ, Francis JM, Neubauer S, Taggart DP. Effects of off-pump versus on-pump coronary artery bypass grafting on early and late right ventricular function. Circulation. 2008:117:2202-2210. Malouf PJ, Madani M, Gurudeva.

[31] Stucchi R, Poli G, Fumagalli R. Hemodynamic monitoring in ICU. Minerva Anestesiol 2006, 72 (6) :483-7.

[32] Bigatello LM, George E. Hemodynamic monitoring. Minerva Anestesiol 2002, 68 (4): 219-25.

[33] Umana E, Ahmed W, Fraley MA, et al. Comparison of Oscillometric and intra-arterial systolic and diastolic Blood Pressure in lean, overweight, and obese Patients. Angiology 2006; 57 (1) :41-5.

[34] Araghi A, Bander JJ Guzman JA. Arterial blood pressure monitoring in overweight Critically ill Patients: invasive or noninvasive? Crit Care 2006, 10 (2): R64.

[35] Pinsky MR, Payen D. Functional hemodynamic monitoring. Crit Care 2005, 9 (6) :566-72.

[36] Hayes MA, Timmins AC, Yau EH, et al. Elevation of systemic oxygen delivery in the Treatment of Critically Ill Patients. N Engl J Med 1994, 330 (24) :1717-22.

[37] Pinsky MR. At the threshold of noninvasive functional hemodynamic monitoring. Anesthesiology 2007; 106 (6) :1084-5.

[38] Michard F, Teboul JL. Predicting fluid responsiveness in ICU Patients: a critical analysis of the evidence. Chest 2002; 121 (6) :2000-8.

[39] Arthur C. St. Andre, MD, FCCM; Anthony DelRossi, MD. Hemodynamic management of Patients in the first 24 hours after-cardiac surgery. Crit Care Med 2005, 33:2082-2093

[40] Matte P, Jacquet L, Van Dyck M, Goen M. Effects of Conventional physiotherapy, continuous positive airway pressure and non-invasive Ventilatory support with bilevel positive airway pressure coronary artery bypass grafting After. Acta Anaesthesiol Scand 2000; 44: 75-81.

[41] Estes RJ, Meduri GU. The pathogenesis of ventilator-associated pneumonia. Intensive Care Med 1995, 21:365-83.

[42] Montner PK, Greene ER, Murata GH, Stark DM, Timms M, Chick TW. Hemodynamic effects of nasal and face mask continuous positive airway pressure. Am J Respir Crit Care Med 1994, 149:1614-8.

[43] Yoshiyuki Takami and Hiroshi Ina. Beneficial effects of bilevel positive airway pressure under cardiopulmonary bypass surgery After. Interactive Cardiovascular and Thoracic Surgery 2 (2003) 156-159.

[44] Anavekar NS, MacMurray JJ, Velazquez EJ, et al. Relation Between Renal dysfunction and cardiovascular outcomes after-myocardial infarction. N Engl J Med 2004; 351:1285-95.

[45] Shamagian LG, Varela A, Pedreira M, Gomez I, Virgo A, Gonzalez-Juanatey JR. Kidney failure is an independent predictor of mortality in patients hospitalized for heart

failure and is associated with a worse cardiovascular risk profile. Rev Esp Cardiol. 2006; 59:99-108.

[46] Easy L, Núñez J, Bodí V, et al. Prognostic value of serum creatinine in acute coronary syndrome without ST-segment elevation. Rev Esp Cardiol. 2006; 59:209-16.

[47] Hillis GS, Croal BL, Buchan KG, et al. Renal function and outcome from coronary artery bypass grafting. Circulation. 2006; 113:1056-62.

[48] Van den Berghe G, Bouillon, R., Mesotten, D., Braithwaite, S. S., Pei, J., Yi, D., Khoo, T. K., Olsen, K. A., Mohammedi, K., Roussel, R., Marre, M., Hall, P., Finfer, S., Chittock, D., the NICE-SUGAR Study Investigators, (2009). Glucose control in Critically ill Patients .. NEJM 361: 89-90 2009.

[49] Griesdale, D. G.S., de Souza, R. J., van Dam, R. M., Heyland, D. K., Cook, D. J., Malhotra, A., Dhaliwal, R., Henderson, W. R., Chittock, D. R., Finfer, S., Talmor, D. (2009). Intensive insulin therapy and Mortality Among Critically Ill Patients: a meta-analysis study Including NICE-SUGAR data. CMAJ 180: 821-827.

[50] Stamou SC, Hill PC, Dangas G, Pfister AJ, Boyce SW, Dullum MK, et al. After coronary artery bypass Stroke: Incidence, predictors, and clinical outcome. Stroke. 2001; 32:1508-13.

[51] Hogue CW Jr, Barzilai B, Pieper KS, Coombs LP, DeLong ER, Kouchoukos NT, et al. Sex Differences in Mortality and neurological outcomes after-cardiac surgery: a Society of Thoracic Surgery National Database Report. Circulation. 2001; 103:2133-7.

[52] CHW Hogue, Murphy SF, Schechtman KB, Davila-Roman VC. Risk factors for early or delayed stroke after-cardiac surgery. Circulation. 1999, 100:642-7.

[53] Libman RB, Wirkowski E Neystat M, Barr W, Gelb S, Graver M. Stroke associated with cardiac surgery. Determinants, timing, and stroke subtypes. Arch Neurol. 1997; 54:83-7.

[54] Perez-Vela JL, Ramos-González A, López-Almodóvar LF, Renes-Carreño E, type-Bárcena A, Rubio-Regidor M, et al. Neurological complications in the immediate postoperative period of cardiac surgery. Contribution of brain MRI. Rev Esp Cardiol. 2005; 58:1014-21.

[55] Williams GD, Bratton SL, Riley EC, et al. Coagulation tests cardiopulmonary bypass correlate with DURING blood loss in children undergoing cardiac surgery. J Cardiothorac Vasc Anesth 1999, 13:398-404.

[56] Despotism GJ, Filos KS, TN Zoysa, et al. Factors associated with Excessive Postoperative Blood Loss and hemostatic transfusion requirements: multivariate analysis in cardiac surgical Patients. Anesth Analg 1996; 82:13-21.

[57] Kessler C, Szurlej D, Von Heymann C. Management of refractory cardiac post-op bleeding with rFVIIa: Cases Reported to hemostasis.com registry [abstract]. J Thromb Haemost 2003:1131.

[58] Gomes WJ, Carvalho AC, Honorio Palma J, Concalvez I, Buffolo E. Vasoplegic Syndrome: A new dilemma. J Thorac Cardiovasc Surg 1994; 107: 942-3

[59] Ricardo Levin , Marcela Degrange. Síndrome vasopléjico en postoperatorio de cirugía cardíaca. Rev CONAREC Mayo-Junio 2006; (22), 84:78-81

[60] Czerny M, Baumer H, Kilo J. Inflammatory response and myocardial injury following coronary artery bypass grafting with or without cardiopulmonary bypass. Eur J Cardiothorac Surg 2000; 17: 737-42.
[61] Argenziano M, Choudhri AF, Mozami N, Levin H, Landry DH, Oz MC. A prospective randomized trial of arginine vasopressine in the treatment of vasodilatadory shock after left ventricular assist device placement. Circulation 1997; 96(suppl 2): II 286-290.
[62] Leyh, RG. Kofidis T, Strüber M, Fischer S, Knobloch K, Wachsmann B et al. Methylene blue: the drug of choice for catecholamine-refractory vasoplegia after cardiopulmonary bypass. J Thorac Cardiovasc Surg2003; 125: 1426-31
[63] Yiu P, Robin J, Pattison W. Reversal of refractory hypotension with single-dose methylene blue after coronary artery bypass surgery. JThorac Cardiovasc Surg 1999; 118: 195-6.
[64] Evora PRB. Should methylene blue be the drug of choice to treat vasoplegias caused by cardiopulmonary bypass and anaphylactic shock ?.J Thorac Cardiovasc Surg 2000; 119: 632-3.
[65] Pagni S, Austin E. Use of intravenous methylene blue for the treatment of refractory hypotension after cardiopulmonary bypass. J Thorac Cardiovasc Surg 2000; 119: 1297-8.
[66] Kofidis T, Struber M, Wilhelmi M et al. Reversal of severe vasoplegia with single-dose methylene blue after heart transplantation. J Thorac Cardiovasc Surg 2001;122: 823-4.
[67] Levin RL, Degrange MA, Bruno GF, Del Mazo CD, Griotti JJ and F.J. Boullon, Methylene blue reduces mortality and morbidity in vasoplegic patients after cardiac surgery. Ann Thorac Surg 2004; 77: 496-9.
[68] Gomes W, Carvalho AC, Palma JH, Teles CA, Branco JN, Silas MG et al. Vasoplegic syndrome after open heart surgery. J Cardiovasc Surg(Torino) 1998; 39: 619-23.
[69] Talbot MP, Temblay I, Denault AY, and Belisle S. Vasopressin for refractory hypotension during cardiopulmonary bypass. J Thorac Cardiovasc Surg 2000; 120: 401-2.
[70] Landry DW and Oliver JA. The pathogenesis of vasodilatory shock. N Engl J Med 2001; 345: 588-95.
[71] Mekontso-Dessap A, Houel R, Soustelle C, Kirsch M, Thebert D and Loisance DY, Risk factors for post-cardiopulmonary bypass vasoplegia in patients with preserved left ventricular function. Ann Thorac Surg 2001; 71:1428-32.
[72] Ozal E, Kuralay E, Yildirim V, Kilic S, Bolcal C, Kucukarslan N et al. Preoperative methylene blue administration in patients at high risk for vasoplegic syndrome during cardiac surgery. Ann Thorac Surg 2005; 79: 1615-19.
[73] shock after cardiac surgery: identification of predisposing factors and use of a novel pressor agent. J Thorac Cardiovasc Surg 1998;116(6):973—80.
[74] Goldhaber SZ, Visani L, De Rosa M. Acute pulmonary embolism: clinical outcomes in the International Cooperative Pulmonary Embolism Registry (ICOPER). Lancet 1999;353:1386-9.
[75] Georghiou GP, Brauner R, Berman M, Stamler A, Glanz L,Vidne BA, Erez E. Successful resuscitation of a patient with acute massive pulmonary embolism using emergent embolectomy. Ann Thorac Surg 2004;77:697-9.

[76] Yalamanchili K, Fleisher AG, Lehrman SG, Axelrod HI, LafaroRJ, Sarabu MR, et al. Open pulmonary embolectomyfor treatment of major pulmonary embolism. Ann Thorac Surg 2004;77:819-23.

[77] Tankut Hakki Akay, MDAtilla Sezgin, MD,Suleyman Ozkan, MD et. al Successful Surgical Treatment of Massive Pulmonary Embolism after Coronary Bypass Surgery. *Tex Heart Inst J 2006;33:498-500*

[78] Douketis JD, Kearon C, Bates S, Duku EK, Ginsberg JS. Risk of fatal pulmonary embolism in patients with treated venous thromboembolism. JAMA 1998;279:458-62.

[79] Roque Ramos, MD; Bakr I. Saiem, MD, FCCP;Maria P. De Pawlikowski, The Efficacy of Pneumatic Compression Stockings in the Prevention of Pulmonary Embolism After Cardiac Surgery CHEST 1996; 109:82-85

[80] John V. Booth, MBChB, FRCA*, Erin E. Ward, BS*, Kelly C. Colgan. Metoprolol and Coronary Artery Bypass Grafting Surgery: Does Intraoperative Metoprolol Attenuate Acute _-AdrenergicReceptor Desensitization During Cardiac Surgery? Anesth Analg 2004;98:1224 -31

[81] Dimitri Kalavrouziotis, *MD; Karen J. Buth, MSc; and Imtiaz S. Ali, MD*. The Impact of New-Onset Atrial Fibrillation on In-hospital Mortality Following Cardiac Surgery*CHEST 2007; 131:833–839*

[82] Roach GW, Kanchuger M, Mangano CM et al, for the multicenter study of perioperative ischemia research group and the ischemia research and education foundation investigators (1996) Adverse cerebral outcomes after coronary bypass surgery. N Engl J Med 335:1857–1864

[83] Hakala T, Hedman A (2003) Predicting the risk of atrial fibrillation after coronary artery bypass surgery ScandCardiovasc J 37:309–315

[84] Maisel WH, Rawn JD, Stevenson WG (2001) Atrial fibrillation after cardiac surgery. Ann Intern Med 135:1061–1073

[85] Siebert J, Rogowski J, Jagielak D, Anisimowich L, Lango R, Narkiewich M(2000) Atrial fibrillation after coronary artery bypass grafting without cardiopulmonary bypass. Eur J Cardiothorac Surg 17:520–523

[86] Tamis-Holland JE, Homel P, DuraniM, Iqbal M, Sutandar A, Mindich BP, Steinberg JS (2000) Atrial fibrillation after minimally invasive direct coronary artery bypass surgery. J Am CollCardiol 36:1884–1888

[87] W. JungU. MeyerfeldtR. BirkemeyerAtrial arrhythmias after cardiac surgeryin patients with diabetes mellitusClin Res Cardiol 95:Suppl 1, I/88–I/97 (2006

[88] Echt DS, Liebson PR, Mitchell LB et al (1991) Mortality and morbidity in patients receiving encainide, flecainide, or placebo: the cardiac arrhythmia suppression trial. N Engl J Med324:781–788

[89] Crystal E, Connolly SJ, Sleik K, Ginger TJ, Yusuf S (2002) Interventions on prevention of postoperative atrial fibrillation in patients undergoing heart surgery. A meta-analysis. Circulation106:75–80

[90] Daoud EG, Snow R, Hummel JD, Kalbfleisch SJ, Weiss R, Augostini R (2003) Temporary atrial epicardial pacing as prophylaxis against atrial fibrillation after heart surgery. J Cardiovasc Electrophysiol 14:127–132

[91] Vijayaraman P, Ellenbogen KA (2003) Postoperative atrial fibrillation: some more answers, some new questions. J Cardiovasc Electrophysiol 14:133–134
[92] Omran H, Jung W, Lüderitz B (1998) Dysfunction of the left atrium after cardioversion of atrial fibrillation. Am J Cardiol 81:837–838
[93] Roger J.F. Baskett, William A. Ghali, Andrew Maitland and Gregory M. HirschThe intraaortic balloon pump in cardiac surgery*Ann Thorac Surg* 2002;74:1276-1287
[94] Kusiak V, Goldberg S. Percutaneous intra-aortic balloon counterpulsion. Cardiovasc Clin 1985;15:281–302.
[95] McCarthy P, Golding L. Temporary mechanical circulatory support. In: Edmunds L, ed. Cardiac surgery in the adult. New York: McGraw-Hill, 1997:319–38.
[96] Dietl C, Berkheimer M, Woods E, Gilbert C, Pharr W, Benoit C. Efficacy and cost-effectiveness of preoperative IABP in patients with ejection fraction of 0.25 or less. Ann Thorac Surg 1996;62:401–9.
[97] Weintraub R, in discussion of Christenson J, Badel P, Simonet F, Schmuziger M. Preoperative intraaortic balloon pump enhances cardiac performance and improves the outcome of redo CABG. Ann Thorac Surg 1997;64:1237–44
[98] Aksnes J, Abdelnoor M, Bere V, Fjeld N. Risk factors of septicemia and perioperative myocardial infarction in a cohort of patients supported with intra-aortic balloon pump (IABP) in the course of open heart surgery. Eur J Cardiothorac Surg 1993;7:153–7.
[99] Creswell L, Rosenbloom M, Cox J, et al. Intraaortic balloon counterpulsation: patterns of usage and outcome in cardiac surgery patients. Ann Thorac Surg 1992;54:11–20.
[100] Naunheim K, Swartz M, Pennington D, et al. Intraaortic balloon pumping in patients requiring cardiac operations. J Thorac Cardiovasc Surg 1992;104:1654–61.
[101] Downing T, Miller D, Stinson E, et al. Therapeutic efficacy of intraaortic balloon pump counterpulsation: analysis with concurrent "control" subjects. Circulation 1981;64(suppl II):108–13.
[102] Tedoriya T, Kawasuji M, Sakakibara N, Takemura H, Watanabe Y, Hetzer R. Coronary bypass flow during use of intraaortic balloon pumping and left ventricular assist device. Ann Thorac Surg 1998;66: 477–81.
[103] Antiplatelet Trialists' Collaboration. Collaborative overview of randomised trials of antiplatelet therapy—II: maintenance of vascular graft or arterial patency by antiplatelet therapy. BMJ 1994;308:159-68.
[104] Burger W, Chemnitius JM, Kneissl GD, et al. Low-dose aspirin for secondary prevention—cardiovascular risks after its perioperative withdrawal versus bleeding risks with its continuation—review and meta-analysis. J Intern Med 2005;257:399-414.
[105] Ferraris VA, Ferraris SP, Moliterno DJ, et al. The Society of Thoracic Surgeons practice guideline series: aspirin and other antiplatelet agents during operative coronary revascularization (executive summary). Ann Thorac Surg 2005;79:1454-61.
[106] Sadony V, Korber M, Albes G, et al. Cardiac troponin I plasma levels for diagnosis and quantitation of perioperative myocardial damage in patients undergoing coronary artery bypass surgery. Eur J Cardiothorac Surg 1998;13:57-65.

[107] Thielmann M, Massoudy P, Schmermund A, et al. Diagnostic discrimination between graft-related and non-graft-related perioperative myocardial infarction with cardiac troponin I after coronary artery bypass surgery. Eur Heart J 2005;26:2440-7.

2

Intra-Aortic Balloon Counterpulsation Therapy and Its Role in Optimizing Outcomes in Cardiac Surgery

Bharat Datt, Carolyn Teng, Lisa Hutchison and Manu Prabhakar
Southlake Regional Health Centre
Canada

1. Introduction

Several discoveries and inventions in medicine have revolutionized it's practice. Examples would include the discovery of Insulin by Dr William Banting in 1920. The discovery of Heparin by Dr Jay McLean and its first clinical use in Toronto in 1933-36, the advent of the membrane oxygenator, heart lung machines with progressively smaller footprints, intra aortic balloon (IAB) pumps and VAD's (ventricular assist device) would be some of the devices which significantly impacted outcomes in cardiac surgery.
The fundamentals of IAB technology were first tested by Harken in 1958, who is credited with the first use of diastolic augmentation. The pump for Harken's system was a failure due to massive hemolysis. Moulopoulous (in the 1960's) from the Cleveland Clinic developed the first successful prototype of an Intra-aortic balloon pump (IABP) which could be timed to the cardiac cycle.
The IABP device as we know it was reported by Dr Adrian Kantrowitz (Fig 1) and his team from Grace Sinai hospital in Detroit. The first clinical implant was performed at Maimonides Medical Centre, Brooklyn, NY in Oct 1967 for a 48 yr old woman in cardiogenic shock unresponsive to traditional therapy. The IAB was inserted through a cut down of the left femoral artery (LFA) and pumping performed for 6 hrs. The shock was reversed and the patient discharged. The device was further developed for cardiac surgery by Dr David Bregman at New York Presbyterian Hospital in 1976.
Studying the history of counterpulsation elucidates the great strides in IAB technology and its clinical applications. The size of the balloons initially inserted were as large as 15 Fr. Two operations were required for balloon usage, one to insert the balloon by cut down in a femoral artery, and a second operation to remove the balloon. Advances in technology afforded progressively smaller IAB catheter sizes and eventually 8 and 9Fr. balloons were developed. Current IAB catheter sizes are 7 and 7.5Fr.
In 1968 -Kantrowitz and his group began to use the IABP regularly in clinical practice.
Since 1979 balloon placement utilizes the Seldinger (percutaneous) technique.
The wrapped IAB was developed in 1985. Advances in technology facilitated graduating from cut down insertions to percutaneous and sheathless insertions going from cut down insertions to percutaneous and finally sheathless insertions. Smaller diameter catheters permitted this along with user friendly consoles with automated and real time timing algorithms.

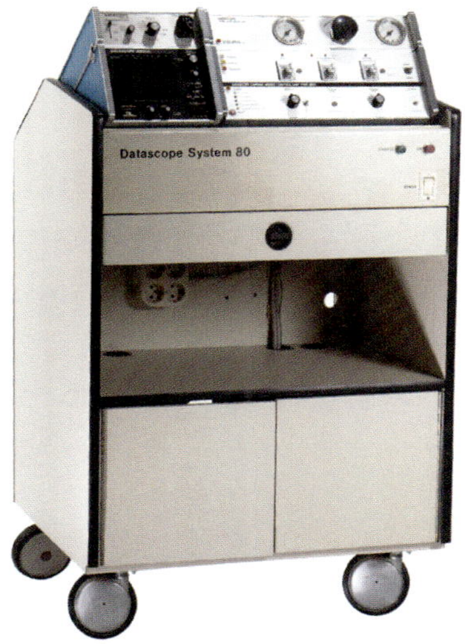

Fig. 1. Datascope System 80

2. Fundamentals of cardiac physiology

Understanding of counterpulsation, requires a knowledge of relevant cardiovascular physiology. The heart works as a series circuit of pumps, the left system and the right system.

The right atrium (RA) receives blood from the inferior and superior vena cava and coronary sinus, most of which flows passively into the right ventricle (RV) through the tricuspid valve. An additional 20% of ventricular filling occurs through the atrial kick corresponding to the "p" wave of the Electrocardiogram (ECG). *(Quaal 1993)*

The right system feeds the low pressure pulmonary vasculature which offers little resistance to the blood ejected from the right ventricle (RV). Consequently the right ventricular musculature is one third the girth of the Left Ventricle. The left atrium receives blood from four pulmonary veins and passively empties the blood into the left ventricle through the mitral valve. Since there are no valves in the pulmonary veins, elevation of left atrial pressure results in an increase in pulmonary vascular resistance (PVR).

Generation of high pressure is required by the left ventricle, most of the pressure being generated occurs during isovolumetric contraction (Fig2-phases of contraction-electrical and mechanical) in order to open the aortic valve, and overcome SVR and aortic end diastolic pressure (AEDP), which is a function of the systemic vascular resistance.

The intraventricular septum also contributes to the left ventricular ejection along with the thick circular posterior and lateral walls.

Some of the energy imparted to the blood through ventricular ejection is stored in the proximal aorta and large arteries as potential energy during their peak expansion. This is known as the Windkessel effect. In diastole, this energy is transformed into kinetic energy by the aorta and large arteries causing a recoil, which maintains a pressure head in the aorta. This in turn maintains a runoff during diastole into the peripheral arteries. It's important to note that coronary arteries fill during diastole.

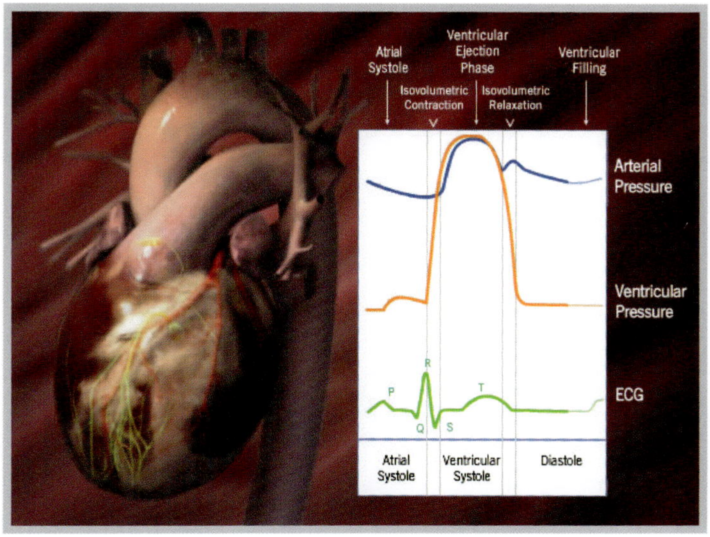

Fig. 2. Phases of electrical and mechanical contraction

3. Cardiac output

Cardiac output is the product of stroke volume and heart rate. Stroke volume is the amount of blood ejected by the Left Ventricle with every beat.
Stroke volume is dependent on

1. Preload
2. Afterload
3. Inotropy or (ventricular contractility) and
4. Heart rate

4. Preload

This concept suggests that the length of ventricular muscle fiber determines the magnitude of contraction. The length of the LV muscle fiber in turn is dependent upon the left ventricular end diastolic volume (LVEDP). In other words increase in left atrial filling would increase the magnitude of LV contraction. The ability of the LV to vary the strength of its contraction as a function of the LVEDP and end diastolic muscle fiber length is defined as Frank Starling law (fig 3). This gain in contractility is impaired when the stretch goes beyond physiological limits. In clinical practice the length of the muscle fiber is proportional to the LVEDP 'which is measured indirectly as the pulmonary artery wedge pressure (PAWP) by means of a Swan Ganz catheter. In a normal LV, very slight changes in PAWP or LVEDP, produces significant increases in stroke volume.

5. Afterload

Afterload is defined as the resistance to LV ejection. Major components are SVR and AEDP. AEDP is the resistance the LV has to overcome in order to open the aortic valve. Ninety percent of myocardial oxygen consumption takes place during the isovolumetric

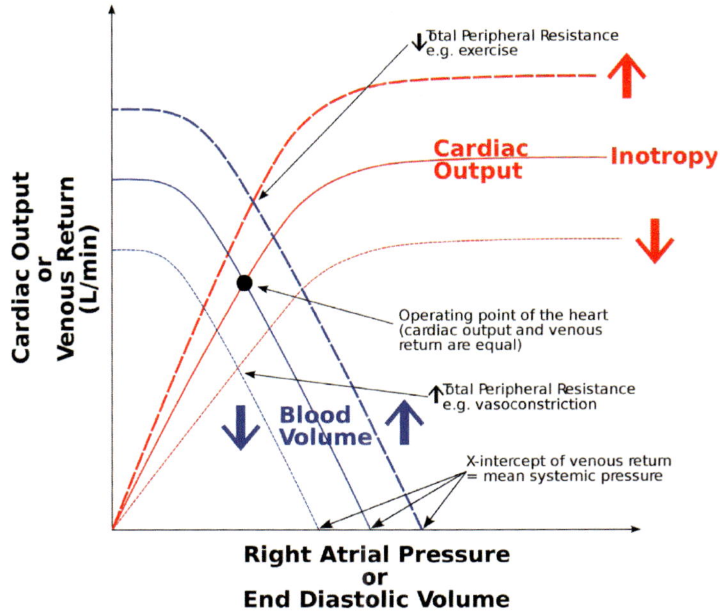

Fig. 3. Starling Law

contraction phase when the LV is trying to overcome the resistance caused by the AEDP in order to open the Aortic valve. The aim of counterpulsation is to lower AEDP, thereby reducing afterload and myocardial oxygen consumption during isovolumetric contraction (fig 4).

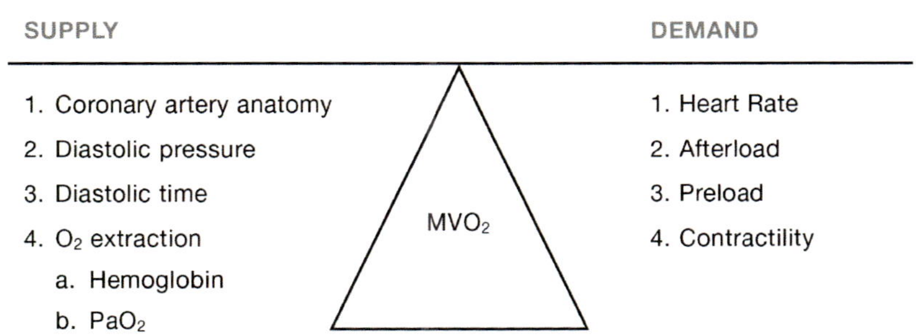

Fig. 4. Myocardial Oxygen Supply and Demand

6. Contractility

Contractility is defined as the change in the force of contraction, independent of myocardial fiber length. Contractility inotropic performance can be increased by endogenous production of catecholamines or exogenous administration of vasopressors like norepinephrine (NE), dopamine, calcium etc. Myocardial contractility decreases wuth hypoxemia and drugs like barbiturates, procainamide, lidocaine, propranolol etc.

7. Ventricular function

In order for us to appreciate the need for the IAB, we need to understand ventricular function, end diastolic volume and the Fick equation. Ventricular function in critical care is assessed by the Ejection Fraction (EF). EF is defined as the volume of blood ejected per beat (stroke volume or SV) divided by the volume in the LV prior to ejection, end diastolic volume (EDV). Stroke vol equals EDV minus end systolic volume (ESV). The equation for EF would then be:

$$EF = EDV\text{-}ESV/EDV = SV/EDV$$

Ventricular function is graded into four groups by two dimensional echocardiography according to ejection fraction as shown in fig 5 (*Conolly HM & Kohl J 2012*).

LV Grade	Ejection Fraction
Grade 1 LV	≥ 55%
Grade 2 LV	45 to 54%
Grade 3 LV	30 to 44%
Grade 4 LV	≤ 30%

Fig. 5. LV Grade and Corresponding Ejection Fraction

Diastolic volume index: EDV indexed to the patients body surface area (BSA) is another measure of ventricular performance. A normal index is considered less than $100ml/m^2$. In patients with regurgitant valves and volume overload, the end diastolic volume index (EDVI) may be high despite preserved LV function.
The Fick Equation: Defines the relationship between C.O and oxygen extraction.

$$O2\ consumption = C.O \times O2\ content\ difference\ (sao2\text{-}svo2)$$

$$C.O = O2\ consumption / O2\ content\ difference\ (sao2\text{-}svo2)$$

Therefore CO is inversely proportional to O2 content difference, assuming that O2 consumption remains constant. A normal value for arterio-venous oxygen difference would be less than 5 ml/dl or 50ml/L. A low cardiac output state would encourage increased oxygen extraction, resulting in widening of arterio-venous o2 content of greater than 5ml/dl. *(Hensley et al.,1995)*

8. Heart rate

Increase in the frequency of contraction increases C.O at a given filling pressure. This is called the staircase (Bowditch) effect. Reduction in diastolic time can result in reduction of ventricular filling, thus limiting C.O increase with tachycardia. An important corollary to remember is that the filling of coronary arteries takes place in diastole and tachycardia can compromise diastolic coronary filling.

9. Coronary circulation and anatomy

The myocardium is perfused during diastole through the coronary system (fig 6).
The major vessels of the coronary circulation are the left main coronary that divides into left anterior descending and circumflex branches, and the right main coronary artery. The left and right coronary arteries originate at the base of the aorta from openings called the coronary ostia located just distal to the aortic valve leaflets.

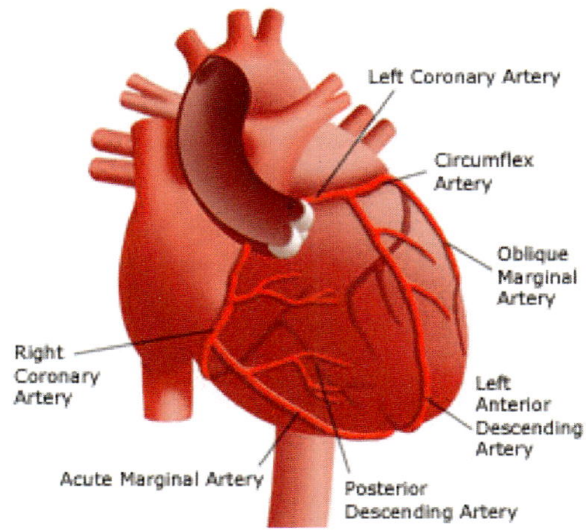

Fig. 6. The Coronary System

The left and right coronary arteries and their branches lie on the surface of the heart, and therefore are sometimes referred to as the epicardial coronary vessels. These vessels distribute blood flow to different regions of the heart muscle. When the vessels are not diseased, they have a low vascular resistance relative to their more distal and smaller branches that comprise the microvascular network. As in all vascular beds, it is the small arteries and arterioles in the microcirculation that are the primary sites of vascular resistance, and therefore the primary site for regulation of blood flow. The arterioles branch into numerous capillaries that lie adjacent to the cardiac myocytes. A high capillary-to-cardiomyocyte ratio and short diffusion distances ensure adequate oxygen delivery to the myocytes and removal of metabolic waste products from the cells (e.g., CO_2 and H^+). Capillary blood flow enters venules that join together to form cardiac veins that drain into the coronary sinus located on the posterior side of the heart, which in turn drain into the right atrium. There are also anterior cardiac veins and thebesian veins that drain directly into the cardiac chambers. The LAD supplies blood to the front (anterior-septal) portion of the heart and the LCX supplies the side (anterio-lateral) and back (posterior) of the left ventricle. The right coronary artery supplies blood to the ventricles, the right atrium (RA), the inferior portion of the myocardium and the sino-atrial node. The LAD give rise to various branches called the diagonals and marginal's while the RCA bifurcates into the posterior descending artery (PDA) and the acute marginal artery. The RCA supplies blood to the inferior portion of the myocardium.

10. Heart failure

Forward heart failure or congestive heart failure is defined as the inability of the heart to keep up with its demand. Forward heart failure can lead to backward heart failure. Heart failure can be caused by structural heart disease, coronary artery disease, Cardiomyopathy or conduction disorders, more often than not requiring surgical correction. Conduction disorder can impair C.O by causing a too slow/fast heart rate, loss of atrial kick or loss of conduction. Left ventricular failure is directly related to the need for an IAB. Heart failure can be manifested as angina, crescendo or unstable angina or exercise induced angina. Heart failure causes ischemia and myocardial ischemia can be silent. Ninety seven percent of peri-operative ischemia has been found to be silent (Hensley 1995). Silent ischemia can translate into peri-operative infarct or ischemia both of which could cause heart failure. Left Ventricular failure can be divided into three stages. Stage 1 (fig 7) is manifested as vasoconstriction leading to decreased pumping efficiency, increased LV volume and pressure. These physiological events activate baroreceptors leading to increased heart rate, increased afterload (SVR), increased myocardial oxygen demand and ultimately an increase in preload (LVEDP).

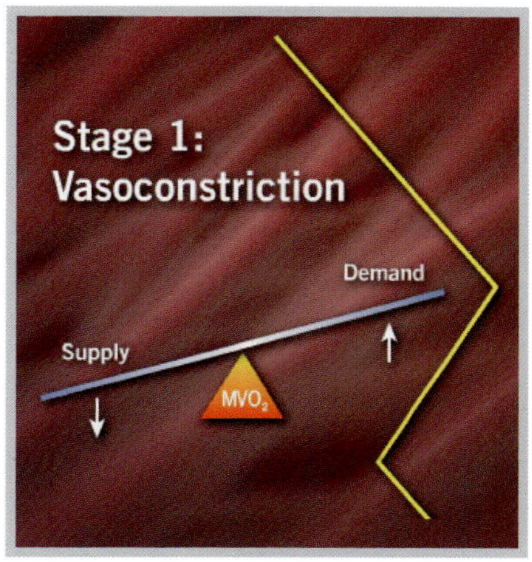

Fig. 7. Stage 1 Vasoconstriction

Stage two (Fig 8) leads to hypervolemia as the heart tries to compensate with the additional afterload. There is a decrease in cardiac output and glomerular filtration pressure, further activating the Renin-Angiotensisn system. There is an increase in sodium and water reabsorption leading to an increase in preload and afterload. There is a decrease in cardiac

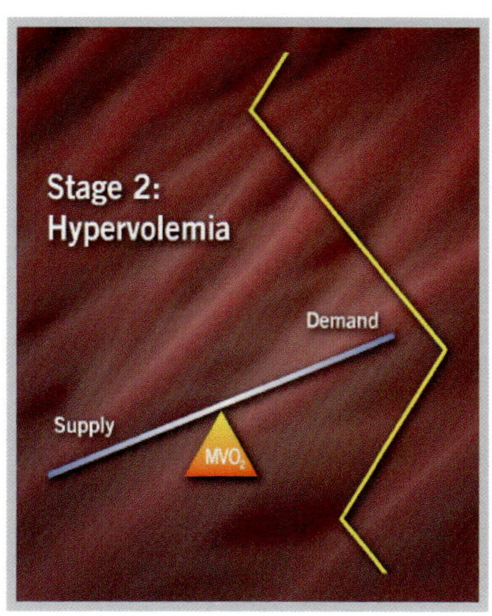

Fig. 8. Stage 2 - Hypervolemia

output, decrease in oxygen supply, increase in heart rate and increase in oxygen demand. There is an increase in pulmonary artery wedge pressures.
The final stage of LV failure (Fig 9) is the manifestation of tissue hypoxia. Decreased cardiac output, decreased MAP, decreased oxygenation coupled with pulmonary edema causes acceleration of anaerobic metabolism, lactic acid production, Tissue anoxia and finally tissue death. Its ideal to insert the IAB in stage one or by stage two, so that we prevent the final stage of heart failure.

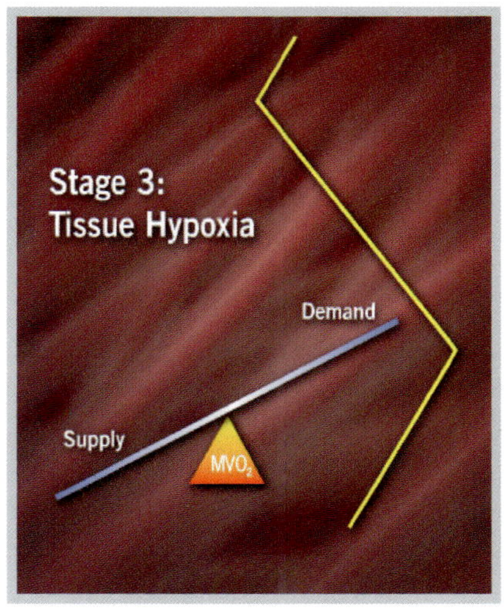

Fig. 9. Stage 3 - Tissue Hypoxia and Apoptosis

11. Indications for mechanical circulatory support

Before we cite specific indications for IAB insertion, we should discuss indications for mechanical circulatory support. In other words, we should be able to delineate or define ventricular failure. LV failure would be defined as cardiac index (CI) of less than 1.8 L/min/m² with a systolic blood pressure of less than 90 mmhg (ref: Hensley Martin) despite maximized preload (mean atrial pressure > 20 mmhg), optimized heart rate (> 80) and normalized ionized calcium. This could be extrapolated to RV failure except for the systolic blood pressure. RV work is the function of the difference between the RA and PA mean pressure. As the difference between the two approaches zero, pulmonary blood flow is passive and RV failure is present. RV failure can occur with or without pulmonary hypertension.
Mechanical support is suggested when the above criteria are present despite maximum inotropic support. Maximum inotropic support can be defined as any two or more (*High et al., 1995*) of the following combinations:

1. > 10 µg/kg/min of Dopamine
2. > 10 µg/kg/min of Dobutamine
3. > 0.2 µg/kg/min of Epinephrine
4. > 0.75 µg/kg/min of Milrinone after loading dose
5. > 10 µg/kg/min of Nor-epinephrine

For patients with severe forms of LV failure, ventricular assist devices (VAD) are indicated. The initial indicated mechanical support in these scenarios is the IABP. Large and prolonged inotrope infusion will only tend to increase the workload of the ventricle. The IABP does the exact opposite, decreases the workload of the heart.

12. Indications for IAB insertion

In cardiac surgery the IAB is indicated for the following situations:

A. Pre-op predictors:
   1. Grade 3 to 4 LV dysfunction or ejection fraction (EF) of less than 0.30 (*Dietl CA et al.,1996*)
   2. Severe and/or multiple valvular disease with end stage myocardial impairment not including aortic regurgitation
   3. Anticipated prolonged CPB time
   4. Coronary artery disease (CAD) only partially correctible by grafting with concomitant LV dysfunction
   5. Persistent ST Changes before, during or after induction of general anesthesia
   6. Coronary obstruction via clot or otherwise

B. Intra/post-op predictors:
   1. Pre/post CPB ischemia
   2. Incomplete repair or bypass
   3. Prolonged CPB time
   4. Large ventriculotomy or LV resection for LV aneurysm repair.
   5. Particulate or air embolus in coronary arteries.
   6. Persistent ST changes post CPB.

Clinical indications for the IAB are listed below (fig 10 showcases benchmarks in 2005 for IAB use)

1. Ventricular failure after myocardial infarction (MI) - (*Barron et al., 2001*) or acute myocardial infarction (AMI). As in all other cases the IAB will would decrease afterload and increase coronary perfusion. Early insertion is recommended to ameliorate the threatening extension of MI.
2. Angina- chest pain is usually the initial stages of an MI and here again early insertion is recommended
3. Unstable angina with or without ST segment elevation
4. Cardiomyopathy- In the majority of cases when cardiomyopathy occurs the patient suffers from dilated cardiomyopathy and the IAB assist in raising mean blood pressure and reducing afterload. In a very few cases of initial stages of hypertrophic cardiomyopathy, where the ventricle tends to be a small volume ventricle (extremely thick myocardial wall), a sudden decrease in AEDP would result in insufficient volume left to fill the increased capacitance . This would actually result in a drop in MAP and systolic blood pressure, especially at an augmentation of 1:1
5. Acute mitral valve regurgitation (*Abid et al.,2002*) and/or stenosis with LV rupture
6. Aortic stenosis without aortic insufficiency (AI) or accompanied by mild AI
7. Congestive heart failure
8. Intractable ventricular arrhythmias secondary to ischemia or otherwise. In these cases IAB's with fibre optic technology can be used to track rapid or irregular heart rhythms
9. Ventricular irritability
10. Bridge to transplant or destination therapy
11. Support in the catheterization laboratory (*Stone GW et al.,1997*) for stenting or PTCA (Percutaneous Transluminal Coronary Angioplasty)

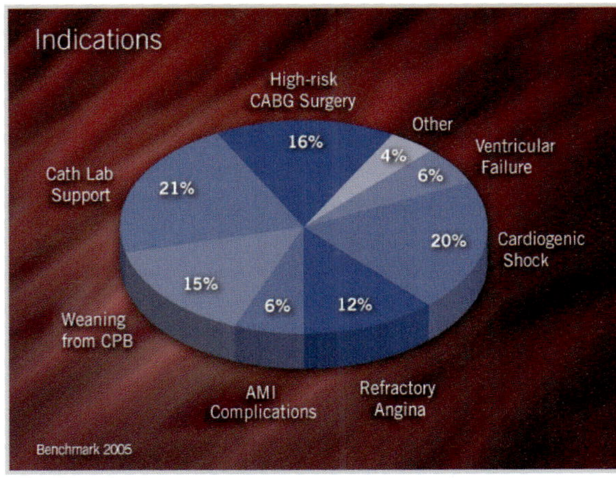

Fig. 10. BENCHMARK for IAB use (2005)

12. Myocardial ischemia or stunning of the heart- In this scenario much of the myocardium has suffered reversible damage and scarring has occurred only in a portion of the heart.
13. VSD (ventricular septal defect) - particularly post MI. This may be accompanied by papillary muscle rupture and acute mitral regurgitation
14. Support in the General OR for patients with ongoing heart disease or a history of heart disease
15. Transport (*Sinclair TD & Verman HA,2009)*for unstable patients
16. Left main disease
17. Cardiac contusion and/or trauma
18. Septic shock or pre-shock syndrome
19. Pulsatile flow (*Onorati F et al.,2009*)during CPB

Freedman coined the term "Myoconservation" (*Quaal 1993*). It is defined as the hemodynamic support provided within the crucial window of opportunity, ensuring that enough myocardium remains viable to permit normal function of the heart following definitive coronary therapy-whether it be CABG or coronary stenting/PTCA. The IAB is one of the very important modalities available to the cardiac surgeon/cardiologist which supports myoconservation by supporting the coronary circulation, supporting the systemic circulation, reduction in LV stress and reduction in LV workload.

Miller et al in 1986 summarize "The result of our clinical experience suggest that more aggressive use of IAB is likely to save lives of coronary disease patients who develop severe complications of their disease. There have been no deaths reported among our patients with refractory unstable angina who had an IAB inserted and all evidence suggests that short of actually opening the vessel to obtain relief from angina, IAB insertion is the most effective method to treat these patients"

More recent studies (*Christenson JT 1999*) have confirmed the efficacy of pre-operative IAB use in high-risk coronary patients.

13. Absolute contraindications for IAB insertion

1. Aortic regurgitation or insufficiency. In this physiology, raising AEDP would result in increase of regurgitant factor thereby increasing workload of the heart. In instances of mild AI a decision can be made if the benefits outweigh the risks.

2. Aortic dissection. Precludes IAB insertion. Attempting to Place an IAB in this situation may lead to placement in the false lumen or at the very least increase circulation into the false lumen.

14. Relative contraindications for IAB insertion

1. Severe peripheral vascular disease (PVD). Although this sometimes precludes insertion, we have had some experience with this. A discussion on PVD patients will be conducted a little later.
2. Unresected thoracic, abdominal or thoraco-abdominal aneurysm. An insertion of a mechanical device like the IAB and the counterpulsation of such a device against a diseased aortic wall may result in aortic dissection
3. Sepsis or infection
4. Severe thrombocytopenia
5. Coagulopathy or coagulopathic disorder
6. End stage terminal disease
7. End stage cardiomyopathy unless bridge to transplant/destination therapy
8. Severe atherosclerosis

15. Pre-insertion predictors of risks associated with IAB insertion

1. Age- Increased age appears to be an increased risk. It is probably because of increased atherosclerosis associated with increased age (*Goldberger 1986*). There are other studies reporting inconsistent results.
2. Gender- women tend to have a greater risk of complication due to their smaller stature. This is probably due to the smaller lumen size of the femoral artery in women. The IAB catheter was expected to occupy greater lumen space in women thereby increasing the likelihood of ischemia and/or thrombus formation. Women are 1.6 to 1.8 more likely to experience limb ischemia/vascular complications than men (*Skillman JJ et al, 1988*).
3. Peripheral vascular disease (PVD) - These patients have higher likelihood for IAB complications due to insertion difficulties. Gottlieb suggested a three times likelihood for complications (*Gottlieb SO et al.,1984*), others have suggested less (*Skillman JJ et al,.1988*).
4. Type-II diabetes- Due to severe and diffuse atherosclerotic disease, higher incidence of hypertension and dampened resistance to bacterial contamination, diabetics tend to have a higher risk of complication post IAB. Some investigators found that diabetics (*Wasfie T et al.,1988*) had a 22% incidence of complications post IAB insertion as compared to 14% for non-diabetics. For insulin dependent diabetes a higher complication rate of 34% (*Alderman JD et al., 1987*) was suggested.
5. Duration of IAB therapy- Findings for the duration of safe use of IAB therapy remain inconclusive (*Quaal 1993*)

16. Complications of IAB insertion

1. Loss of pedal pulses- Occurs in 15 – 25% of patients (*funk M et al.,1989*). Asymptomatic loss occurs transiently without resulting in limb ischemia and usually returns spontaneously or after IAB removal.

2. Limb ischemia- Occurs in 12 - 47% patients and is the most frequently reported complication (*Curtis JJ et al., 1988*). This may result from decreased cardiac output subsequent to heart failure, elevated SVR, low output syndrome, intimal injury or dissection, vessel catheter discrepancy, catheter occlusion or distal thrombo-embolism. Limb ischemia usually preceded by pain in the affected limb, change in pallor, cyanotic color changes, mottling, decreases in sensation, motor function loss, decrease in temperatures in extremity and loss of pedal pulses. Treatment is usually done by removal of IAB, thrombectomy, femoro-popiteal grafting and/or papaverine administration.
3. Thromboembolism- Percutaneous insertion/removal of IAB may result in dislodging of plaques or clots into the renal, splanchnic, hepatic or peripheral arteries. Clots can be seen while removing IAB catheters. It is our institutional policy to have some sort of anti-coagulation during IAB therapy. Although Low molecular weight Dextran has been used, heparin is preferable as it can be reversed with protamine. Generally maintaining the **aPTT 1.5 - 2** times normal is sufficient to prevent formation of thrombin, thereby protecting from subsequent embolism. It is also recommended to flush the IAB catheter with heparinized saline prior to insertion. The only incidence where this may not be necessary is when the patient is fully heparinized and on CPB. It is always a good practice even in this situation to flush with heparinized saline. At Southlake we use pre-mixed heparinized saline bags with 5000 units of heparin in 500ml of saline.
4. Compartment syndrome- The legs and thighs of humans are made up of compartments containing bone, muscle, nerve tissue and blood vessels, surrounded by a fibrous membrane or fascia. Compartment syndrome is caused by an increased pressure within the non-distensible fascial space reducing capillary blood flow which in turn compromises enclosed fascial tissue. A fasciotomy can be performed to relieve the pressure.
5. Aortic Dissection- Is the most serious of complications from IAB insertion. Often unrecognized until removal or until IAB therapy is discontinued resulting in hemodynamic instability and death. Diagnosis is confirmed upon autopsy. Isner in 1980 found an incidence of aortic dissection in 36% of IAB patients (*Isner JM et al,. 1980*).With the advent of smaller French sizes in IAB catheters and better techniques and training, incidence of aortic dissection as a direct consequence of IAB insertion has drastically reduced .Symptoms of aortic dissection include severe back and/or abdominal pain, falling hematocrit and mediastinal enlargement. Aortic Dissection has to be treated aggressively and immediately by attempting to repair the dissection in the operating room.
6. Local injury- False aneurysm formation, hematoma, lymphedema, lymph fistula, wound hemorrhage, laceration of the femoral/iliac artery or the aorta are common complications and can be treated by evacuation and/or arterial repair.
7. Infective complication- Local wound infection is possible necessitating debridement, drainage, systemic antibiotics and rare cases removal. Sterility is very important while inserting the IAB whether in the peri-operative setting or otherwise. Generally the thigh is prepared by applying betadine prior to insertion and is covered by sterile dressing after insertion and anchorage of the catheter by two sutures.

8. IAB rupture/entrapment- IAB rupture is rare but immediate removal/replacement is required. Rupture is more likely in women and patients with smaller size and usually occurs because of the constant contact between IAB membrane and atherosclerotic plaque on the femoral arterial/Aorta walls. The most common sign of IAB leak is blood in the drive line (fig 11). IAB leak can cause either a helium embolus (in instants of patient hypotension where helium pressure within the IAB exceeds blood pressure in the aorta) or entrapment of the catheter. The leak can cause a clot to form within the catheter resulting in prevention of removal of the catheter at the time of IAB removal. This may necessitate a cut down removal of the IAB catheter.

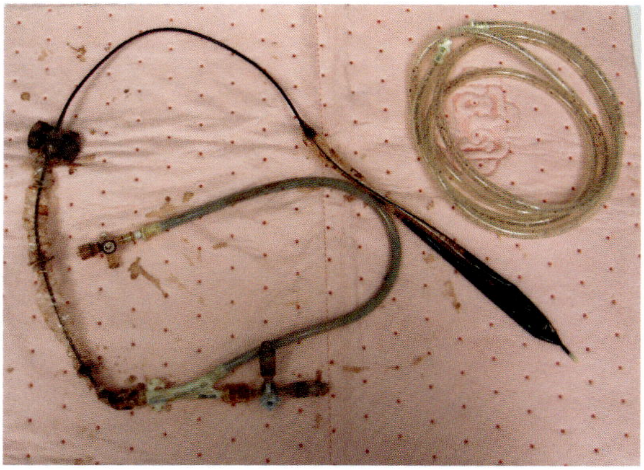

Fig. 11. IAB Catheter with Blood in Drive Line and Balloon

9. Hematologic effects- Long term use of IAB has been associated with increased destruction of red cells and thrombocytopenia. The degree of decrease appears to be related to the duration of therapy (*McCabe 1978*)
10. Malposition of the IAB catheter- If positioned too high, the IAB may occlude blood flowing to the head vessels causing cerebral ischemia and or embolism. If positioned too low it may occlude the renal arteries thereby causing renal ischemia/perfusion and non-optimal coronary perfusion/afterload reduction.

17. Insertion techniques

1. Cut down technique- By 1978 the IAB was a 12fr catheter and prior to that year, cut down insertion was common. Initially, the common femoral artery is dissected and the vascular fascia is opened. With a retractor the femoral artery can be dissected up to a length of 5 cms and umbilical tapes are placed around and behind the femoral artery. Heparin 5000u is administered and the IAB catheter is introduced at an angle to the femoral artery. Placement is confirmed and augmentation initiated. This technique can also be used in patients where femoral pulse is not palpable or where difficulty of insertion is anticipated as in patients suffering from PVD.
2. Percutaneous (Seldinger) technique: An 18 gauge cannula is introduced into the common femoral artery at a 45 degree angle or less. The guide wire is advanced through the needle and the needle removed. The tissue tract around the arterial

puncture is then dilated by the dilator provided in the IAB catheter set. The introducer-dilator set is advanced over the guidewire. Finally the dilator is removed and the IAB catheter advanced over the guidewire. The IAB is introduced over the guide wire and placed in the second or third intercostal space. It is recommended to maintain a continuous flush of the IAB catheter with heparinized saline (1000u in 500ml) after placement. It is also recommended to periodically flush the arterial line from the IAB in order to prevent clotting of the arterial line coming from the IAB catheter. The manufacturer recommends the IAB catheter to be anchored with two sutures to the subcutaneous tissue of the thigh (Fig 12) at the anchors provided on the side of the base of the catheter or by the sutureless securement device provided.

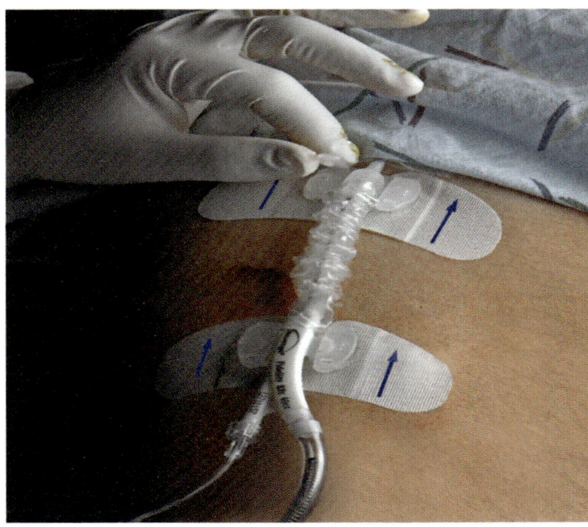

Fig. 12. Proper Anchoring of the IAB Catheter

3. Sheathless insertion- Initially IAB catheters were enveloped by sheaths with bigger French sizes. E.g. The 8Fr IAB catheter has a sheath whose outer diameter is 10Fr. By not using the sheath, the practitioner is reducing trauma to the groin and femoral artery. Current IAB catheters of 7 and 7.5Fr are inserted in our institution without the sheath. Sheathless insertion also reduces the length of catheter indwelling in the tissue, thereby reducing limb ischemia.
4. Subclavian insertion- Currently the manufacturer and FDA (Food and Drug Administration) recommends (in their IFU-instruction for use manual) femoral insertion of all IAB catheters. IAB catheters have regulatory clearance for femoral insertion and are labeled as such. There are situations where the subclavian artery has been used in order to avoid an aorto-iliac stenosis. A subclavicular incision is done and the subclavian artery isolated via cut down. An IAB catheter is placed antegrade down the descending thoracic aorta.
5. Brachial insertion- The brachial artery can be used as a point of insertion where the patients have bilateral obstructive femoral and iliac disease and/or the patient has bilateral femoro-popliteal graft. Due to discomfort associated with positioning, the authors would recommend only in patients who are intubated and on a ventilator. Care

should be taken to insert the IAB on the left rather than the right side. As right sided insertion would not give the IAB enough length to cross the aortic arch and lie in the descending Aorta. We came across a 74 years female diagnosed with coronary artery disease (CAD) and triple vessel disease (TVD) who had aorto-bifemoral grafts inserted in 2004. Her risk factors included hypertension, active smoking history, type 2 Diabetes and previous MI. Her EF was only 28%, she had moderate MR, moderate PAH and left carotid bruit. She was turned down for surgery. She presented in emergency with angina. Had a syncopal episode with rapid atrial fibrillation. She was cardioverted twice and transported to the cath lab for IAB insertion. An IAB (Fig 13) was initially inserted through the right brachial artery and was observed via fluoroscopy to lie in the aortic arch. The IAB was then removed and re-inserted via the left brachial artery and inserted antegrade down the thoracic aorta. Augmentation was initiated, the patient survived the hypotensive episode, was placed in the CCU and discharged on the 9th post-procedure day.

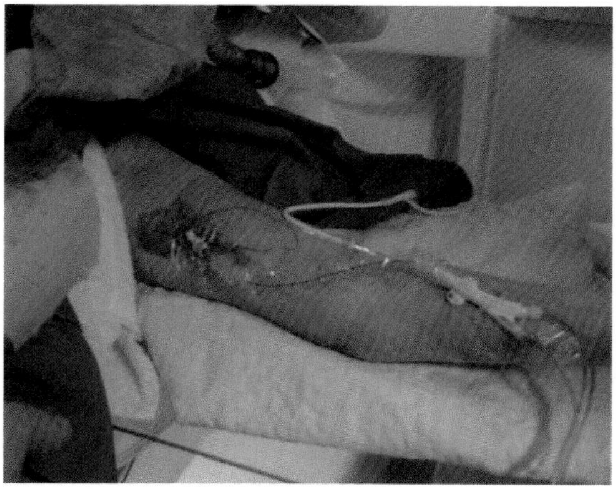

Fig. 13. Transbrachial Insertion

6. Transthoracic Insertion- In instances where the IAB insertion is precluded due to severe PVD or has been tried and failed, The IAB catheter can be introduced down the aorta in operative room situations. We had one such patient- a 65 year old male with active smoking history, no hypertension/daibetic history and a history of pericarditis in 2003. He had a history of severe PVD with bilateral femoral claudication and severe pain in his legs. Angiogram was facilitated through the right radial approach. He underwent CPB and uneventful CABG to his LAD and PIV (posterior interventricular artery). The patient had a hypotensive episode during sternal closure, CPB was re-initiated, mammary spasm suspected and a vein graft anastomosed distal to the previous mammary artery anastomosis. We were unable to separate from CPB, at this time a decision was made to insert an IAB transfemorally. Transfemoral insertion failed and an IAB catheter (Fig 14) was placed antegrade down the thoracic aorta. At this point the patient was able to separate from CPB. Due to suspicion of myocardial edema, late sternal closure was decided upon, the skin closed, dressing placed and patient transported to the CVICU. The patient was taken back to the OR post-op day 3, the IAB

removed and the chest closed. The patient was extubated post-op day 9 and discharged after 25 days. No post-operative morbidity noted other than associate with his history of peripheral vascular disease (*Datt B 2007*)

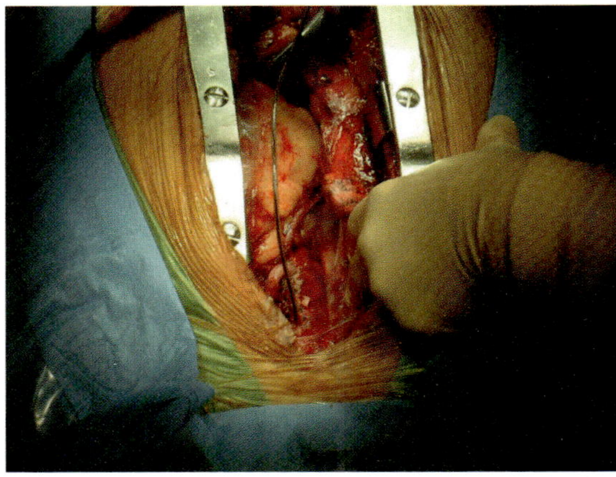

Fig. 14. Trans-thoracic Insertion of IAB Catheter

18. Mechanics of IAB functioning

IAB therapy is often referred to as counterpulsation therapy as the balloon inflates in diastole or counter to the hearts contraction (systole). The IAB is a polyethylene balloon catheter placed percutaneously in the thoracic aorta through the groin (Fig 15).

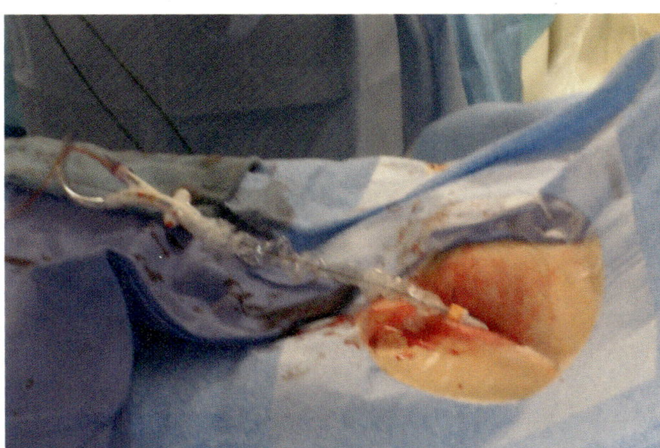

Fig. 15. Femoral Insertion of IAB Catheter

Balloon inflation actively pushes blood into the coronary arteries, increasing myocardial oxygen supply. Balloon deflation decrease AEDP thereby directly reducing myocardial work load and myocardial oxygen consumption by reducing the time period for isovolumetric contraction. This gives the heart time to rest and gives a chance for hibernating myocardium to recover.

The IAB is connected by a driveline to a helium chamber or pressurized gas reservoir which is connected to the IAB catheter via a solenoid valve. The inflation or helium supply is linked to a trigger for the balloon which is usually a synchronized ECG (Electrocardiogram) or the patient's blood pressure. Earlier on in IAB development CO2 was used due to its high solubility and safety in case of balloon leak/rupture and gas embolization. Helium started being used due to its smaller Reynold's number (lower density), thereby allowing a smaller drive line/catheter. Smaller balloon catheters improved gas shuttle speeds, reduced trauma to the groin and resulted in fewer complications post-insertion.
The balloon is usually placed 2 cms below the subclavian artery in the second to third intercostals space. This optimizes coronary perfusion and decreases the chances for renal artery occlusion. Balloon placement is verified in the OR by TEE or post-operatively by CXR (Fig 16).

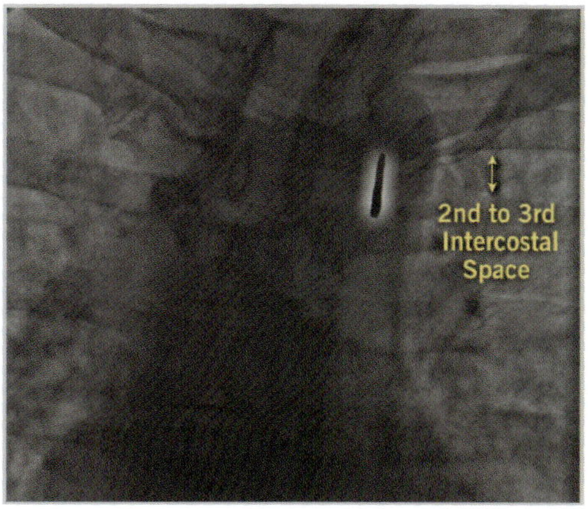

Fig. 16. Chest X-ray Confirmation of IAB Placement

Synchronization of the IAB is achieved usually by using the R wave of the QRS complex to deflate the IAB catheter. In the operating room some practitioners tend to use pressure trigger to circumvent electrical interference from the cautery or other devices. If the patient is pacer dependent, the pacer spike can also be use to trigger IAB deflation. Correct timing is verified by observing the dicrotic notch on the arterial pressure waveform on the balloon console and making sure that balloon inflation takes place just after the dicrotic notch (aortic valve closure) and deflates prior to LV ejection (R wave on QRS complex-Fig 17 & Fig 18)
While using the pressure trigger, it's important to use the dicrotic notch as the marker for inflation. This will prevent the balloon from impinging on LV ejection and adding to the hearts afterload.
At Southlake we use the Maquet IAB console (fig 19) CS 100 which has an auto feature for timing. Another IAB console which the reader may come across would be the ACAT II WAVE console (fig 20) marketed by Arrow international.
The console uses a unique algorithm to establish the initial timing using the ECG or arterial pressure waveforms. It will also automatically readjust the inflation and deflation timing for changes in heart rate or rhythm. This allows for ease of nursing care post-operatively and decreases the necessity of the perfusionist except for troubleshooting. The IAB has three choices for augmentation. 1:1, 1:2 and 1:3. The IAB is generally initiated at 1:2 in order to be

able to check the timing of the IAB catheter. The timing can be verified by using the inflation interval option on the console. Generally at a higher heart rate (>100), a better augmentation pressure is achieved by lowering the ratio to 1:2 or 1:3. The (stroke) volume of the balloon used is dependent on the size of the balloon and is chosen based on the height of the target patient (fig 21).

Recently, due to the reduction in french size of the IAB catheters to 7Fr, it is possible to insert 40cc balloons in most patients, except those very small or very large.

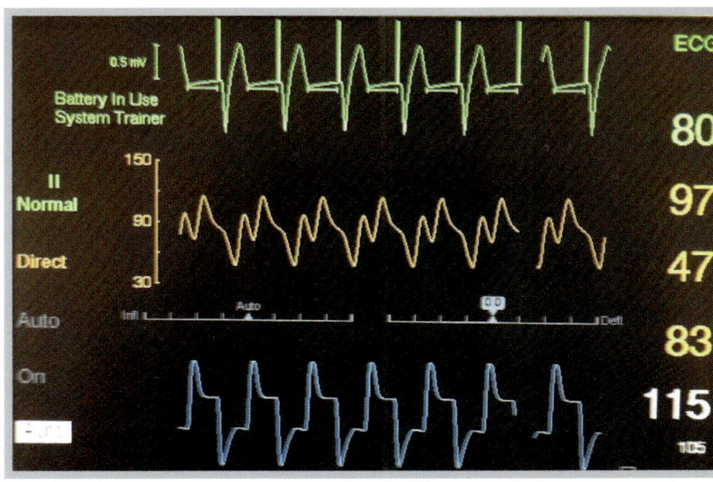

Fig. 17. Inflation (1:1) After timing IAB (pacing trigger)

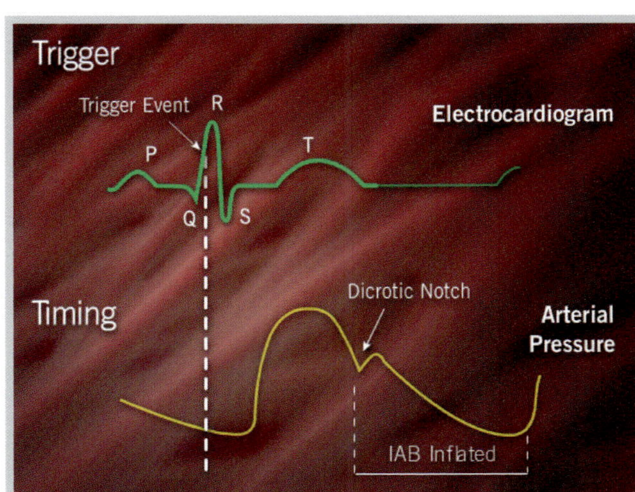

Fig. 18. Proper IAB Timing

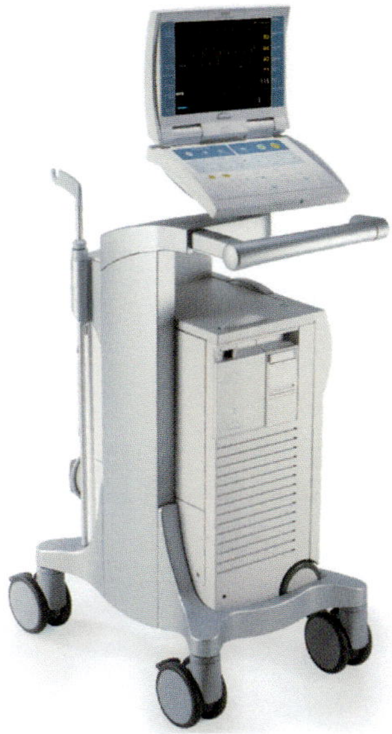

Fig. 19. CS100 MAQUET IABP

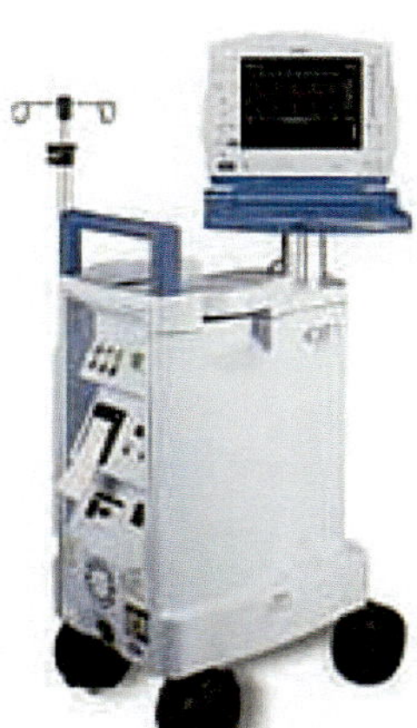

Fig. 20. ACAT II WAVE Arrow IABP

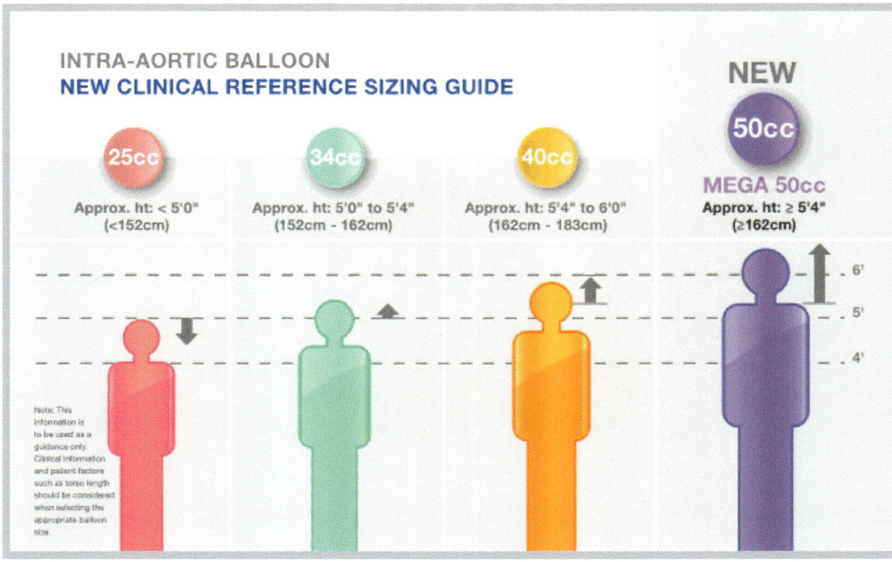

Fig. 21. Size Selection Criteria for IAB Catheter

19. Timing errors

There are four major timing errors with the IAB. The IAB is usually timed at a 1:2 ratio (one inflation every second heart beat) and the deflation is triggered off the R wave in the QRS complex. If the IAB is timed improperly, it can actually add to the afterload of the heart by inflating prior to the closure of the aortic valve. In this situation the cardio-vascular hemodynamics can deteriorate quickly and it is important for the practitioner to understand and avoid these errors.

1. *Early inflation*: The waveform shows inflation of IAB prior to dicrotic notch, diastolic augmentation encroaches into systole (fig 22) and is not hard to miss. The physiological effects would be potential premature closure of aortic valve, increase in LVEDP, LVEDV (Left Ventricular End Diastolic Volume) and PCWP (Pulmonary Capillary Wedge Pressure). The net effect would increase afterload, myocardial oxygen consumption and possibility of adding to Aortic regurgitation.
2. *Late inflation*: Inflation of IAB after the dicrotic notch, indicated by the lack of a sharp "V" on the waveform (fig 23). The physiological effects include sub-optimal coronary perfusion and decreased diastolic augmentation.
3. *Early deflation*: Viewed as a sharp drop in the waveform after diastolic augmentation. Assisted AEDP can be equal to the unassisted AEDP (fig 24). There may be little or no decrease in assisted systolic pressure. There is an absence of a sharp"v" or pore-systolic dip. This error will also lead to sub-optimal coronary perfusion, mvo2 and afterload reduction. There is also a potential for causing retrograde coronary and carotid blood flow with the latter causing an increase in angina.
4. *Late deflation*: Possibly the most dangerous of all timing errors. Rate of rise of assisted systolic pressure may be prolonged. Assisted AEDP may be equal to unassisted AEDP. Diastolic augmentation waveform may be dampened (fig 25), depending on how late

the deflation is. Physiologically, afterload reduction is absent. IAB is actually impeding LV ejection and increasing afterload. Isovolumetric contraction phase increases along with myocardial oxygen consumption. Hemodynamics deteriorate rapidly.

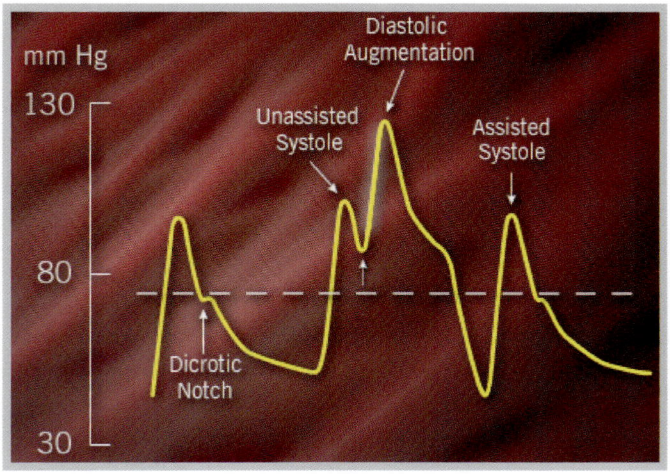

Fig. 22. Early Inflation

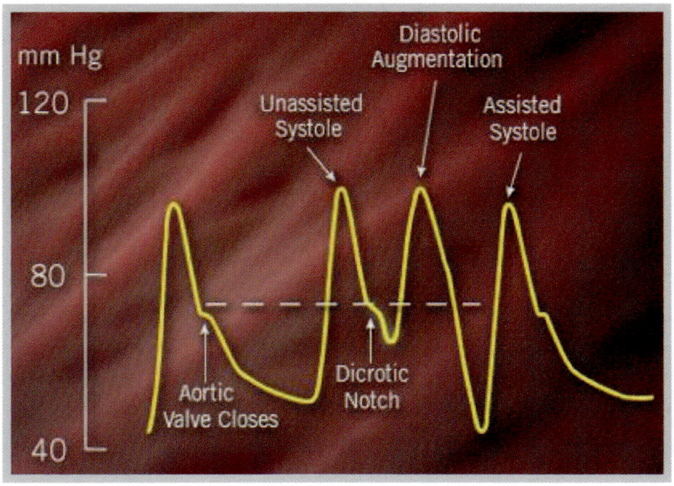

Fig. 23. Late Inflation

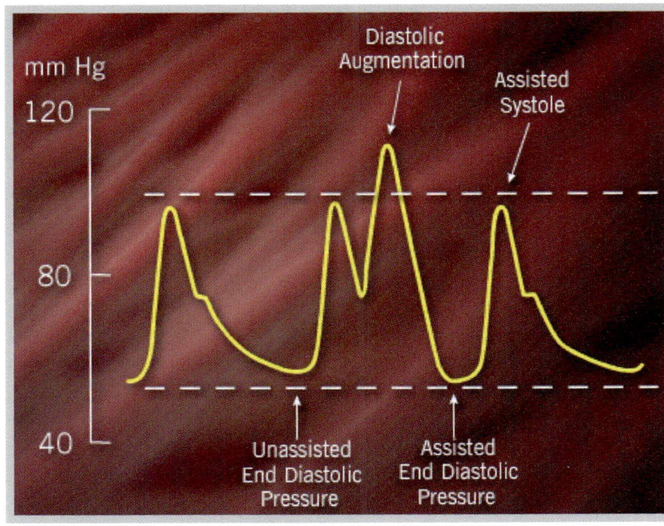

Fig. 24. Early Deflation

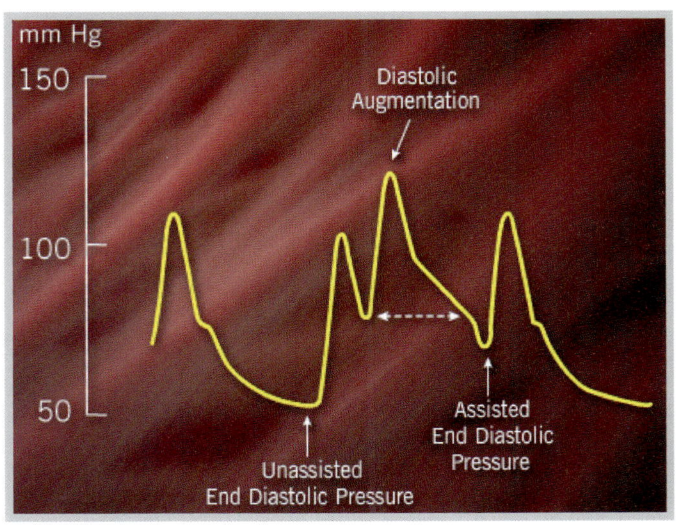

Fig. 25. Late Deflation

20. IAB weaning

IAB weaning is usually done when the following physiological parameters are observed in target patients.

1. No afterload reduction as seen on balloon waveform
2. Increased urine output
3. Improved LV function and hemodynamics

4. Cessation and/or improvement of ventricular and/or atrial arrhythmias
5. Cessation or reduction of angina
6. When transportation or operative procedure (revascularization of left main or aortic/mitral valve repair/replacement) is completed and the patient hemodynamics appear to be stable
7. When the shock phase has been successfully tided over

The IAB is generally weaned by reducing the ratio from 1:1 to 1:3, after which the augmentation volume of the balloon catheter can be reduced. If the IAB volume is being decreased as a part of the weaning process, ensure adequate movement of the IAB catheter in order to minimize clotting or thrombus formation. The IAB is never turned off when the IAB catheter lies in the aorta due to the risk of thrombus formation. Afterload reduction by the IAB can be explained via numbers. The stroke volume of an average sized patients in normal health is usually 70 to 80 ml. In a patient in compromised cardio-vascular state, this stroke volume is reduced to 40 or 50ml. What a 40cc IAB catheter does is to complement the native stroke volume of 30-40ml until hibernating myocardium recovery and myocardial rest result in an increased stroke volume of that patient.

21. Advancements in IAB catheter and IAB console technology

Considerable improvements have been made in IAB catheter and console technology in the more than 40 years since counterpulsation was introduced to clinical practice. Early IABP consoles required intensive user intervention, as all aspects of console operation were manually controlled. Early IAB catheters were 12 Fr. and required surgical insertion via a cutdown to the femoral artery. Surgical insertion could take 1-2 hours and complication rates were high. In 1979, IAB catheter insertion improved significantly with the development of percutaneous IAB insertion. Insertion time was reduced, typically to 15 minutes.

Additional improvements to the catheter in the early years included the addition of an inner lumen to facilitate wire-guided insertion and the lumen could then be used to monitor the arterial blood pressure. Prefolding of the membrane during manufacturing eliminated the need for the clinician to wrap the membrane prior to insertion through the introducer sheath. Catheters were also made smaller, from 12 Fr. to 10.5 Fr. and then to 9.5 Fr. Catheters are now 7 and 7.5 Fr. and this has helped reduce the incidence of limb ischemia to less than 3%. Reducing the catheter shaft diameter required a significant change to the way catheters were designed. With early dual lumen catheters, the inner lumen used for wire guiding the insertion and monitoring the arterial pressure was a separate catheter within the balloon catheter gas lumen. With the development of a co-lumen design where the two lumens of the catheter were extruded together with the inner and outer lumens sharing a common wall, the catheter diameter was reduced while maintaining the gas shuttle lumen and maximizing the inner lumen to accommodate the largest guide wire possible. The range of balloon membrane sizes was also expanded over the years from 40 cc in the early days of counterpulsation to 25 cc, 34 cc, 40 cc, and 50 cc IAB membranes. The size of balloon used is determined by patient height. The most recent improvement in IAB catheter technology has been the addition of a fiber optic pressure sensor to acquire the arterial pressure signal. This technology is immune to artifact, resulting in a high fidelity arterial pressure waveform for accurate IAB timing.

While innovations in IAB catheter technology were being developed, improvements in IAB console technology were also occurring. Major improvements to the console over the years have been aimed at making the algorithms smarter, the pneumatics faster, and the consoles smaller and lighter. Early consoles required constant operator intervention to maintain optimal triggering and timing. Improvements to the algorithms in the console resulted in the automation of timing so that once the operator established the initial timing, the console could adjust the timing for changes in patient heart rate and rhythm. Console pneumatic improvements reduced IAB inflation and deflation time, which was important for tracking tachycardic rhythms. Consoles were made smaller and lighter to facilitate transport by aircraft or ambulance.

The most significant improvement to console design occurred with the development of fully automated operation. With this capability, the console can automatically select the most reliable trigger and establish initial timing. It will then automatically readjust timing for changes in heart rate and rhythm, using advanced algorithms to track predictable (regular) as well as unpredictable (irregular) rhythms. The algorithms will also select an alternate trigger if the current trigger is lost. This automation, along with smaller fiber optic catheters offers the clinician the most advanced IAB counterpulsation system for optimal patient benefit.

22. Intra-aortic balloon pump use during percutaneous coronary angioplasty

The Intra-aortic balloon pump (IABP) can also provide important hemodynamic support during complex percutaneous coronary intervention (PCI), both in the elective setting, and for acute coronary syndromes, including ST segment elevation myocardial infarction. Modern coronary interventions can generally be performed to a wide array of patient subsets with low risk of procedural complications. However, optimal patient outcomes in PCI require identification of higher risk patients, and attempts to modify those risks. One of the main predictors of outcomes in PCI is Left Ventricular dysfunction, i.e. Ejection fraction <30%. The availability of mechanical support helps provide "backup" or reserve during the procedure and decreases the risk of hemodynamic compromise. Typically, mechanical support is initiated prior to commencing PCI, and removed shortly after successful PCI. Intra-aortic balloon pump use results in the dual benefits of increased peak diastolic pressure, while lowering the end-systolic pressure. There is a resultant reduction in after-load (*Perera D et al,2010*) and improved coronary perfusion, which leads to improved myocardial oxygen supply, with decreased myocardial energy demands.

The common scenarios for IABP use in PCI include:

1. Acute Coronary Syndromes (ACS) / ST elevation Myocardial Infarction (STEMI), complicated by cardiogenic Shock, due to LV systolic dysfunction or a mechanical complications such as acute mitral regurgitation or ventricular septal defect.
2. PCI in a coronary artery supplying a large territory of myocardium, typically with underlying Left ventricular dysfunction (practically speaking, Grade 3 or worse - EF < 30%). Specific scenarios include i) coronary intervention on a diseased vessel that also supplies flow to another occluded vessel (via channels, called collateral arteries, that fill that territory in retrograde fashion), ii) unprotected left main stenting, iii) PCI to the only patent artery iv) PCI with concomitant valvular disease, if anticipated deterioration in the valvular disease (ex. patients with at least moderate ischemic mitral regurgitation, and planned PCI that could worsen degree of regurgitation).
3. If patients have clinical signs of abnormal resting hemodynamics, prior to PCI: low systolic blood pressure (SBP) <100, with objective or clinical suspicion of elevated left heart filling pressures - pulmonary capillary wedge pressure >20mmHg.

4. Survival Dependent vessel: Any one artery supplying a sufficient amount of myocardium such that (in the opinion of the cardiologist) closure of the vessel would be fatal.

It should be noted that there is considerable practice variation with Intra-aortic balloon support during high risk coronary intervention. Recognizing the higher risk of access related and other vascular complications with its insertion, some clinicians prefer to have the IABP readily available and use it only if hemodynamic compromise develops. . One trial conducted in centers in the United Kingdom, The Balloon Pump-Assisted Coronary Intervention Study, assessed whether routine intra-aortic balloon pump insertion, prior to PCI, reduced the risk of major adverse cardiac and cardiovascular events in patients with severe left ventricular dysfunction and advanced coronary disease. The results of this trial involving just over 300 randomized patients did not support routine use, given no difference between the groups. Clinical judgment is certainly exercised in situations (such as those described above) where the IABP is inserted "pre-emptively", with anticipated hemodynamic stress during PCI.

23. Counterpulsation – An anesthesiologists perspective

As an anaesthetist, working in the perioperative care of cardiac surgery patients for the last 20 years, I have observed a significant change in the attitudes and uses of the intra aortic balloon pump. I have watched the use of the IABP change from a last resort salvage technique for the patient on maximal inotropes with low output syndrome and a dismal prognosis, to a first line tool aiming for preservation of myocardial tissue in unstable cardiac surgery patients. The presumed IABP's favorable myocardial oxygen supply/demand profile and the ease of percutaneous insertion have been instrumental in this change (*Trost JC 2006*).

In our institution IABPs are often inserted in preoperative cardiac surgery patients: who are experiencing unstable angina, especially post myocardial infarction, not responsive to standard non-invasive therapies; that have low output syndrome or congestive heart failure secondary to severe left ventricular dysfunction or mechanical complications such as a ventricular septal defect or mitral regurgitation induced by a myocardial infarction ; and rarely who have acute myocardial ischemia causing intractable arrhythmias. It appears that the earlier the balloon is placed in a hemodynamically struggling patient, the more stable the patient is in the post-operative period. This practice is consistent with the Task Force on Practice Guidelines of the American Heart Association and American College of Cardiology (*Ryan TJ 1999*). Frequently, IABPs are inserted for preoperative cardiac surgery patients with symptomatic left main disease. The intention of the IABP is the preservation of viable ïschemic myocardial tissue. The mechanism of the preservation may relate more to decreased myocardial demand and collateral flow as Kimura showed that in the presence of a coronary artery stenosis of greater than 90% the IABP diastolic augmentation did not result in an increased post-stenotic pressure (*Kimura A 1996*). The insertion of the IABP into the aforementioned patients facilitates the anaesthetist's ability to maintain cardiovascular stability and a favourable myocardial oxygen supply/delivery ratio at induction, maintenance and release from bypass. Replace with" The importance and validity of the IABP in maintaining a favorable myocardial oxygen supply/demand ratio is realized in the post-operative period (*Christenson 1997*).

Intraoperatively, IABPs are inserted into our patients when difficulty to wean from the bypass machine is anticipated due to instability in the pre-bypass or bypass period or for failure to wean from the bypass machine, once reversible causes for the failure are ruled out. There may be a survival advantage to placing the IABP prior to coming off bypass based on one review. Delaying insertion of the IABP in the unstable perioperative patient who is unresponsive to reasonable doses of inotropes or who has rapidly accelerating inotropic requirements may have deleterious effects. Theoretically this is supported by the following facts. High inotropic doses increase myocardial inotropy and tension resulting in increased myocardial oxygen demands. Impaired diastolic relaxation and increased ectopy and afterload, as seen with certain inotropes, may further tip the myocardial supply/demand balance in favour of demand (*Katz AM 1990*). Myocardial injury may be further exacerbated by the inotropes increased delivery of calcium to the cell, overcoming the ischemic myocardium's presumed protective attempt at limiting available calcium. Early insertion of the IABP in the unstable post-bypass patient appears to theoretically and anecdotally improve outcome (*Poole Wilson PA 1990*).
Postoperative insertion of the IABP in the majority of our cases is for myocardial failure or signs of ischemia. Many times there is a dramatic improvement post balloon insertion. The mechanism producing this improvement is often not clear .Possibilities include a heightened diastolic pressure overcoming decreased coronary flow secondary to low mean arterial pressure, left internal mammary spasm or air within a coronary artery, improved collateral flow (Kern MJ 1991), or decreased demands secondary to decreased afterload and preload resulting in decreased myocardial wall tension. The IABP often assists in stabilization of the patient, although more definitive therapy may be required. The location of the ischemia, as visualized by the electrocardiogram and often echocardiogram, the magnitude of the failure, the surgical knowledge of the coronary disease and surgery and the response to the IABP determine the need for further management.
We have come to use IABP's earlier, and the indications have broadened to include all stages of the perioperative care. The theoretical protective effect of the IABP with respect to the myocardial supply/demand ratio, the ease of insertion of the IABP by the percutaneous route clinical observations and limited studies support this practice.

24. Conclusion

The IABP since its advent in 1960 has progressively become an indispensable technology available to the healthcare team in cardiology and cardiac surgery. Improvements in membrane technology have reduced the french sizes required to be used for femoral percutaneous insertion. This has minimized trauma caused by femoral insertion of the IAB catheter.
Earlier on in my training as a perfusionist, old school cardiac surgeons always inserted IAB's later rather than sooner. Counterpulsation technology was always thought to be a last ditch effort and mortality was thought to be higher once the IAB was inserted. This perception has changed radically over the last twenty years.
The ease of insertion (compared to VAD's and artificial lungs), ease of removal, low risk of complications and availability in the peri/post and pre-operative environment in a hospital setting has made counterpulsation an ideal choice to treat acute or chronic heart failure. There is no doubt at this point of the positive effects of counterpulsation on early mortality and post-operative morbidity in cardiac surgery. In instances where IAB insertion is

precluded or insertion has failed, transthoracic (in a peri-operative setting), transbrachial or subclavian insertion can also be performed with a positive impact on survival. Morbidity and mortality however are higher in these kinds of cases and may have to do with the pre-operative risk factors these patients come into surgery for. The cardiac surgeon has to tread the fine line between deciding the optimal timing for IAB insertion by weighing the benefits of counterpulsation vs the low risk of complications. It is increasingly being understood that for a poor LV and /or a patient with a risk of peri-operative infarct, it is optimal to insert an IAB sooner rather than later. The catheter can easily be removed first or second post-operative day after the surgery has performed and the risk for infarct been mitigated.

At Southlake, a 380 bed community hospital, we perform approximately 1000 heart surgeries and 3000 PTCA's annually. In support we insert 250 IAB catheters annually and are the largest IAB user in Ontario-Canada. We are a comparatively new heart centre, having started our cardiac surgery program in 2004. Aggressive use of counterpulsation reflects the new belief in early IAB insertion in cardiac patients at risk of pre, peri or post-operative infarct. Transfusion rates at SRHC for CABG in the first half of 2009 approximate 26% (Fig 26).

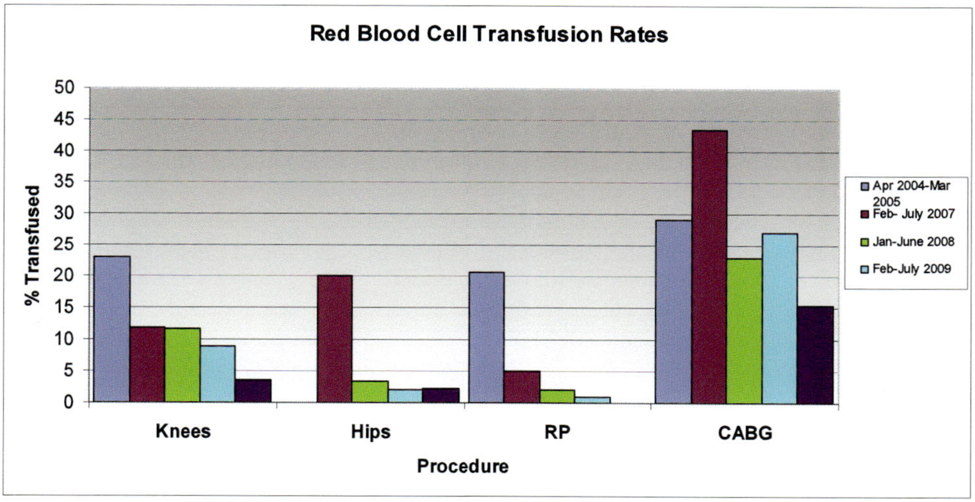

Fig. 26. Red Blood Cell Transfusion Rate for 2009 at SRHC.

Mortality at SRHC for late 2009 (July to Dec 2009) was based on Toronto Risk Score (TRS). The observed mortality ranged from 0.5% (TRS 2-4) to 8.5% (TRS >8) as shown in fig 27.

	TRS 0-2 (n=286)	TRS 3-4 (n=420)	TRS 5-7 (n=432)	TRS >8 (n=236)
Incidence of Observed Mortality	0	0.5%	2.1%	8.5%
Incidence of Observed Mortality by Count	0	2	9	20
Calculated Expected Mortality	1.52%	2.17%	3.95%	10.16%

Fig. 27. Observed and Expected Mortality at SRHC by Toronto Risk Score

It is the opinion of the authors that the above average results in morbidity and mortality for our cardiac patients may partly be due to the aggressive use of IAB in cardiac procedures. Aggressive use of counterpulsation therapy preempts infarction for the cardiac patient and in turn improves outcomes in cardiac surgery.

25. Acknowledgement

I would like to thank Maquet cardiovascular LLC (formerly Datascope) for providing most of the figures and pictures from their educational archives. I would also like to thank Maquet International who funded the editing costs of printing this chapter.

26. References

Abid Q,et al.(2001).Use of Intraaortic balloon pump in left ventricular rupture after mitral valve replacement.*Annals of thoracic surgery*.74(6),(dec 2002),2194-5,12643426.

Alderman JD,Gabliani GI,McCabe CH et al.(1987). Incidence and management of limb ischemia with percutaneous wire-guided intraaortic balloon catheters.*Journal of the American college of Cardiology*.Vol 9,issue:3,(mar 1987),524-530, doi:10.1016/S0735-1097(87)80044-X .

Barron HV,et al. (2001). The use of Intra-aortic balloon counterpulsation in patients with cardiogenic shock complicating acute myocardial infarction:Data from the national registry of myocardial infarction 2.*American Heart Journal*,141(6),(jun 2001),889-892,11376306.

Christenson JT,Simonet F,Badel P,et al.(1999).Optimal timing of Intra-aortic balloon pump support in high risk coronary patients.*The annals of thoracic surgery*.vol 68,issue:3,(nov 1999),934-939, 1097-1103, doi:10.1016/S0003-4975(99)00687-6.

Conolly HM,Koh j.(2012) Echocardiography,In: Braunwalds heart disease,atext book of cardiovascular medicine,2012,Bonozo R,Mann DL,Zipes DP,Libby P,200-276,Saunders Elsevier,ISBN 978-0-8089-2436-4,Philadelphia,PA,USA

Curtis JJ,Boland M,Bliss D et al.(1988). Intra-aortic balloon cardiac assist: complication rates for the surgical and percutaneous insertion techniques.*American Surgery*.(mar 1988),54(3),142-147, PMID 3348547

Datt B, Hutchison L, Peniston C. *(2007)*. Trans-Aortic Counterpulsation:A viable alternative? *Journal of extracorporeal technology*.(jun *2007);*vol 39,issue:2,91-95. PMID17672190.

Dietl CA,et al.(1996).Efficacy and cost effectiveness of pre-operative IABP in patients with ejection fraction of 0.25 or less. *The annals of thoracic surgery*, vol: 62, issue: 2, (aug 1996), 401-409, ISSN 00034975.

Funk M,Gleason J,Foel D.(1989). Lower limb ischemia related to use of the intraaortic balloon pump.*Heart lung*.18(6),(Nov 1989),542-552,PMID 2584053

Goldberger M,Tabak SW,Shah PK.(1986).Clinical experience with intraaortic balloon pump counterpulsation in 112 consecutive patients.*American Heart journal*. Vol 111,issue:3,(march 1986),497-502,doi:10.1016/0002-8703(86)90054-2.

Gottlieb SO,Brinker JA,Borkon AM., et al.(1984). Identification of patients at high risk for complications of intraaortic balloon counterpulsation: A multivariate risk factor analysis.*TheAmerican journal of cardiology*.Vol 53,Issue:8,(Apr 1984),1135-1139, doi:10.1016/0002-9149(84)90650-7.

Hensley FA,Martin DE,Chambers CE,Luck JC.(1995). The cardiac patient,In:*A practical approach to cardiac anesthesia*,1995,Hensley FA,Martin DE,3-31,Little Brown and company,ISBN-0-316-35786-3,Toronto,Ontario

High KM,Pae WE,Pierce WS,Circulatory assist devices,In:*A practical approach to cardiac anesthesia*,1995, Hensley FA,Martin DE,499-515, Little Brown and company,ISBN-0-316-35786-3,Toronto,Ontario.

Isner JM et al,.(1980). Complications of the intraaortic balloon counterpulsation device: Clinical and morphologic observations in 45 necropsy patients.*The American journal of Cardiology*.Vol 45,issue:2,(Feb 1980),260-268, doi:10.1016/0002-9149(80)90644-X.

Katz AM (1990): Future perspectives in basic science understanding of congestive heart failure, Am J Cardiol, (1990) 468-471, 66:468.

Kern MJ, Aguirre F, Penick D et al, (1991): Enhanced intracoronary flow velocity during intra-aortic balloon counterpulsation in patients with coronary artery disease, Circulation 84 (suppl II): II-359-368, 1991).

Kimura A, Toyota E, Songfang L, et al (1996). Effects of intraortic balloon pumping on septal arterial blood flow velocity waveform during severe left main coronary artery stenosis. J Am Coll Cardiol 1996; 810-816, 27: 810

McCabe JC,Abel RM,Subramaniam VA et al.(1978). Complications of Intra-Aortic Balloon pump insertion and counterpulsation. *Circulation*. Vol 6,issue:10,(Apr 1978), 769-773, PMID 630686

Onorati F et al. (2009).Body perfusion during adult cardiopulmonary bypass is improved by Pulsatile flow with intraaortic balloon pump. *International journal of artificial organs*.32 (1), (jan 2009), 50-61, 19241364

Perera D, Stables R, Thomas M, et al (2010). Elective intra-aortic balloon counterpulsation during high-risk percutaneous coronary intervention: a randomized controlled trial. JAMA..304(8), (aug 2010),867-874. Cardiovascular Division, King's College London,BCIS-1.

Poole-Wilson PA,(1990). Future perspectives in the management of congestive heart failure, Am J Cardiol,(1990) 66: 462-467.

Quaal,Susan. (1993).Indications In:*Comprehensive Intraaortic Balloon Counterpulsation, 1993,* Conti CR, Janicki JS,Kantrowitz A, Moulopolous S, 118-143, Mosby, ISBN 0-8016-6656-2,St Louis, Missouri

Quaal,Susan. (1993).Physiological fundamentals relevant to balloon counterpulsation, In:*Comprehensive Intraaortic Balloon Counterpulsation, 1993,* Conti CR, Janicki JS,Kantrowitz A, Moulopolous S, 3-24, 74-75, Mosby, ISBN 0-8016-6656-2, St Louis, Missouri.

Ryan TJ, Antman EM, Brooks NH et al. (1999). Update: ACC/AHA guidelines for the management of patients with acute myocardial infarction: a report of the American College of Cardiology/American Heart Association Task Force on Practice Guidelines (Committee on Management of Acute Myocardial Infarction). J Am Coll Cardiol 1999, 34: 890-911.

Sinclair TD & Verman HA.(2009).Transfer of patients dependent on an intraaortic balloon pump utilizing critical care services.*Air medical journal*.28(1),(jan-feb 2009),40-46,19131025.

Skillman JJ,Kim D,Baim DS.(1988).Vascular complications of percutaneous femoral cardiac interventions.Incidence and operative repair.*Arch Surgery*.123(10),(Oct 1988),1207-12,PMID 2972269

Stone GW,et al.(1997). A prospective, randomized evaluation of prophylactic intraaortic balloon counterpulsation in high risk patients with acute myocardial infarction treated with primary angioplasty. Second Primary Angioplasty in Myocardial Infarction (PAMI-II) Trial Investigators.Journal of American college of cardiology.29 (7), (jun 1997), 1459-67, 9180105.

Trost JC, Hillis LD,(2006). Intra-Aortic Balloon Counterpulsation. Am J Cardiol (2006); 97: 1391-1398.

Wasfie T,Freed PS,Rubenfire M., et al.(1988). Risks associated with intraaortic balloon pumping in patients with and without diabetes mellitus.*The American journal of Cardiology*.vol 61,issue:8,(mar 1988),558-562, doi:10.1016/0002-9149(88)90764-3.

3

The Hybrid Operating Room

Georg Nollert, Thomas Hartkens, Anne Figel,
Clemens Bulitta, Franziska Altenbeck and Vanessa Gerhard
Siemens AG Healthcare Sector, Forchheim
Germany

1. Introduction

The integration of interventional and surgical techniques is demanding a new working environment for an interdisciplinary cardiovascular team: the hybrid operating room, where angiographic imaging capabilities are integrated in an operating suite. A deep understanding of the clinical applications, the current and future technology, and their implications on workflows is needed for a sound room design.

2. Clinical applications in cardiovascular therapy

2.1 Definition of hybrid procedures

The definition of hybrid procedures in the literature varies widely. A strict definition of a hybrid procedure is a major procedure that combines a conventional surgical part including a skin incision with an interventional part using some sort of catheter-based procedure guided by fluoroscopic or MRI imaging in a hybrid room without interruption. Wider definitions include procedures where the interventional and surgical parts are done in sequence, where a surgical part is only necessary in case of emergency or even minor procedures as venous cut downs. Sometimes, fluoroscopy guided interventions performed by surgeons (e.g. endovascular aortic repair in aortic abdominal aneurysms) are referred to as hybrid procedures. The term hybrid procedure in the radiology world may also refer to the combination of two imaging modalities for diagnostics or therapeutic purposes. In this chapter, the strict definition of hybrid procedures is applied and only procedures with fluoroscopic imaging are included, as interventional MRI still is in its very early stage.

2.2 Pediatric cardiac surgery

Although surgery remains the treatment of choice for most congenital cardiac malformations, interventional cardiology approaches are increasingly being used in simple and even complex lesions. The percutaneous approach can be challenging due to low patient weight or poor vascular access, induced rhythm disturbances and hemodynamic compromise (Bacha et al., 2007). Difficult and complex anatomy as in double-outlet right ventricle or transposition of the great arteries, or acute turns or kinks in the pulmonary arteries of tetralogy of Fallot patients can make percutaneous procedures challenging if not impossible (Sivakumar et al., 2007). However, surgery also has its limitations. Examples are operative closure of multiple apical muscular ventricular septal defects, adequate and lasting relief of peripheral pulmonary artery stenosis, or management of a previously implanted stenotic stent. Combining interventions and surgery into a single therapeutic procedure potentially leads to reduction of complexity, cardiopulmonary bypass time, risk, and to improved outcomes. The hybrid approach to hypoplastic left heart syndrome serves as a role model of the hybrid concept for congenital heart disease. Extracorporeal circulation and deep hypothermic circulatory arrest in infants can be avoided (or at least shortened), as shown in the extensive experience of several groups (Bacha et al., 2006; see Fig. 1).

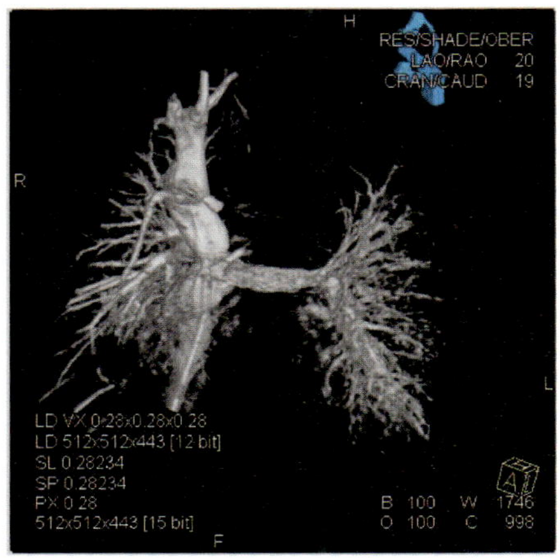

Fig. 1. Hypoplastic left heart syndrome. Intraoperative post-Fontan evaluation of the superior and inferior venae cavae as well as the stented pulmonary arteries. Imaging: Courtesy of Prof. Berger, Dr. Ewert German Heart Center, Berlin, Germany (Nollert et al., 2010)

Completion angiography in congenital heart diseases is another important concept. Residual structural lesions after cardiac surgery for congenital heart disease may complicate the postoperative recovery and result in poor outcomes. Therefore, intraoperative assessment of the newly created anatomy in 2D with fluoroscopy may help to avoid these complications. Rotational angiography with 3D reconstruction of the soft tissues (DynaCT) results in an even better delineation of the 3D anatomy and may change surgical strategy in a substantial subgroup of patients with CHD. Holzer and colleagues (R.J. Holzer et al., 2009) reported their experience with this imaging modality with 31 patients (median age and weight: 7.5 months and 6.5 kg, respectively) who underwent 32 complex surgical procedures, most of them involving pulmonary artery and/or aortic arch reconstructions. The angiograms were performed with regular catheters in a dedicated hybrid suite. Unexpected disorder was identified in 18 procedures (56%), including right and left pulmonary artery and coronary stenoses. The therapeutic strategy was modified in nine of 32 procedures (28%) and included surgical revision, hybrid therapy, early catheterization and a change in medical management. No major adverse events were noted. These advantages may be achieved in the operating room rapidly with fast image processing and even a reduction of contrast media and ionizing radiation dose (Pedra et al., 2011). The combination of an angiography system in the OR with magnetic resonance imaging may even further reduce dose and contrast and add additional functional data (Lurz et al., 2009).

2.3 Coronary artery disease

Routine evaluation of bypass grafts is the first indication for imaging in coronary artery bypass grafting. In a study designed and published by the Vanderbilt Heart and Vascular Institute (Zhao et al., 2009), routine intraoperative completion angiography performed in a fully functional hybrid operation room detected important defects in 97 of 796 (12% of the grafts) venous coronary artery bypass grafts in 366 adult patients (14% of the patients) with complex coronary artery disease. Their findings in completion angiography at the end of the operation included suboptimal anastomoses, poor lie of the venous bypass graft, and bypasses to not diseased vessels. The angiography findings led to a change in the management, including minor adjustments of the graft, traditional surgical revision or percutaneous coronary interventions, resulting in optimal bypass outcomes.

Surgical bypass grafting and percutaneous coronary artery revascularization are traditionally considered isolated options. A simultaneous hybrid approach may allow an opportunity to match the best strategy for a particular anatomic lesion. Revascularization of the left anterior descending artery with the left internal mammary artery is by far the best treatment option in terms of long term results. Integrating this therapy with percutaneous coronary angioplasty (hybrid procedure) offers multi-vessel revascularization through a mini-thoracotomy. Particularly in high risk patients, morbidity and mortality decreases in comparison to conventional surgery (Kon et al., 2008; Bonatti et al., 2008). A study from FuWai Hospital in Beijing (Hu et al., 2011) reports on 104 patients with multivessel coronary artery disease who were compared with the same sized group of patients undergoing off-pump surgery matched by propensity scores. The patients treated with the hybrid approach had a significantly lower ICU stay and intubation time and experienced less complications in terms of bleeding and transfusions needs. At a median follow up of 18 months, patients undergoing the hybrid procedure also had a significantly higher freedom from major adverse cardiac or cerebrovascular events (99 % vs. 90.4 %; $p = 0.03$). The hybrid procedure was also less costly than an exclusively percutaneous strategy.

2.4 Transcatheter aortic valve implantation (TAVI) procedures

Conventional aortic valve replacement for aortic stenosis is based upon standardized guidelines with excellent outcomes particularly in younger patients at relatively low-risk and will remain the gold standard for aortic valve replacement in the upcoming years. However, transcatheter techniques have developed to valid alternatives in high-risk patients in whom conventional surgical techniques are considered too invasive and risky. The Partner trial (Leon et al., 2010) using the Edwards Sapien valve demonstrated that patients with severe aortic stenosis, who are not eligible for conventional aortic valve replacement because of too high risk, benefit overwhelmingly from TAVI in comparison to standard therapy including valvuloplasty at one year in terms of survival (Cohort B, Leon et al., 2010). In addition, 700 enrolled very high risk patients undergoing TAVI for severe aortic stenosis had comparable mortality rates to those receiving conventional aortic valve replacements at one year (Cohort A, 25% vs. 26%). The transfemoral approach was used on approximately two-thirds of TAVI patients, while the transapical approach was used in the remaining third, unlike Cohort B where only the transfemoral approach was used.

Joint recommendations of the European Society of Cardiology and the European Association of Cardio-thoracic Surgery consider the hybrid operating room the optimal environment for these new therapeutic options (Vahanian et al., 2008). In Germany, joint recommendations of the German Society of Cardiology and the German Society of Cardiac,

Thoracic and Vascular Surgery demand a hybrid operating room or hybrid cathlab as a prerequisite for a TAVI program.

Currently two valves, the Corevalve (Medtronic, Minneapolis, MN) and the Sapien valve (Edwards, Irvine, CA) have been granted CE mark in 2007 and are successfully being implanted. Several newer generation valves aim to improve the results by more sophisticated designs to decrease the common current TAVI complications of aortic regurgitation, misplacement, and heart block. Advanced image guidance by dedicated 2D and 3D applications (e.g. syngo Aortic Valve guide, Siemens; Heart Navigator, Philips; C-THV, Paieon) may further simplify navigation and deployment of the devices. Some of the upcoming TAVI valves (e.g. Symetis Acurate, Jena Valve, Embracer, Medtronic) have dedicated mechanisms to anchor in the sinuses. Therefore, anatomically correct rotation of the valve within the aortic annulus is needed to optimally deploy the devices. 3D imaging may prove highly valuable to understand the correct relationships between the valve and the annulus.

2.5 Mitral valve repair

For repair of mitral regurgitation, various devices are currently under investigation and await FDA approval. Currently, it is also not quite clear which of the devices will be used in a hybrid operating room, because some approaches will most likely be performed in regular cathlabs. In Europe, only the MitralClip Mitral valve repair system (Abbott Vascular, Santa Clara, CA) has received CE mark in 2008. Studies for FDA clearance are ongoing. The MitralClip is creating a double orifice mitral valve by connecting the free edges of the anterior and posterior leaflets at the A2 / P2 level. The Everest II trial (Feldman et al., 2011) compared the MitralClip with surgical mitral valve with repair in patients with moderate or severe mitral valve surgery, who were candidates for mitral valve surgery and demonstrated superior safety at the expense of inferior efficacy. Experimentally, prostheses for mitral und tricuspid valve replacement are under development and certainly will be available within the next years. Complex hybrid procedures may arise where the various parts of the mitral valve apparatus (e.g. chordae, leaflet and ring) are repaired on a beating heart in combination with purely interventional techniques (e.g. MitralClip). For imaging purposes, fluoroscopy will most likely be combined with 2D and 3D ultrasound and a fusion of these modalities may become helpful. The reason is that the metal devices are optimally imaged without artifacts by fluoroscopy whereas the valve itself is better evaluated with ultrasound. As an alternative to transesophageal echocardiography, the use of intracardiac 2D and 3D echo (Accunav and Accunav V, Siemens AG Healthcare, Montainview, CA) may prove useful, because it would allow avoiding general anesthesia in selected patients.

2.6 Thoracic endovascular aortic repair (TEVAR)

Thoracic endovascular aortic repair (TEVAR) has become a valid alternative to open repair. In selected cases, EVAR, in combination with open surgery, is even applied for pathologies of the aortic arch and distal ascending aorta (Walsh et al., 2008). Endoleaks are common complications of EVAR and may be missed by angiographic evaluation. CT-like imaging with the angiographic C-arm enables the surgeon to diagnose this complication intraoperatively and correct it. A group from University of London (Biasi et al., 2009) demonstrated in a study of 80 patients undergoing EVAR that 3D imaging with DynaCT in the operating room was able to detect endoleaks in 5 patients. These endoleaks were not detected by conventional completion angiography. In addition, conventional CT evaluations before discharge did not reveal any endoleak which was not previously seen in DynaCT. In addition, the hybrid operating room allowed for immediate treatment of the endoleaks, if required. In the near future, off the shelf fenestrated aortic stents will become available for the treatment of extensive aortic disease. These fenestrated stents have to be rotated in the aorta, such that the fenestrations cover the branches of the aorta. For these highly complex procedures, 3D imaging in a hybrid operating room may be extremely helpful for the navigation of wires and devices.

2.7 Hybrid surgery for rhythm disturbances

The combination of the surgical epicardial approach with the interventional endocardial approach for the treatment of rhythm disturbances in particular atrial fibrillation offers theoretically advantages over conventional endocardial or epicardial therapy alone. First reports emphasized the potential benefit. Krul and coworkers from Amsterdam (Krul et al., 2011) reported on 31 patients with atrial fibrillation (AF); thereof 13 with persistent and two with permanent AF. A minimally-invasive approach combining thoracoscopic pulmonary vein isolation (PVI) and ganglionated plexus (GP) ablation with intraoperative electrophysiological confirmation of PVI was performed in order to decrease recurrences of AF during follow-up. Results at one year follow-up were very encouraging, with 86% of the patients without recurrence of AF. A hybrid approach for drug-refractory ventricular tachycardia was described by Michowitz (Michowitz et al., 2010). Fourteen patients (most of them after previous cardiac surgery) underwent surgical ablation with an epicardial approach with concomitant electrophysiological mapping. The authors conclude that the surgical access with subxiphoid window and limited anterior thoracotomy in the electrophysiology lab is feasible and safe.

Pacemakers and implantable cardioverter defibrillators (ICD), particularly bi-ventricular systems, may be optimally implanted in a hybrid OR environment, because the hybrid operating theatre offers the required superior angulation and imaging capabilities in comparison to mobile C-arms, and the higher hygienic standards compared to cathlabs. DynaCT angiographic 3D imaging may prove useful for imaging the venous system of the heart. The coronary sinus can be depicted in 3D and than be overlaid over the fluoroscopy image to better guide placement of the left ventricular lead.

2.8 Other applications outside cardiovascular therapy

Hybrid operating rooms outside cardiovascular therapies are currently more and more used in neurosurgery, traumatology, orthopedics, urology, and general surgery. Interdisciplinary usage may be considered.

The need for hybrid operating theatres is not restricted to cardiac surgery. Vascular surgeons and neurosurgeons have equally developed hybrid procedures necessitating angiography systems in the OR. Furthermore, hybrid operating rooms are already in use by abdominal surgeons, traumatologists, orthopedic surgeons, and even urologists. Imaging needs, hygienic requirements, and room set up - particularly for neurosurgery - may be considerably different. Other surgical disciplines may want to introduce navigation systems, magnetic resonance imaging, endoscopy, biplane angiography systems, or a lateral position of anesthesia equipment. However, the hybrid operating rooms are more commonly shared with interventionalists including cardiologists, interventional radiologists, electrophysiologists, neuroradiologists, and pediatric cardiologists. Their specific needs have to be carefully considered and weighted when planning the hybrid theatre.

3. Imaging techniques in the hybrid operating room

The imaging capabilities of modern, fixed C-arms have dramatically changed in the last five years. Traditionally, fixed C-arms have been used either for simple 2D fluoroscopy or 3D rotational angiography. Nowadays, C-arms, which are able to acquire CT-like 3D images, are used for image-based guidance and even provide intra-operative functional imaging, like flow analysis.

3.1 Fluoroscopy

Traditional fluoroscopy provides real-time, high resolution, low-contrast images in two dimensions through the use of an image intensifier. With ultrasound and endoscopy it is the main imaging modality to guide devices in real time through the body (see Fig. 2a). Brilliant image quality is needed to depict fine anatomic structures and devices. In particular, in cardiac interventions, imaging the moving heart requires a high frame rate (30f/s, 50Hz) and high power output (at least 80kW). Thus, the image quality needed for cardiac applications can only be achieved by high powered fixed angiography systems. In modern fluoroscopy devices image intensifiers have been replaced with digital flat panel detectors which enabled fluoroscopy to transition into three dimensions, producing CT-like images (see below). Fluoroscopy is performed with continuous X-ray to guard the progression of a catheter or other devices within the body in live images. To minimize the doses for the patient and the surgeon, dose saving measurements are essential in modern fluoroscopy devices (see section 3.4).

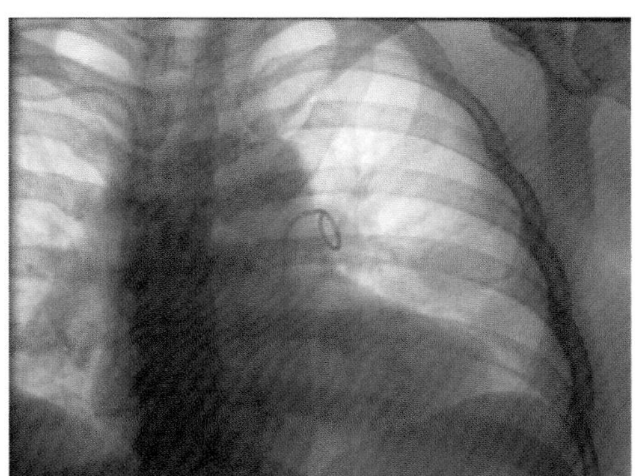

Fig. 2a. 2D fluoroscopic image

3.2 Data acquisition

Angiographic systems provide a so-called *acquisition mode,* which stores the acquired images automatically on the system to be uploaded into an image archive later. While standard fluoroscopy is predominantly used to guide devices and to re-position the field of view, data acquisition is applied for reporting or diagnostic purposes. In particular, when contrast media is injected, a data acquisition is mandatory, because the stored sequences can be replayed as often as required without re-injection of contrast media. To achieve a sufficient image quality for diagnoses and reporting, the angiographic system uses up to 10 times

higher x-ray doses than standard fluoroscopy. Thus, data acquisition is not recommended as long as fluoroscopy is sufficient or the images do not need to be stored.
Data acquisition can be combined with specific imaging protocols, for example, to enhance blood vessels while removing background structures (see section 3.3) or to acquire 3D images (see section 3.5).

3.3 Digital subtraction angiography

Over the past three decades, digital subtraction angiography (DSA) has become a well-established 2D imaging technique for the visualization of blood vessels in the human body (Katzen, 1995). With this technique, a sequence of 2D digital X-ray projection images is acquired to show the passage of an injected contrast agent through the vessels of interest. Background structures are largely removed by subtracting an image acquired prior to injection (usually called the mask image) from the live images (often referred to as contrast images). It is obvious that in the resulting subtraction images, background structures are completely removed only if these structures are exactly aligned and have equal grey-level distributions (see Fig. 2b). Therefore, various motion correction algorithms are applied to reduce such artifacts in the image.

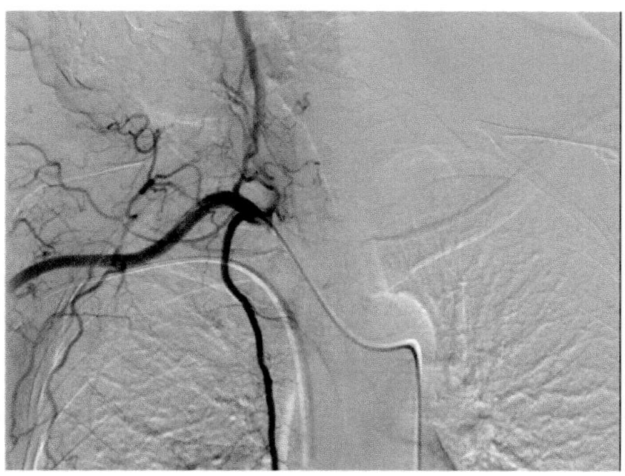

Fig. 2b. 2D digital subtraction angiography shows the difference between an initial fluoroscopic acquisition and a fluoroscopic acquisition after injecting contrast agent. Thus, the vessels are clearly depicted in these images. Other remaining structures (white next to black structures) caused by motion, are considered artefacts, and can be partly compensated by modern angiography devices.

DSA is clinically used for diagnostic and therapeutic applications of vessel visualization throughout the entire body. During complex interventional procedures, DSA is often combined with so-called *road mapping*. In this mode, a DSA sequence is performed and the frame with maximum vessel opacification is identified, which becomes the road map mask. The road map mask is subtracted from subsequent live fluoroscopic images to produce real-time subtracted fluoroscopic images overlaid on a static image of the vasculature. Road mapping is useful for the placement of catheters and wires in complex and small vasculature, because fluoroscopy alone may not adequately show the vessels and may not visualize small wires in the distracting underlying tissue. It is also possible to combine the road mapping feature with a feature called image fade, which allows the user to manually adjust the brightness of the static vessel road-map overlay.

3.4 Radiation dose and dose reduction

Ionizing radiation may, depending on the dose, cause damage to organic tissue. The mechanisms by which radiation damages the human body are two-fold: (1) radiation directly destroys the DNA of the cells by ionizing atoms in its molecular structure and, (2) radiation creates free radicals, which are atoms, molecules, or ions with unpaired electrons. These unpaired electrons are usually highly reactive, so radicals are likely to take part in chemical reactions that eventually change or harm the DNA of the cells.

The human body can repair damaged cells to a certain extent, but if exposed to a high amount of radiation beyond a given threshold in a short period of time, "deterministic" damage will occur. Deterministic radiation damage includes changes of the blood count, hair loss, tissue necrosis or cataract. Exposure levels of typical medical diagnostic imaging procedures are far below the threshold for deterministic radiation damage. However, deterministic effects are an important consideration in external radiation therapy and radionuclide therapy.

In order to assess the risk of radiation exposure, quantitative measurements of dose were introduced:

- *Absorbed dose D* (also called "energy dose"), measured in Gray (Gy) units, characterizes the amount of energy deposited in tissue. It is defined as the amount of radiation required to deposit 1 Joule (J) of energy in 1 kilogram of any kind of matter.
- *Equivalent dose H*, measured in Sievert (Sv) units, takes in account the damage caused by different types of radiation. It is the absorbed dose multiplied by a weighting factor characteristic for the particular type of radiation. For X-ray, H = D.
- *Effective dose E*, measured in Sievert (Sv) units, includes the sensitivity of different organs to radiation. It is the sum of the equivalent doses in all irradiated organs multiplied by the respective tissue weighting-factors.

Determining the effective dose in angiography depends on several factors, primarily on the variability in organ sensitivity to radiation. For instance, bone marrow is far more sensitive to radiation than the liver. The degree to which organs are affected by radiation also depends on the angle of the beams. Because dose distribution in angiography is not as "homogeneous" as it is for CT, these factors must be considered when estimating the damage caused by irradiation. The effective dose includes the sensitivity to radiation of the different organs. It is the sum of the equivalent doses in all irradiated organs multiplied by the respective tissue weighting-factors.

Effective dose provides a good comparison with natural background radiation, which is on average about 2.4 mSv per year. Typically, during a cardiac diagnostic intervention with 15 p/s, the effective dose per minute is 0.6 mSv (Cusma et al., 1999).

In general, low dose goes hand in hand with less visibility, while higher image quality requires, among other factors, a higher dose. To obtain a specific image quality, it is necessary to choose the "right" dose for the tissue being penetrated.

Because guidance of endovascular devices requires continuous X-ray, modern angiographic systems include several measures for dose reduction (Balter et al., 2010). There are three parameters which can be adapted by the user to reduce the radiation exposure:

1. *Footswitch on-time:* footswitch on-time controls how long the body is exposed to X-ray beams, thus how long the body is irradiated: less time means less radiation.
2. *Frame rate:* high frame rates are used to visualize fast motion without stroboscopic effects. However, the higher the frame rate, the more radiation. Therefore, it is best to keep the frame rate as low as possible, according to the clinical need. Modern

angiographic systems can adjust the frame rate downward in various steps, from 60 pulses per second (p/s) used in pediatric cardiology to 0.5 p/s in some systems for slowly moving objects. A reduction to half pulse rate reduces dose by about half. The reduction from 30 p/s to 7.5 p/s results in a dose saving of 75%.

3. *Source-Image- Distance (SID)*: according to the quadratic law and a requested constant dose at the detector, a greater distance between the source and the imager increases the skin dose. Rising SID from 105 cm (=SID 1) to 120 cm (=SID 2) increases skin dose (i.e. the dose at the IRP) by approximately 30%, if C-arm angles, table position, patient, and requested dose at the detector do not change. Fig. 3 illustrates the setup including the lower (SID = 105 cm) and the upper (SID = 120 cm) position of the detector.

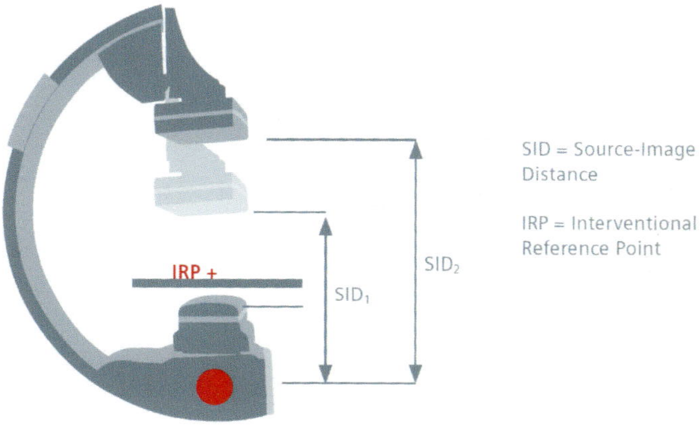

Fig. 3. C-arm, two different SIDs, constant table height, location of the IRP

Additionally, modern angiographic systems provide some inherent features to reduce dose. For example, variable copper filters reduce the skin dose by filtering the low-energy photons out of the X-ray, called *beam hardening*. Some systems adjust the thickness of such filters automatically according to the absorption of the patient entrance dose along the path of the X-ray beam through the patient. This automatic filter insertion maintains low skin dose without degrading image quality and can result in a dose saving of up to 50%.

Other measurements include radiation-free collimation or radiation-free object positioning. Using the last image hold (LIH) as a reference, the system allows radiation-free collimation and semitransparent filter parameter setting to precisely target the region of interest (see Fig. 4). A similar approach is implemented for optimal patient positioning for imaging: graphic display of the outline of the upcoming image allows translation of the table without fluoroscopic radiation exposure and provides an indication of which anatomy is in the field-of-view of the detector. For specific cardiac interventions, such measurements can reduce the overall fluoroscopy time by 0.5 to 3 minutes. Under typical fluoroscopy conditions, this may result in a dose reduction of 20 to 120 mGy.

More and more countries and authorities require the reporting of patient exposure to radiation following an intervention. To meet current and future regulations, modern angiographic systems allow effective reporting of dose exposure, thus enable enhanced in-house dose reporting and analysis.

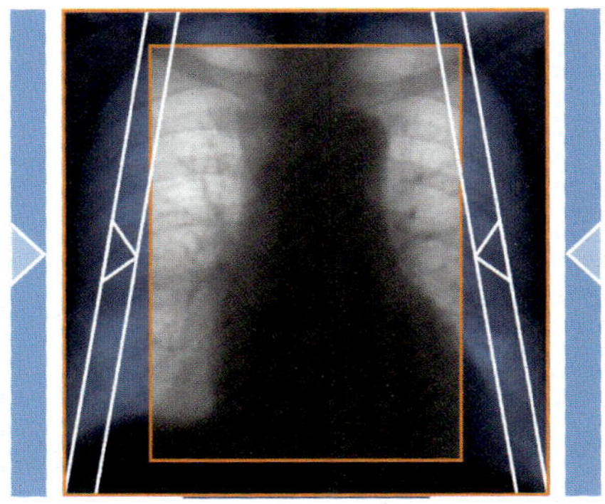

Fig. 4. Radiation-free collimation: The collimator position is indicated on the last image hold (LIH) by a white frame.

3.5 3D DynaCT imaging

Three-dimensional (3D) C-arm computed tomography (DynaCT) is a new and innovative imaging technique. It uses two-dimensional (2D) X-ray projections acquired with a flat-panel detector C-arm angiography system to generate CT-like images (Kalender & Kyriakou, 2007). The C-arm sweeps around the patient acquiring up to several hundred 2D views serving as input for 3D cone-beam reconstruction. Usually, a minimum angular scan range of 180 degrees, plus the so-called fan-angle, is required. For typical C-arm CT devices, this results in an angular scan range requirement of at least 200 degrees. Resulting voxel data sets can be visualized either as cross-sectional images or as 3D data sets using different volume rendering techniques.

Thanks to a detector optimized for high-resolution 2D fluoroscopic and radiographic imaging, the spatial resolution provided by DynaCT can be very high. For example, a common FD for large-plate C-arm systems, such as the 30 cm × 40 cm Pixium 4700 flat-panel detector (Trixell, Moirans, France) offers a native pixel pitch of 154 µm in a 2480 ×1920 matrix. Due to read-out bandwidth limitations, such detectors are operated in 2 × 2 binning mode during DynaCT, which means the smallest high contrast object that can be resolved has a size of about 0.2 mm (Strobel et al., 2009).

Initially targeted at neuroendovascular imaging of contrast enhanced vascular structures, 3D C-arm imaging has been continuously improved over the years. It is now possible to acquire CT-like soft-tissue images directly in the hybrid OR (see Fig. 5). Beyond their use for trans-arterial catheter procedures, these 3D data sets are also valuable for guidance and optimization of percutaneous treatments. In combination with 2D fluoroscopic or radiographic imaging, information provided by DynaCT can be very valuable for therapy planning, guidance, and outcome control - in particular for complicated interventions (Doelken et al., 2008).

There are low-dose DynaCT protocols that achieve acceptable image quality for radiosensitive patients, such as pediatric patients, and provide adequate diagnostic image quality. In clinical practice, the balance between image quality and dose has to be considered. For the prerequisites mentioned above, a five second high contrast DR rotational 3D run applying 0.36 µGy/f can be reduced to 0.1 µGy/f resulting, in a dose saving of 72%. Low-dose DynaCT can be achieved with an effective dose of 0.3 mSv.

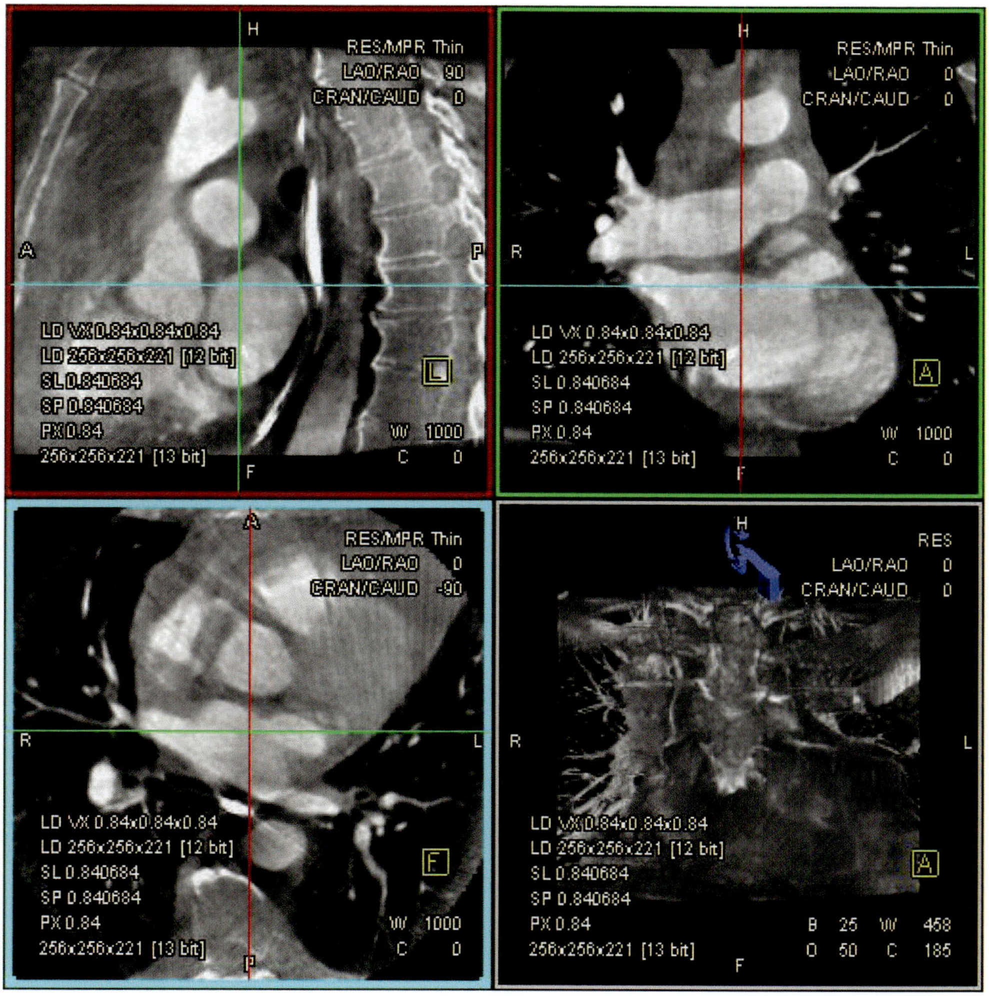

Fig. 5. Cardiac DynaCT image: the C-arm CT results were obtained with syngo DynaCT running on a syngo X-workplace (Siemens AG, Healthcare Sector, Forchheim, Germany)

3.6 Advanced visualization

Recent post-processing algorithms analyse an entire digital subtraction angiography (DSA) sequence at once and represent the sequence in one single colour-coded image. In order to obtain a colour-coded image, the algorithm takes the time to maximum opacification of each individual pixel, starting with the injection and subsequently visualising the distribution of the contrast medium through the vessels. These time measurements are then represented by a colour, allowing visualisation of the complete vessel tree in one image. Thus, the colours represent the contrast agent from its initial entry into the blood vessels to its flow throughout the anatomy of interest in one image.

Such dynamic flow evaluations provide a greater understanding of the contrast flow within the pathology, greater ease in visualizing the success of a procedure, and they assist the

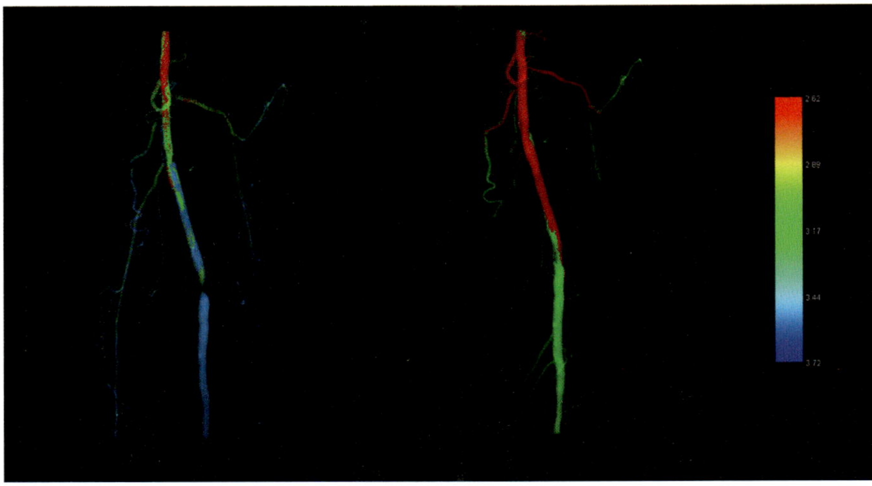

Fig. 6. Advanced visualization of an entire DSA sequence (iFlow): Colour-coded pre and post-procedural results visualize the improvement of flow

clinicians in image review by showing a complete Digital Subtraction Angiography (DSA) run in a single image (Ahmed et al., 2009). For example, this technology can be used to enhance pre-procedural and post-procedural imaging of patients under treatment for stenoses of peripheral vessels (see Fig. 6). Flow deviations and the increased utilisation of collaterals can more easily be detected prior to intervention, since anomalies more readily attract the physician's attention due to their specific colours. Following the intervention, the success of a balloon dilatation or stent implantation of a stenosis is readily visible due to the improved flow.

3.7 Fusion imaging and 2D/3D overlay

Modern angiographic systems are not just used for imaging, but support the surgeon also during the procedure by guiding the intervention based on 3D information acquired either pre-operatively or intra-operatively. Such guidance requires that the 3D information is registered to the patient. The next sections illustrate why 3D images acquired by an angiographic system are inherently registered with the patient and show new applications based on this fundamental feature of modern angiographic systems.

3.7.1 Information flow between workstation and angiographic system

3D DynaCT images are calculated from a set of projections acquired from different angles around the patient. The volume is reconstructed on a separate workstation. Even though the workstation and the angio system can be considered as separate systems, there is a close link and a continuous information flow between these systems. For example, when the user virtually rotates the volume on the workstation to view the anatomy from a certain perspective, the parameter of this view can be transmitted to the angio system, which then drives the C-arm to the exact same perspective for fluoroscopy. In the same way, if the C-arm angulation is changed, this angulation can be transmitted to the workstation which updates the volume to the same perspective as the fluoroscopic view (see Fig. 7).

The information flow between the angiographic system and the workstation ensures that an anatomical structure in the fluoroscopic image can be related to an anatomical structure in the 3D image and vice versa: that means the images are registered with each other. Even pre-operatively acquired images can be related to the patient by image-to-image registration of the pre-operative image with the intra-operative acquired DynaCT. Information in the pre-operative image (e.g. a surgical plan) can be directly overlaid on top of a live fluoroscopy.
Inherent registration of 3D images of the angiographic systems to the patient triggers new applications which go beyond just simple imaging, but towards image-driven guidance based on 3D information as illustrated in the next sections.

3.7.2 Overlay of 3D information on top of 2D fluoroscopy

Any 3D information extracted from the image in the workstation can be overlaid on the live fluoroscopic image. Firstly, the 3D image itself can be overlaid colour-coded on top of the fluoroscopic image. For example, in Fig. 8, a 3D angiography is colour-coded in orange and overlaid on the live fluoroscopy. Any change of the angulations of the C-arm will cause the workstation to re-calculate in real-time the view on the 3D image to match exactly the view of the live 2D fluoroscopy image. Without additional contrast agent injection the surgeon can observe device movements simultaneously with the 3D overlay of the vessel contours in the fluoroscopy image.
Fig. 7 illustrates an alternative way to add information from the workstation to the fluoroscopic image. After either manual or automatic segmentation of the anatomical structures of interest in the 3D image, the outline can be overlaid as a contour onto the fluoroscopic image. In this example, an AAA aneurysm has been segmented in the DynaCT image. The contour of the 3D segmentation is shown in the fluoroscopic view and provides additional information which is not visible in the fluoroscopic image. Overlaid landmarks do not necessarily need to be extracted from images directly, but might be added by the

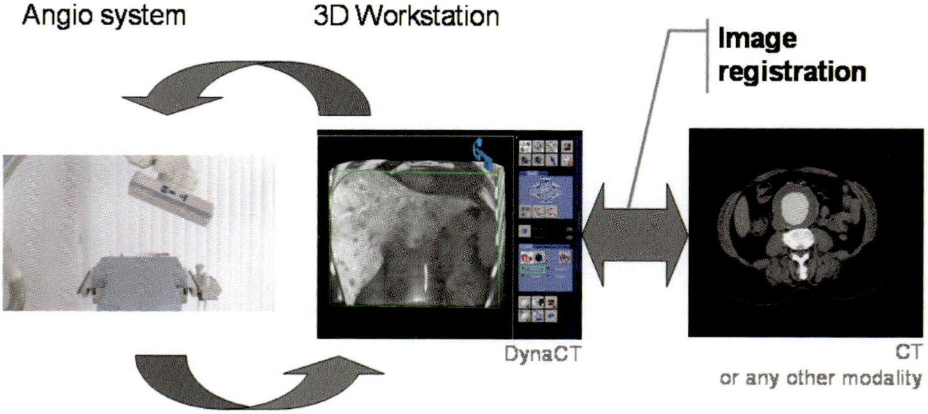

Fig. 7. Linkage between a modern angio system and its workstation. The corresponding information flow guarantees the registration between the 3D DynaCT image in the workstation and a 2D fluoroscopic live image and is the prerequisite of true 2D/3D image fusion

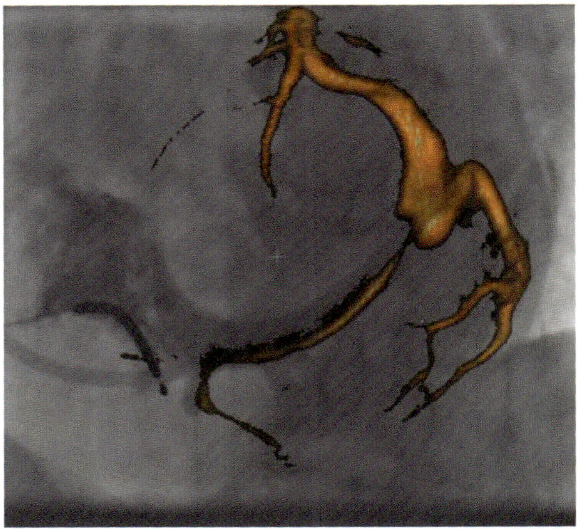

Fig. 8. Overlay of 3D DynaCT image (orange) on top of a fluoroscopic image during cardiac resynchronization therapy. Courtesy of K.-J. Gutleben, M.D., G. Nölker, M.D. A. Sinha, M.D., J. Brachmann, M.D., Department of Cardiology, Klinikum Coburg, Germany.

surgeon. For example to place fenestrated stents, a pre-operatively acquired CT image could be used to mark the ostia of the visceral arteries manually by the surgeon. By aligning the pre-operative CT image with the intra-operatively acquired DynaCT image, the ostia can be displayed (beside the contour of the arteries) in the fluoroscopic image. Notably, this truly is 3D information, i.e. any change in the C-arm position or angulations will update the view on the marks to perfectly match the live fluoroscopy image.

3.7.3 Guidance during Trans-Aortic Valve Implantation (TAVI)

Trans-Aortic Valve Implantation requires exact positioning of the valve in the aortic root to prevent complications. A good fluoroscopic view is essential, whereby an exact perpendicular angle to the aortic root is considered to be optimal for the implantation. Recently, applications have been released which support the surgeon in selecting this optimal fluoroscopy angulation or even drive the C-arm automatically into the perpendicular view to the aortic root (see Fig. 9).

Some approaches are based on pre-operative CT images, which are used to segment the aorta and calculate optimal viewing angles for valve implantations. CT images must be registered with DynaCT or fluoroscopic images to transfer the 3D volume to the actual angiographic system. Errors during the registration process might result in diversification from the optimal angulations of the C-arm and must be manually corrected. Additionally, anatomical variations between the acquisition of the pre-operatively CT image and surgery are not accounted for. Patients are generally imaged with hands-up in a CT scanner while surgery is performed with arms aside the patient, which leads to substantial errors.

Algorithms purely based on DynaCT images acquired in the OR by the angiographic system are inherently registered to the patient and show the present anatomy structures. With such an approach, the surgeon does not rely on pre-operative CT images acquired by the radiological department which simplifies the workflow in the OR and reduces errors in the process.

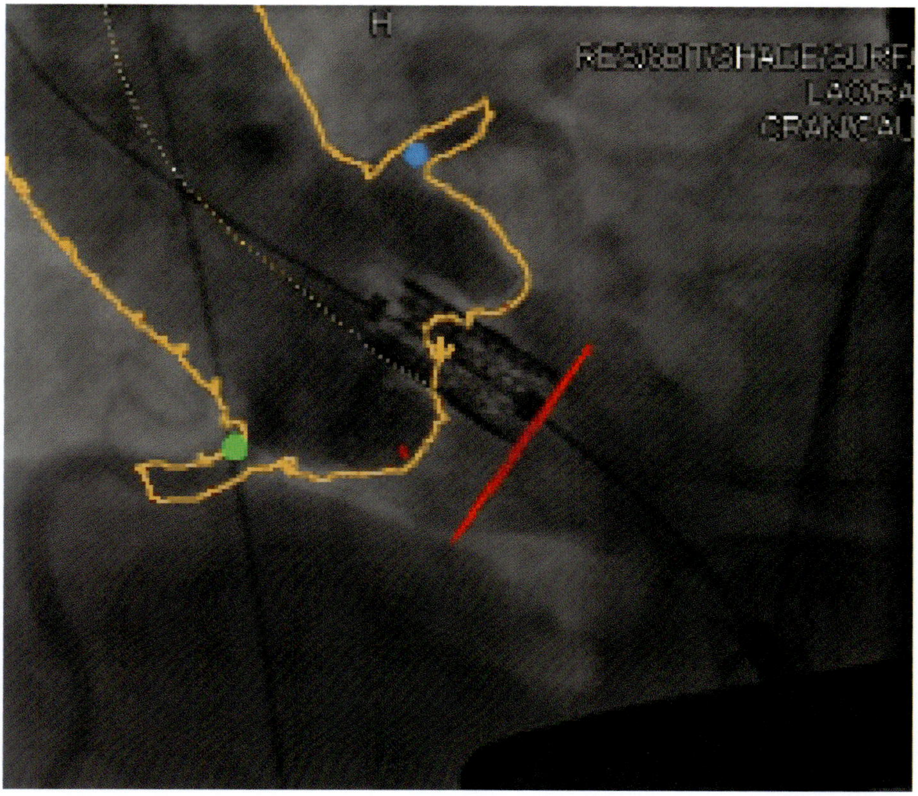

Fig. 9. Image-driven guidance during Trans-Aortic Valve Implantation (TAVI). Contours were automatically segmented from a 3D DynaCT image and the C-arm was positioned perpendicular to the aortic root for live fluroscopy based on anatomical landmarks extracted from the DynaCT image without user interaction. (Siemens AG, Forchheim, Germany)

4. Planning the hybrid room

Careful planning and professional expertise is a key factor for every hybrid room project. Before planning a hybrid operating room a clear vision for the utilization should be established (Benjamin, 2008).

Today's operating rooms require concepts that address the requirements and needs of different surgical specialties and procedures. Workflow efficiency is a key success factor for the hospital and the surgical program. Minimal turnover times and optimal processes throughout the entire surgical workflow and the actual surgical procedure are required (Tomaszewski, 2008). Therefore, a hybrid operating room should ideally be integrated into an existing OR suite. All aspects and steps starting with patient transfer from the ward to anesthesia and operating room preparation are important. Addiontional aspects for planning are material supply processes, i.e. of materials necessary for the procedure, and postoperative intensive care surveillance and treatment.

Due to high cost, OR facilities are commonly shared by different disciplines. A very flexible room layout and design allow for the necessary repositioning of devices and changes of the

OR configuration (Tomaszewski, 2008). This is especially important with the increasing utilization of novel technologies and with space limitations in most OR suites. Layout and design should be ergonomic and workflow driven. For the hybrid OR with the addition of an angiography system to the room it becomes even more important, because this oftenly involves non-standard installations, or non-standard functionality, or non-standard products. During the entire planning and implementation process clear, frequent and comprehensive communication of all parties involved is vital.

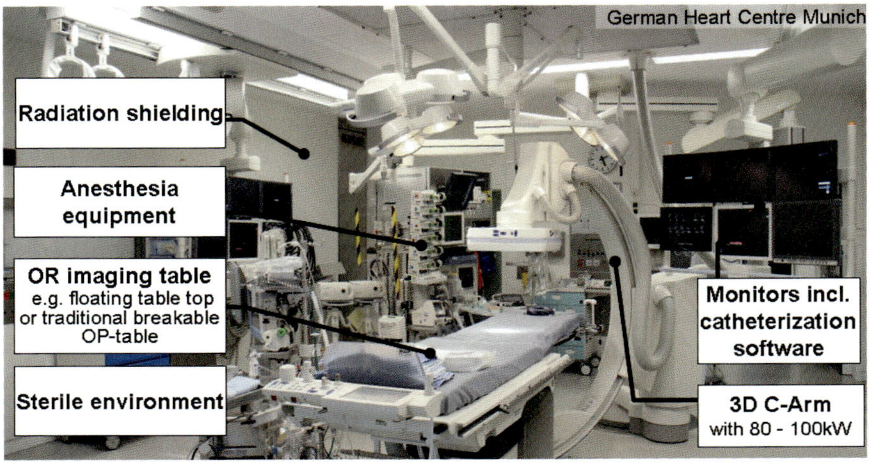

Fig. 10. Example of an hybrid OR highlighting relevant major equipment for planning

4.1 Team

Hybrid operating rooms are used by different surgical disciplines, interventionalists, cardiologists and anesthesiologists. Further staff working in these rooms includes nurses and technicians, resulting in a multitude of requirements impacting the room design and determining various resources like space, medical, and imaging equipment. Building a hybrid operating room needs a team approach with joint effort of customers and vendors (Tomaszewski, 2008; Benjamin, 2008).

Hybrid operating rooms are always individual solutions tailored to the needs and preferences of the team and the hospital. Several planning iterations with experienced technological support from equipment and imaging vendors lead to an optimal solution. Hybrid OR projects involve renovation, new construction, or a little of both. OR equipment layout planning and implementation strategies are challenging. A clear understanding of the project scope and customer objectives is critical and qualified, multidisciplinary hospital team is needed to ensure success of this complex endeavour.

All team members should be committed to the project. To that end, a clearly defined and agreed project organization including all stakeholders with clearly defined roles and responsibilities is necessary.

4.2 Choosing the angiographic system

Choosing the imaging system for a hybrid OR depends on the intended utilization of the room (Bonatti et al., 2007; Ten Cate et al., 2004).

Team member	Topics
Surgeon(s)	Working positions, clinical applications, procedural descriptions, imaging and equipment requirements
Nursing staff (circulating and scrub nurses)	Working positions, patient and material logistics
Surgical technicians (i.e. perfusionist)	Working positions, equipment requirements
Anesthetist	Working positions, equipment requirements
Anesthesia nurses	Working positions, equipment requirements, material logistics
OR manager	Scheduling, general workflow management
Biomedical engineers	Technical room planning
Equipment planners, Architects	Technical room planning, construction, drawings, project management
Vendors	Installation requirements and schedule

Table 1. Team members of an OR and the issues they care about

Expert consensus rates the performance of mobile C-arms in hybrid ORs as insufficient and recommends floor-mounted systems for hygienic reasons (Bonatti et al., 2007). In fact, some hospitals do not allow operating parts directly above the surgical field, because dust may fall in the wound and cause infection. Since any ceiling-mounted system includes moving parts above the surgical field and impairs the laminar airflow, such systems are not the right option for hospitals enforcing highest hygienic standards. Ceiling-mounted systems require substantial ceiling space and, therefore, reduce the options to install surgical lights or booms.

Nonetheless, many hospitals choose ceiling-mounted systems because they cover the whole body with more flexibility and - most importantly - without moving the table. The latter is sometimes a difficult and dangerous undertaking during surgery with the many lines and catheters that must also be moved. Moving from a parking to a working position during surgery, however, is easier with a floor-mounted system, because the C-arm just turns in from the side and does not interfere with the anesthesiologist. The ceiling-mounted system, by contrast, during surgery can hardly move to a parking position at the head end without colliding with anesthesia equipment. In an overcrowded environment like the OR, biplane systems add to the complexity and interfere with anesthesia, except for neurosurgery, where anesthesia is not at the head end. Monoplane systems are therefore clearly recommended for rooms mainly used for cardiac surgery. There are certainly exceptions: especially if pediatric cardiologists or electrophysiologists are important stakeholders in room usage, a biplane system may also be considered (Bonatti et al., 2007; Tomaszewski, 2008).

3D imaging may become more and more important for OR planning and postoperative evaluation of the operative site. Therefore, a large detector would offer greater options, including portrait imaging. The preference for a detector may vary, although the majority opts for a large detector (Nollert & Wich, 2008).

In summary, mobile C-arms are generally considered insufficient for cardiovascular imaging and do not comply with international standards for cardiac imaging (Bonatti et al., 2007). For hybrid rooms, fixed monoplane and biplane angiographic systems are available which are either mounted on the ceiling or on the floor. Beside conventional C-arm systems, a dedicated robotic surgical C-arm is available, which allows maximal flexibility in the operating room.

4.3 Tables

The selection of the OR table depends on the primary use of the system. Interventional tables with floating table tops and tilt and cradle compete with fully integrated flexible OR tables. Identification of the right table is a compromise between interventional and surgical requirements (Bonatti et al., 2007; Nollert & Wich, 2008).

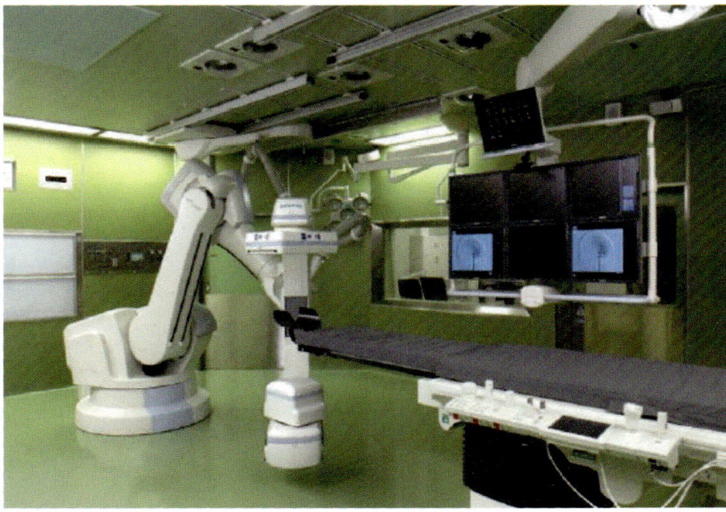

Fig. 11. Siemens robotic surgical C-Arm system Artis zeego

Surgical and interventional requirements may be mutually exclusive. Surgeons, especially orthopedic, general and neurosurgeons usually expect a table with a segmented tabletop for flexible patient positioning. For imaging purposes, a radiolucent tabletop, allowing full body coverage, is required. Therefore, non-breakable carbon fibre tabletops are used.

Interventionalists require a floating tabletop to allow fast and precise movements during angiography. Cardiac and vascular surgeons, in general, have less complex positioning needs, but based on their interventional experience in angiography may be used to having fully motorized movements of the table and the tabletop. For positioning patients on non-breakable tabletops, positioning aids are available, i.e. inflatable cushions. Truly floating tabletops are not available with conventional OR tables. As a compromise, floatable angiography tables specifically made for surgery with vertical and lateral tilt are recommended (Ten Cate et al., 2004). To further accommodate typical surgical needs, side rails for mounting surgical equipment like retractors or limb holders should be available for the table. The position of the table in the room also impacts surgical workflow. A diagonal position in the OR may be considered in order to gain space and flexibility in the room, as well as access to the patient from all sides.

Alternatively, a conventional surgery table can be combined with an imaging system if the vendor offers a corresponding integration. The operating room can then be used either with a radiotranslucent but not breakable tabletop that supports 3D imaging, or with a universal breakable tabletop that provides enhanced patient positioning, but restricts 3D imaging. The latter are particularly suited for neuro- or orthopedic surgery, and these integrated solutions recently also became commercially available. If it is planned to share the room for hybrid and open conventional procedures, these are sometimes preferred. They provide greater workflow flexibility because the tabletops are dockable and can be easily exchanged, but require some compromises with interventional imaging.

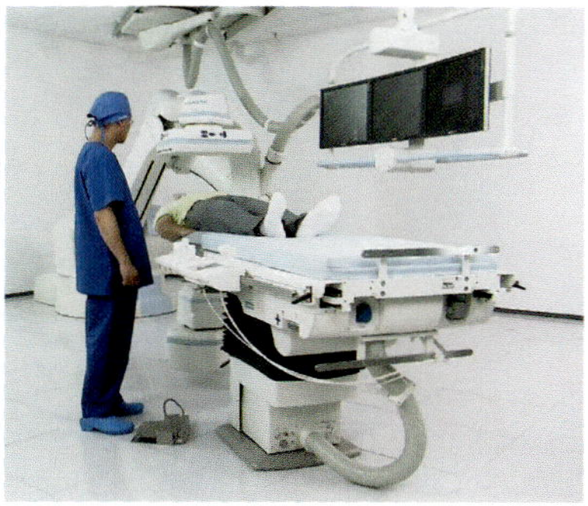

Fig. 12. Example Siemens OR angiography table with a free floating tabletop

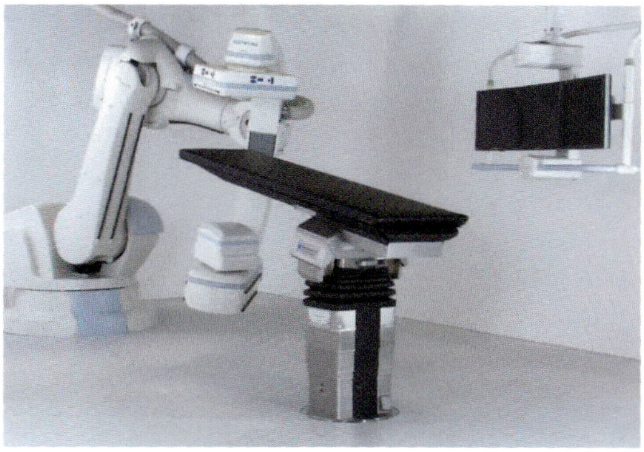

Fig. 13. Integrated Trumpf OR table with a radiolucent carbon fibre tabletop

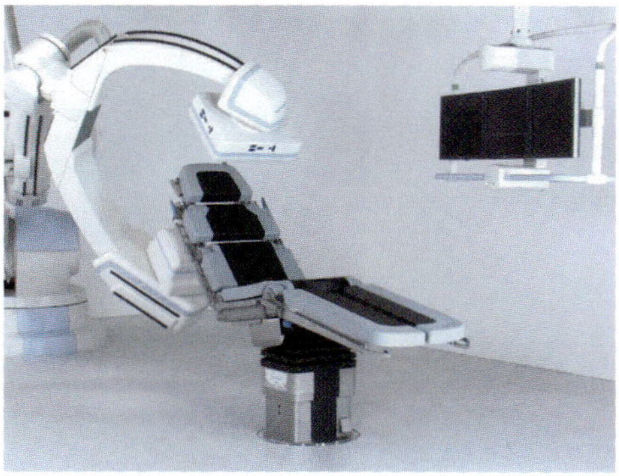

Fig. 14. Integrated Trumpf OR table with breakable tabletop and metal parts that impair image quality

In summary, important aspects to be included considered are the position in the room, radiolucency (carbon fiber tabletop), compatibility, and integration of imaging devices with the operating table. Further aspects include table load, adjustable table height, and horizontal mobility (floating) including vertical and lateral tilt. It is important to also have proper accessories available, such as rails for mounting special surgical equipment (retractors, camera holder). Free floating angiography tables with tilt and cradle capabilities are best suited for cardiovascular hybrid operating rooms.

4.4 Lights

Ceiling space in a hybrid OR may be limited, particularly if a ceiling mounted system is preferred. Thus, OR lights need special attention, because they may collide with the imaging systems, pendants or display booms (Tomaszewski, 2008).

In general, two different light sources are needed in an operating room: the surgical (operating) lights used for open procedures and the ambient lighting for interventional procedures. Particular attention should be paid to the possibility to dim the lights. This is frequently needed during fluoroscopy or endoscopy.

For the surgical lights it is most important that they cover the complete area across the operating room table. Moreover, they must not interfere with head heights and collision paths of other equipment. The most frequent mounting position of OR-lights is centrally above the OR table. If a different position is chosen, the lights usually are swivelled in from an area outside the OR table. Because one central axis per light head is necessary, this may lead to at least two central axes and mounting points in order to ensure sufficient illumination of the surgical field. The movement range of the angiography system determines the positioning of the OR lights. Central axes must be outside of moving path and swivel range. This is especially important as devices have defined room height requirements that must be met. In this case, head clearance height for the OR-light may be an issue. This makes lights a critical item in the planning and design process (Tomaszewski, 2008).

Other aspects in the planning process of OR lights include avoidance of glare and reflections. Modern OR lights may have additional features, like build in camera and video capabilities. For the illumination of the wound area, a double-arm OR-light system is required. Sometimes even a third light may be required, in cases where more than one surgical activity takes place at the same time, e.g. vein stripping of the legs.

In summary, the key topics for planning the surgical light system include:

- Central location above the OR table (impossible with ceiling mounted systems).
- Usually three light heads for optimal illumination of multiple surgical fields
- Suspension accommodating unrestricted, independent movement and stable positioning of light heads
- Modular system with options for extension, e.g. video monitor and/or camera

4.5 Hygiene

The operating room has different and stricter hygienic requirements and standards to meet than an interventional suite. Recently, hygiene has become a strong focus in addressing quality of healthcare delivery (Kerr, 2009; Hirsch, 2008; Sikkink et al., 2008; Peeters et al., 2008). Several workflow related aspects are crucial for achieving optimal hygienic conditions in operating rooms. A surgical scrub facility immediately outside of the OR is mandatory to allow proper scrubbing in for all procedures. Hats, gloves, facemasks and proper gowns are

mandatory, as well as access sterile processing facilities for the disposal of soiled material from open procedures. Finally, clean air, air conditioning and ventilation technologies play an important role in achieving these hygienic standards.
Today, this is mainly achieved with dedicated air-conditioning and ventilation solutions that create a limited protection zone, usually called "Laminar Airflow", even though this terminology might sometimes be technically misleading. These ventilation systems need to cover the entire aseptic environment of surgery in operating rooms, including the tables for materials and instruments. This zone allows for clean-room handovers of sterilized materials and shields the surgical team in sterilized garb, usually by a sufficiently large low-turbulence displacement air flow. Recent guidelines, e.g. in Germany, emphasize the importance of low turbulence. To meet the requirements of air cleanliness for operating theatres or other surgery rooms with strict hygienic requirements, very high volume flows of clean air are necessary. There are different solutions available to do so in an energy-efficient way. Usually, low-turbulence displacement circulating air canopies are employed.
Local requirements for the hygienic aspects of Heat, Ventilation, Air Conditioning (HVAC) vary significantly. Experts knowing the local requirements need to be involved in order to ensure clearance of the hybrid OR at the end of the project. This topic is to be discussed in detail with the responsible individuals and authorities in order to avoid non compliance with local regulations.

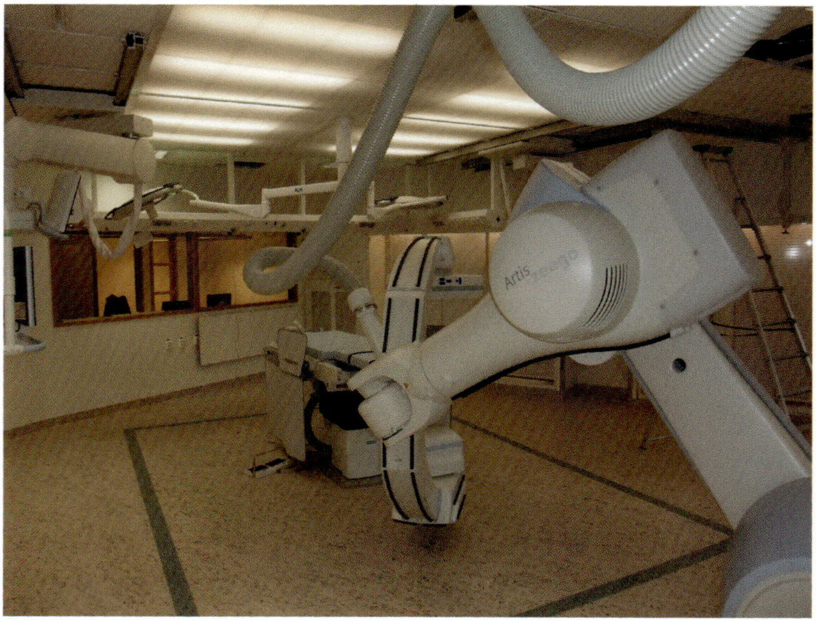

Fig. 15. Example for a Laminar Airflow ceiling ensuring a clean environment above the surgical area

4.6 Room layout

The main objective of OR design is to improve the OR workflow and enhance safety by ensuring good access and clear walkways. This sets the stage for equipment and equipment planning in the OR. Devices should be easy and quick to position and park. The limited space must be utilized optimally. Ergonomic aspects are to be considered for layout and design, which should enable flexible device management to cater to the needs of the various users and procedures. A clear floor and optimized cable management allow for efficient cleaning and easier maneuvering of devices. Moreover, this avoids tripping hazards. Camera and monitor systems for displaying patient data, for educational purposes or for telemedicine, may be necessary. Thus, and because of the complex needs for viewing during hybrid procedures, a good understanding of the visualization needs is vital. Data integration and IT are becoming more and more prominent for documentation, archiving and information provision.

Interventional rooms have excellent imaging capabilities, but frequently lack the prerequisites required for formal operating rooms. Operating rooms meet those required standards, but usually lack high-level imaging capabilities. Therefore, the hybrid operating room has different space requirements. The larger the better should be the basic principle for planning. Staff calculations have shown that, in hybrid procedures, up to 18 people are in the hybrid room. Current recommendations for hybrid operating rooms suggest > 70 m^2 in comparison to 40-60 m^2 for conventional operating rooms (space for a control and a technical room has to be added). The room has to fulfill radiation safety requirements as any other angiography room.

A key part of any conceptual design is to visit other institutions that have built a hybrid OR (Benjamin, 2008). Thereby, customers learn from best practice and understand what works best for others and what other sites would have done differently if they could do it again. Topics include type of storage space, type of angiography system, handling of the patient flow and anesthesia services, control room concept, sufficiency of space, the type of inventory control and storage they have, and usage of barcodes or infrared technology. Storage capabilities are especially important. Oftentimes there will be no personnel available to fetch devices stored outside the OR. Build-in glass cabinets have proven to be particularly useful because they allow the nurses to quickly locate materials. Design includes the following steps and activities (Tomaszewski, 2008):

- Define your current and future workflow and setup
- Start with a generic standard/sample layout of a hybrid room with the considered imaging system as a general guideline
- Involve all stakeholders (scrub nurses, technicians, surgeons, anesthesiologist, etc.)
- Cooperate with all vendors involved in the project

Centres with close proximity of intervention rooms and ORs probably have better prerequisites than hospitals with the classic separation of interventional rooms located in the internal medicine building and operating theatres located in the surgery building. In this situation, we recommend installing the hybrid room in the surgical wing for two reasons:

1. Immediate readiness of all OR equipment and personnel (e.g., heart-lung machine and perfusionists) and access to all surgical supply chain processes, especially in emergency situations
2. Availability of anesthesia and surgical intensive care

4.7 Planning process

The standard OR-layout is defined by the centrally positioned OR table and required access areas to the patient for anesthesia and surgery. In the hybrid OR the position of the angiography system and the table set the stage for the workflow inside the room. Other

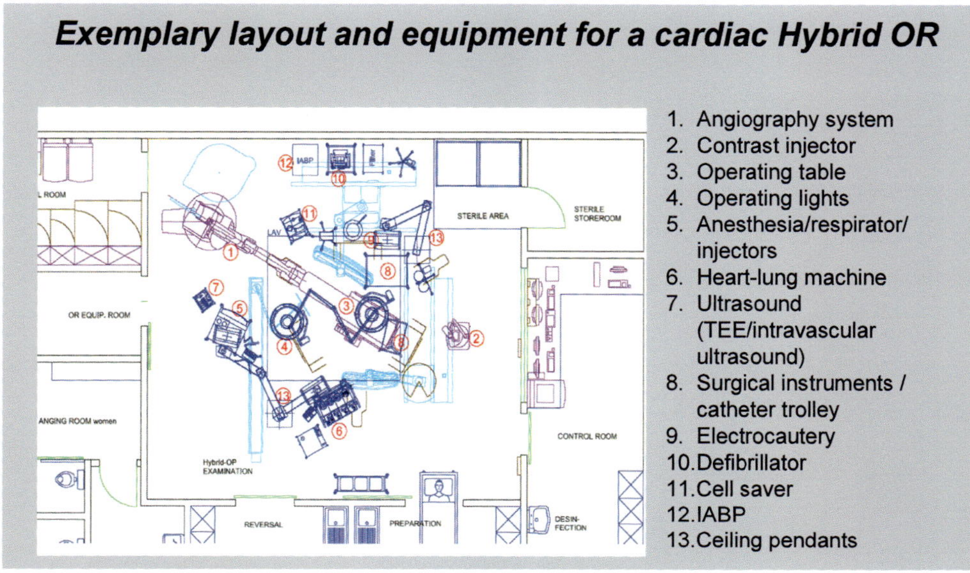

Fig. 16. A schematic room layout and equipment map of a hybrid OR depicts the complexity of planning an OR that allows for efficient workflow for all parties involved

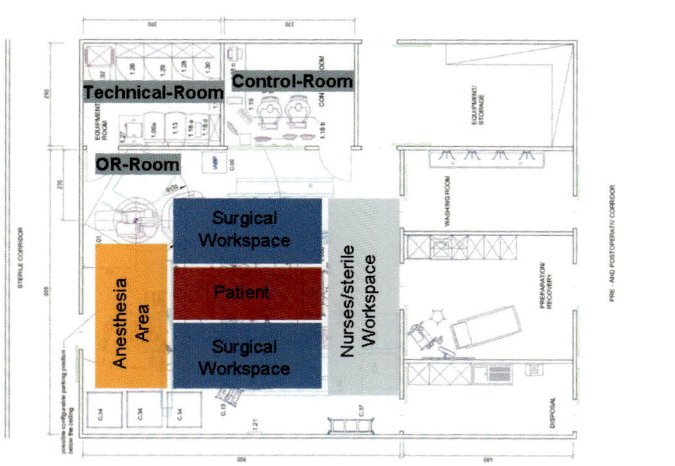

Fig. 17. Schematic Room layout with important areas for workflow considerations highlighted

equipment follows this framework. Planning should always be done in 2D and with CAD, because this is the only way to identify all technical interdependencies and to allow for a reliable check of the technical feasibility of the installation. One single master plan across all equipment and vendors has to be created in CAD, while each vendor is meant to provide proper CAD blocks (Tomaszewski, 2008). However, 2D is usually not easy to "read", even for experienced planners. Fig. 18 and Fig. 19 illustrate this issue.

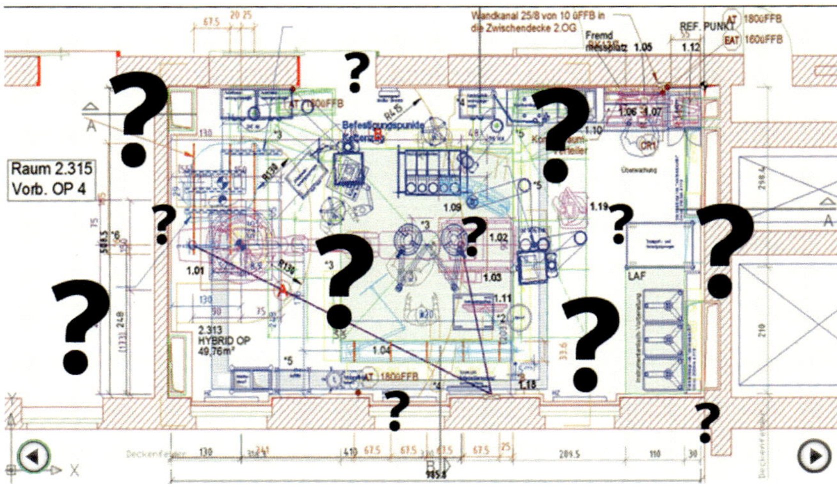

Fig. 18. Example for a 2D drawing of a hybrid OR plan capturing all interdependencies that has limited readability for the parties involved

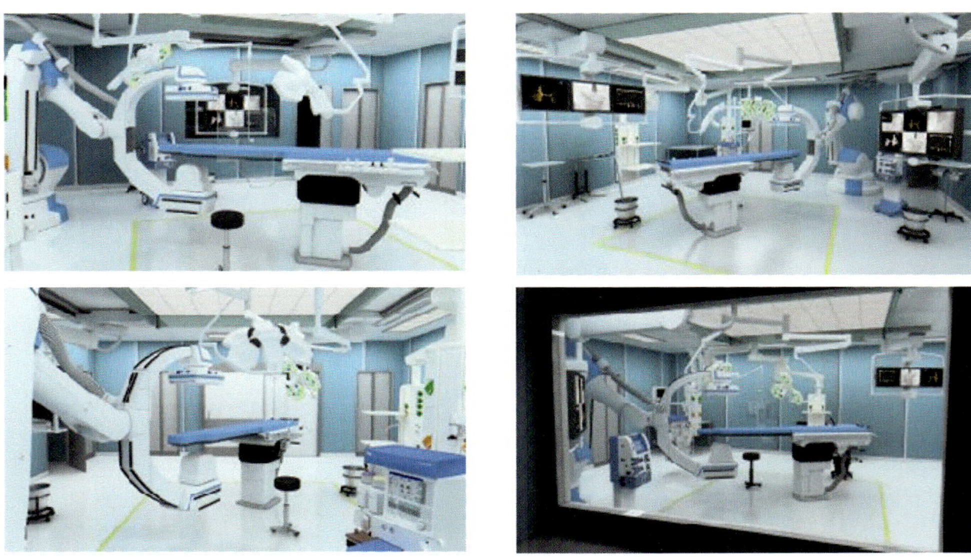

Fig. 19. Examples for 3D presentation of a hybrid OR plan, ensuring a common vision of the future facility across all parties involved

3D visualization helps to illustrate the 2D plan, so that full understanding from all parties involved is ensured. Most medical equipment suppliers and architects have the ability to represent in 3D, such that all elements of the final outcome of the OR can be included in this visualization. The following checklist provides an overview of key aspects for consideration during the planning and design process:

Location and space requirements incl. ancillary spaces for technical room, storage, etc.	Workflow and standard room set-up
Cross-functional team	Angiography system
Surgical versus angiography table	Lights and illumination
Ceiling suspension units and services on these units (number of sockets, gases etc.)	Audio- and video integration including visualization and display placement
Mobile and other equipment, needs and position: anesthesia, monitoring and hemodynamics, injectors, ultrasound, heart and lung machine	IT-integration (HIS, PACS)

Table 2. Overview of key aspects to be considered during the planning and design process

5. Other considerations

5.1 Training for imaging

To take advantage of the multiple advanced imaging capabilities of state-of-the-art fixed angiography systems, extensive training for physicians, nurses and technicians is crucial. Most members of the OR team are not familiar with fixed angiography systems. Only if they are well versed in and comfortable using it, they can take full advantage of the imaging and workflow capabilities of a hybrid OR.

Training of the team can be achieved by different concepts. However, at least one member of the OR team should be trained in very detail in order to use the system to its full potential. This person should serve as a trainer for the other team members and should take responsibility for the imaging. A good possibility is to ask colleagues from the radiology department to take over the training of the OR team member, since they are very familiar with imaging. This specially trained team member should then train several super users, who are also very familiar with the system. By ensuring that multiple OR team members can operate the system very well, 24/7 coverage can be provided in the hybrid OR - also for emergency cases on weekends or during night shifts, if required.

The individual scope of training depends on the responsibility of the OR staff as well as on the workflow set-up. If for example the surgeon himself operates the angiography system, he will be among the ones undergoing training in system handling and operation. If, by contrast, the system is operated by a radiographer, the surgeon will not need to be trained in detail.

Training possibilities are multiple. Principle training may be achieved by training in the hospital's own hybrid OR by the provider of the imaging system (applications training), at other clinical sites by experienced physicians and technicians (mini fellowships), in other departments within the hospital, and at hands-on workshops, usually organized by the industry.

5.1.1 Applications training

When purchasing an angiography system for the hybrid OR, applications training is usually provided by the vendor of the imaging system. This training is generally intended for experienced users and offered for approximately three days. Due to limited experience with imaging systems in the OR team, however, the training needs in surgery are much higher than for example in radiology.

Duration and content of the application training largely depend on how many different clinical disciplines use the system, on their level of experience and on the number of staff to be trained. During these trainings, the users are, depending on their scope of responsibility, being familiarized with system handling, software usage, image processing and archiving, the typical workflow in the hybrid OR and radiation protection. The trainers should be present during different clinical procedures in order to provide training and support system usage in clinical operation. Fig. 20a and Fig. 20b show an example plan for a three weeks applications training.

	Day 1	Day 2	Day 3	Day 4	Day 5
a.m.	-System check **Training for surgeons/ anesthetists** -System and patient positioning depending on surgical request	**Training for surgeons** -System overview -Table/ C-arm -Foot switch -Exam set selection	**Training for nurses** -System overview -Table/ C-arm -Patient Registration -Exam set selection -Foot switch	**Examination** Pacemaker only	**Training for selected staff** -Workflow with 3D imaging -Patient transfer -Post processing at workstation -Archiving datasets
p.m.	**Training for OR nurses** -Collision risks -Sterile covering **Training for cleaning personnel** -System sterility	-Patient browser -Basic post processing -Modification of organ programs	-Patient browser -Post processing (Basic) -Archiving patients (Basic)	**Training for selected staff** -Post processing (Advanced) -Archiving patients (Advanced)	**Training for selected staff** -UPS -Emergency concept

Application support

Fig. 20a. Typical training schedule of the first week of application training for hybrid OR

5.1.2 Mini fellowships at clinical sites

Some experienced clinical sites also offer the possibility to do short fellowships. The fellow is being assigned to an experienced team for 3-5 days. During the fellowship the fellow will experience the typical workflow in a hybrid OR by accompanying the trainer through the different work steps, including treatment decisions and surgery, with the opportunity to discuss the workflow with the whole OR team.

5.1.3 Training in other departments within the hospital

It has also proven to be very beneficial to send a designated Super User to a department in the hospital that is very experienced with angiography systems, for example radiology or cardiology. An internship of about one week helps the user to become familiar with system usage under the guidance of experienced users.

	Day 1	Day 2	Day 3	Day 4	Day 5
a.m.	**Training for complete group** -Repetition of last week's training topics -Checking availability of necessary material	**Training for complete group** -Testing workflow with syngo DynaCT -Last adaptation -First 3D patient	**Training for complete group** -Performing -*syngo* DynaCT -Last adaptations -Second 3D patient	**Training for complete group** -Third 3D patient	**Training for complete group** -Forth 3D patient
p.m.	**Training for complete group** -Performing *syngo* DynaCT run -Testing and improving workflows and positions	**Training for complete group** -Performance check	**Training for complete group** -Performance check	**Training for complete group** -Performance check or -Next Patient	

Application support | Customer's responsibility

Fig. 20b. Typical training schedule of the second and third week of applications training in the hybrid OR

5.1.4 Hands-on workshops

Some device and imaging vendors offer hands-on trainings at conferences or in their factories or showrooms for physicians that are just starting to use imaging systems. During these trainings, experienced cardiac surgeons and cardiologists train less experienced surgeons and fellows on transcatheter procedures and imaging. Corner stone of these trainings are the hands-on sessions. The trainee is guided by an experienced cardiologist or surgeon while practicing the use of devices like catheters and valves under real image guidance by an angiography system. The system and room set-up resembles a real hybrid OR or hybrid cathlab (see Fig. 21).

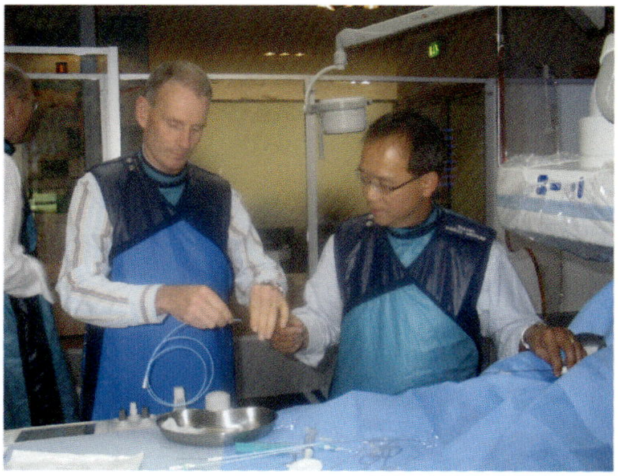

Fig. 21. An experienced interventional cardiologist teaches surgeons in basic wire techniques.

5.2 Financial considerations

Building a hybrid operating room is a considerable economic investment for every hospital. Sound business models and optimal usage of the room are prerequisites to make this endeavour a financial success.

5.2.1 Costs

The costs for hybrid rooms vary considerably depending on whether or not re- or new construction is necessary.

Furthermore, it may be necessary to hire additional staff such as radiology technicians that are familiar with interventional imaging systems. Both new and existing staff may require outside training to be able to use the equipment properly. These decisions depend on the existing knowledge in the hospital and on what procedures will be performed.

A recent study (Neumann, 2009) compared the investment necessary for hybrid suites, cath labs and standard ORs. Room size, construction requirements, angiography system, other equipment, depreciation, maintenance and debt service were taken into account. Overall, investment costs for the standard OR were lowest, followed by the cath lab with a 25% higher price tag. The costs for a hybrid OR were additional 120% of the costs of the standard OR. When comparing the operating costs (maintenance, depreciation, debt service and rent) the same relations applied. The costs for the cath lab were 25% higher than for the OR. Comparing the OR with the hybrid OR, an additional 90% were required per annum.

These figures may differ, depending on system choice, building costs and local requirements but the above mentioned figures give a good indication on the comparative costs. Taking these reasonably high costs into account, the obvious question arises how a hybrid OR can be a profitable investment.

5.2.2 Return on investment

Several US hospitals reported in detail on return on investment. The Vanderbilt group (Greelish, 2009) focused on the growth of a cardiac surgery program through a hybrid room. In the year 2004 the annual case volume of adult cardiac cases was 464. 2004 was also the year when the institution built their first hybrid OR. In the next 3 years the case load almost tripled based upon the hybrid OR set-up.

A similar case load development as in Vanderbilt Heart is to be seen in Beijing's Fu Wai Hospital. The annual report 2008 shows an increase of over 60% of the hybrid procedures a year after their hybrid OR was installed (Fu Wai, 2008).

In an initial pro forma from St. Vincent Heart Center of Indiana (Cronin & Schroyer, 2010) the calculations showed that incremental discharges of 150 patients led to a gross patient revenue of $ 6.2m and net patient revenue of $ 2.4m. Deducting total expenses of $ 0.8, the excess of revenues over expenses was $ 1.6m. The net present value was calculated to be $ 0.8m in 2010 and $ 5.4m in 2015, leading to an internal rate of return of 185% in 2010 and 285% in 2015, respectively.

Data from Cleveland Clinic Foundation showed the return on investment of their cardiac hybrid OR to take only 2 years and 3 months (Cronin & Schroyer, 2010).

The Advisory Board Company reported a detailed investment calculation for a room focusing solely on TAVI procedures in the USA (Katz, 2010). In reality the wide majority of rooms will be used for a multitude of procedures, often from different surgical disciplines in order to make best use of the room capacity. In the Advisory Board Company's pro forma, focussing only on TAVI cases, the cumulated investment came up to $ 3.4m, consisting of $

1.3m for construction work and $ 2.1 for the equipment. In the first year, starting with a very low volume of TAVI patients of 24 and consequently lower revenue of $ 1m, the total net revenue was $ 0.9m after reducing bad debt allowance and billing & collection. Annual total fixed costs accumulated to $ 0.1m, variable costs for devices, labour etc. to $ 0.9m leading to total costs of $ 1m during year one. Consequently the net income was negative by $ 23k in the first year. With an increase in patient volume to 37, however, already in year two a net income of $ 0.4m could be realized.
Table 3 gives an overview and comparison of the cost and return situation (by St. Vincent Heart Center and the Advisory Board Company).

	St. Vincent Heart Center	Advisory Board Company
Gross patient revenue in year 2010 (St. Vincent) / year 1 (Advisory Board)	6200	1000
Net revenue	2400	900
Total expenses	800	1000
Net Present Value (NPV) in year 2010 (St. Vincent) / year 1 (Advisory Board)	800	-23
Net Present Value (NPV) in year 2015 (St. Vincent) / year 5 (Advisory Board)	5400	1300

Rounded figures in k USD

Table 3. Financial comparison of pro forma from St. Vincent Heart Center and The Advisory Board Company (Cronin & Schroyer, 2010)

As a general fact, the set-up of hybrid rooms allows for the treatment of previously untreatable patients. Good examples are TAVIs. Now, patients previously deemed too old or weak for surgery, can be treated by transcatheter valve implantation. With an aging population and developments in medicine, the number of octogenarians and nonagenarians to be treated with new hybrid and minimally invasive procedures that are best performed in a hybrid OR will continue to grow. This will lead to increasing usage of the room capacity and consequently a quicker return on investment. Also, with less invasive treatment the necessity to stay in the ICU and the hospital for a long time in general decreases, along with the risk of infections. This allows discharging patients quicker, which again leads to an improved cost situation in the hospital. Furthermore hybrid rooms help to increase efficiency and decrease turnover time which can lead to additional cases being performed in the hybrid room as compared to a standard OR (Benjamin, 2008). A conventional surgical valve replacement often takes more than three hours, whereas a transcatheter valve implantation can be done in one. Calculations indicate that the mean incremental operating room profit per procedure is about $ 1,500 per hour. If the hospital manages to add only one single hour-long case each day, the hybrid OR could help increase profitability by about $ 300k p.a.
In cardiac surgery, the operating room profit is usually even about 25-30% above the mean incremental OR profit (Resnick et al., 2005).

5.2.3 Positive marketing effects

Another soft factor that can have a positive financial impact is to use the hybrid OR to position the hospital among the technologically most advanced institutions in the area. This

helps to both attract the top medical staff to work in the hospital as well as additional patients that are searching for the best possible treatment.
Also many hospitals make use of the increased publicity they can gain by marketing their hybrid ORs for the public e.g. in TV reports (see Fig. 22).
In summary, to justify the substantial investment in the hospital a detailed business plan needs to be created, taking into account the specific situation in the hospital. Hospital administration usually accepts a start-up phase with a negative margin but will expect positive numbers after. A detailed business plan will enable both users and hospital administration to base the decision for the hybrid OR on solid grounds and make sure it will be used to its full potential.

5.3 Building a hybrid program

One key success factor for a hybrid operating room is the team approach of a committed interdisciplinary team that takes responsibility for the room. Imaging specialists, cross trained physicians, and nurses with the vision to establish new minimally invasive therapies are the cornerstones of a blooming hybrid therapy program.
Bonatti stresses the importance of a dedicated workflow coordinator (Bonatti et al., 2007) to direct the workflow. Since the workflow in a hybrid OR has major differences to the one in a conventional OR it is mandatory that the whole OR team approaches the new concept open-mindedly and willing to change traditional processes fundamentally.
The workflow coordinator or hybrid OR manager takes care of traditional OR management topics such as staffing, ancillary support and inventory management. But he also manages some new tasks such as prioritizing the cases as in giving true hybrid cases priority over standard surgical or cardiologic procedures that can be done in a normal OR or cathlab. He

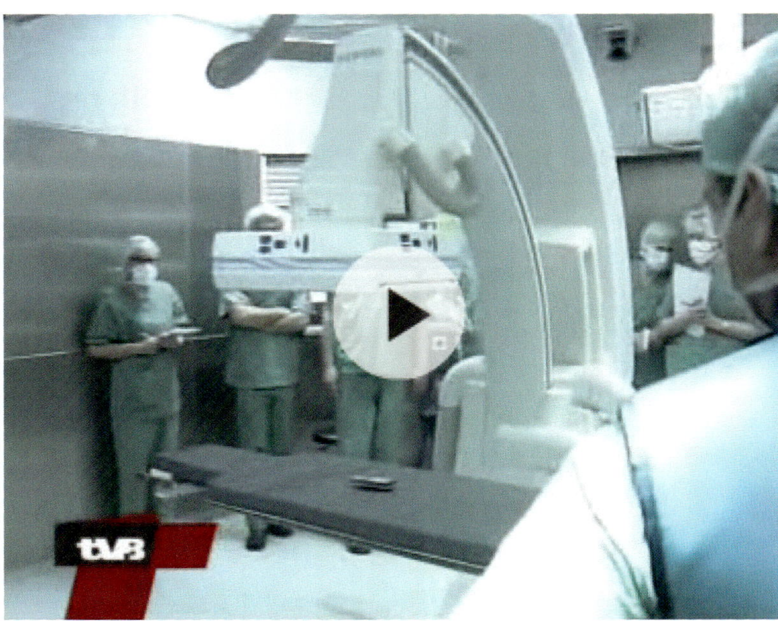

Fig. 22. Coverage on tv.berlin about the hybrid OR at German Heart Center Berlin, Germany

also needs to assure that cross trained physicians are available to work in the new room (Katz, 2010).

A multi-disciplinary approach is necessary to make best use of the hybrid OR and achieve the best patient and hospital outcomes. A key factor herein is a good working relationship between sometimes competing clinical disciplines. For example, cardiac surgeons and interventional cardiologists have to cooperate in numerous cardiac procedures such as TAVI. Multi-disciplinary case conferences in order to discuss the best treatment options are mandatory. Also, consensus and support from other functions in the hospital, such as anesthesia, intensive care, and hospital administration, are essential (Galantowicz & Cheatham, 2005).

However, not only operational integration is necessary, but also financial integration. Accounting practice needs to change with the usage of a hybrid OR. To start with, some institutions split the charges for hybrid procedures into a percutaneous component performed by the interventionist and billed by the cathlab, as well as a surgical component executed by the surgeon and billed by the OR department (Katz, 2010).

Moving forward, full financial integration is of utmost importance in order to avoid competition between different clinical disciplines. Consequently, all involved cardiovascular departments should be under one profit and loss statement of an integrated cardiovascular center (Katz, 2010).

To support the process of implementing a hybrid program it makes sense to set up best practice teams (cardiac and vascular surgery, cardiology, nurses etc.) who jointly develop the approach in the hospital. Visiting other institutions with a successful hybrid OR in operation is of major help in the planning process. Learning from their experience and understanding their mistakes can help shorten the process for all involved staff considerably.

6. References

Ahmed, A.S.; Deuerling-Zheng, Y.; Strother, C.M.; Pulfer, K.A.; Zellerhoff, M.; Redel, T.; Royalty, K.; Consigny, D.; Lindstrom, M.J. & Niemann, D.B. (2009). Impact of intra-arterial injection parameters on arterial, capillary, and venous time-concentration curves in a canine model. *American Journal of Neuroradiology*, Vol.30, No.7, (August 2009), pp. 1337-1341

Bacha E.A.; Daves, S.; Hardin, J.; Abdulla, R.I.; Anderson, J.; Kahana, M.; Koenig, P.; Mora, B.N.; Gulecyuz, M.; Starr, J.P.; Alboliras, E.; Sandhu, S. & Hijazi, Z.M. (2006). Single-ventricle palliation for high-risk neonates: the emergence of an alternative hybrid stage I strategy. *The Journal of Thoracic and Cardiovascular Surgery*, Vol.131, No.1, (January 2006), pp. 163-171, PII S0022-5223(05)01370-X

Bacha, E.A.; Marshall, A.C.; McElhinney, D.B. & del Nido, P.J. (2007). Expanding the hybrid concept in congenital heart surgery. *Seminars in Thoracic and Cardiovascular Surgery Pediatric Cardiac Surgery* Vol.10, No.1, pp. 146-150, PII S1092-9126(07)00020-8

Balter, S.; Hopewell, J.W.; Miller, D.L.; Wagner, L.K. & Zelefsky, M.J. (2010). Fluoroscopically Guided Interventional Procedures: A Review of Radiation Effects on Patients' Skin and Hair. *Radiology*, Vol.254, No.2, (February 2010), pp. 326-341

Benjamin, M.E. (2008). Building a Modern Endovascular Suite. *Endovascular Today*, Vol.3, (March 2008), pp. 71-78

Biasi, L.; Ali, T.; Ratnam, L.A.; Morgan, R.; Loftus, I. & Thompson, M. (2009). Intra-operative DynaCT improves technical success of endovascular repair of abdominal aortic aneurysms. *Journal of Vascular Surgery*, Vol.49, No.2, (February 2009), pp. 288-295, PII S0741-5214(08)01597-8

Bonatti, J.; Schachner, T.; Bonaros, N.; Jonetzko, P.; Ohlinger, A.; Ruetzler, E.; Kolbitsch, C.; Feuchtner, G.; Laufer, G.; Pachinger, O. & Friedrich, G. (2008). Simultaneous hybrid coronary revascularization using totally endoscopic left internal mammary artery bypass grafting and placement of rapamycin eluting stents in the same interventional session. The COMBINATION pilot study. *Cardiology*, Vol.110, No.2, pp. 92-95, PMID 17971657 [PubMed - indexed for MEDLINE]

Bonatti, J.; Vassiliades, T.; Nifong, W.; Jakob, H.; Erbel, R.; Fosse, E.; Werkkala, K.; Sutlic, Z.; Bartel, T.; Friedrich, G. & Kiaii, B. (2007). How to build a cath-lab operating room. *Heart Surgery Forum*, Vol.10, No.4, pp. E344-348, PMID 17650462 [PubMed - indexed for MEDLINE]

Cronin, G.M. & Schroyer, M. (04.05.2010). Financial aspects of building a hybrid operating suite. In: *American Association for Thoracic Surgery, 90th Annual Meeting 2010*, 14.06.2011, Available from
http://www.aats.org/2010webcast/sessions/player.html?sid=10050227B.03

Cusma, J.T.; Bell, M.R.; Wondrow, M.A.; Taubel, J.P. & Holmes, D.R. (1999). Real-time Measurement of Radiation Exposure to Patients During Diagnostic Coronary Angiography and Percutaneous Interventional Procedures. *Journal of the American College of Cardiology*, Vol.33, No.2, (February 1999), pp. 427-435

Doelken, M.; Struffert, T.; Richter, G.; Engelhorn, T.; Nimsky, C.; Ganslandt, O.; Hammen, T. & Doerfler, A. (2008). Flat-panel detector volumetric CT for visualization of subarachnoid hemorrhage and ventricles: preliminary results compared to conventional CT. *Neuroradiology*, Vol.50, No.6, (June 2008), pp. 517–23

Feldman, T.; Foster, E.; Glower, D.G.; Kar, S.; Rinaldi, M.J.; Fail, P.S.; Smalling, R.W.; Siegel, R.; Rose, G.A.; Engeron, E.; Loghin, C.; Trento, A.; Skipper, E.R.; Fudge, T.; Letsou, G.V.; Massaro, J.M.; Mauri, L. & EVEREST II Investigators (2011). Percutaneous repair or surgery for mitral regurgitation. *The New England Journal of Medicine*, Vol.364, No.15, (April 2011), pp. 1395-1406

Fu Wai Hospital, 08 Outcomes, Department of Cardiovascular Surgery of National Cardiovascular Center and Fu Wai Hospital

Galantowicz, M. & Cheatham, J.P. (2005). Lessons Learned from the Development of a New Hybrid Strategy for the Management of Hypoplastic Left Heart Syndrome. *Pediatric Cardiology*, Vol.26, No.2, (April 2005), pp. 190-199

Greelish, JP (2009). Routine angiography after bypass. TCT

Hirsch, R. (2008). The hybrid cardiac catheterization laboratory for congenital heart disease: From conception to completion. *Catheterization Cardiovascular Interventions*, Vol.71, No.3, (February 2008), pp. 418-428

Holzer, R.J.; Sisk, M.; Chisolm, J.L.; Hill, S.L.; Olshove V.; Phillips, A.; Cheatham, J.P. & Galantowicz, M. (2009). Completion angiography after cardiac surgery for congenital heart disease: complementing the intraoperative imaging modalities. *Pediatric Cardiology*, Vol.30, No.8, pp. 1075–1082

Hu, S.; Li, Q.; Gao, P. et al. (2011). Simultaneous hybrid revascularization versus off-pump coronary artery bypass for multivessel coronary artery disease. *TheAnnals of Thoracic Surgery*, Vol.91, pp. 432–439

Kalender, W. & Kyriakou, Y. (2007). Flat-detector computed tomography (FD-CT). *European Radiology*, Vol.17, No.11, (November 2007), pp. 2767-2779

Katz, D. (2010). Outlook for integrated cardiovascular services, In: American College of Cardiovascular Administrators 2010, 24.06.2011, Available from

http://www.aameda.org/Conference/ACCA/ConfHandouts/documents/Contos 2-per.pdf
Katzen, B. T. (1995). Current Status of Digital Angiography in Vascular Imaging. *Radiologic Clinics of North America*, Vol.33, No.1, (January 1995), pp. 1-14
Kerr, J.F. (2009). Keys to Success in Designing a Hybrid Cath Lab. *Cath Lab Digest*, Vol.17, No.3, (March 2009). pp. 32-34
Kon, Z.; Brown, E.; Tran, R.; Joshi, A.; Reicher, B.; Grant, M.C.; Kallam, S.; Burris, N.; Connerney, I.; Zimrin, D. & Poston, R.S. (2008). Simultaneous hybrid coronary revascularization reduces postoperative morbidity compared with results from conventional off-pump coronary artery bypass. *The Journal of Thoracic and Cardiovascular Surgery*, Vol.135, No.2, (February 2008), pp. 367–375, PII S0022-5223(07)01592-9
Krul, S.P.; Driessen, A.H.; van Boven, W.J.; Linnenbank, A.C.; Geuzebroek, G.S.; Jackman, W.M.; Wilde, A.A.; de Bakker, J.M. & de Groot, J.R. (14.04.2011). Thoracoscopic Video-Assisted Pulmonary Vein Antrum Isolation, Ganglionated Plexus Ablation and Periprocedural Confirmation of Ablation Lesions. First Results of a Hybrid Surgical-Electrophysiological Approach for Atrial Fibrillation, In:*Circulation: Arrhythmia Electrophysiology,In Press*
Leon, M.B.; Smith, C.R.; Mack, M. et al.; for the PARTNER Trial Investigators (2010). Transcatheter aortic-valve implantation for aortic stenosis in patients who cannot undergo surgery. *The New England Journal of Medicine*, Vol.363, No.17, (October 2011), pp. 1597–1607
Lurz, P.; Nordmeyer, J.; Muthurangu, V.; Khambadkone, S.; Derrick, G.; Yates, R.; Sury, M.; Bonhoeffer, P. & Taylor, A.M. (2009). Comparison of bare metal stenting and percutaneous pulmonary valve implantation for treatment of right ventricular outflow tract obstruction: use of an X-ray/magnetic resonance hybrid laboratory for acute physiological assessment. *Circulation*, Vol.119, No.23, pp. 2995-3001, ISSN 1524-4539
Michowitz, Y.; Mathuria, N.; Tung, R.; Esmailian, F.; Kwon, M.; Nakahara, S.; Bourke, T.; Boyle, N.G.; Mahajan, A. & Shivkumar, K. (2010). Hybrid procedures for epicardial catheter ablation of ventricular tachycardia: value of surgical access. *Heart Rhythm*, Vol.7, No.11, (November 2010), pp. 1635-1643, PII S1547-5271(10)00700-9
Neumann, F.J. (2009). The hybrid suite: the future for percutaneous intervention and surgery? - Cost issues. In: *EuroPCR 2009*, 24.06.2011, Available from http://www.pcronline.com/Lectures/2009/Cost-issues
Nollert, G. & Wich, S. (2008). Planning a cardiovascular Hybrid OR - the technical point of view. *The Heart Surgery Forum*, Vol.12, No.3, (June 2008), pp. E125-E130
Nollert, G.; Wich, S.; Figel, A. (12.03.2010). The Cardiovascular Hybrid OR-Clinical & Technical Considerations, In: *The Cardiothoracic Surgery Network*, 14.06.2011, Available from http://www.ctsnet.org/portals/endovascular/nutsbolts/article-9.html
Pedra, C.A.C.; Fleishman, C.; Pedra, S.F. & Cheatham, J.P. (2011). New imaging modalities in the catheterization laboratory. *Current Opinion in Cardiology*, Vol. 26, No.2, (March 2011), pp. 86–93
Peeters, P.; Verbist, J.; Deloose, K. & Bosiers, M. (2008). The Catheterization Lab of the Future. *Endovascular Today*, Vol.3, (March 2008), pp. 94-96
Resnick, A.S.; Corrigan, D.; Mullen, J.L. & Kaiser, L.R. (2005). Surgeon Contribution to Hospital Bottom Line. *Annals of Surgery*, Vol.242, No.4, (October 2005), pp. 530–539
Sikkink, C.J.; Reijnen, M.M. & Zeebregts, C.J. (2008). The creation of the optimal dedicated endovascular suite. *European Journal of Vascular & Endovascular Surgery*, Vol.35, No.2, (February 2008), pp. 198-204, PII S1078-5884(07)00544-8

Sivakumar, K.; Krishnan, P.; Pieris, R. & Francis, E. (2007). Hybrid approach to surgical correction of tetralogy of Fallot in all patients with functioning Blalock Taussig shunts. *Catheterization Cardiovascular Interventions*, Vol.70, No.2, (August 2007), pp. 256-264

Strobel, N., Meissner, O.; Boese, J.; Brunner, T.; Heigl, B.; Hoheisel, M.; Lauritsch, G.; Nagel, M.; Pfister, M. & Rührnschopf, E.P. (2009). Medical Radiology, 3D Imaging with Flat-Detector C-Arm Systems, In: *Multislice CT*, Reiser, M.F.; Takahashi, M.; Modic, M. & Becker C.R., pp. 33-51, Springer Verlag

Ten Cate, G.; Fosse, E.; Hol, P.K.; Samset, E.; Bock, R.W.; McKinsey, J.F.; Pearce, B.J. & Lothert, M. (2004). Integrating surgery and radiology in one suite: a multicenter study. *Journal of Vascular Surgery*, Vol.40, No.3, (September 2004), pp. 494-499, PII S0741-5214(04)00754-2

Tomaszewski, R. (2008). Planning a Better Operating Room Suite: Design and Implementation Strategies for Success. *Perioperative Nursing Clinics*, Vol.3, No.1, (March 2008), pp. 43–54, PII S1556-7931(07)00103-9

Vahanian, A.; Alfieri, O.R.; Al-Attar, N. et al. (2008). Transcatheter valve implantation for patients with aortic stenosis: a position statement from the European Association of Cardio-Thoracic Surgery (EACTS) and the European Society of Cardiology (ESC), in collaboration with the European Association of Percutaneous Cardiovascular Interventions (EAPCI). *European Journal of Cardio-Thoracic Surgery*, Vol.34, No.1, (July 2008), pp. 1-8

Walsh, S.R.; Tang, T.Y.; Sadat, U.; Naik, J.; Gaunt, M.E.; Boyle, J.R.; Hayes, P.D. & Varty, K. (2008). Endovascular stenting versus open surgery for thoracic aortic disease: systematic review and metaanalysis of the results. *Journal of Vascular Surgery*, Vol.47, No.5, (May 2008), pp. 1094-1098, PII S0741-5214(07)01592-3

Zhao, D.X.; Leacche, M.; Balaguer, J.M.; Boudoulas, K.D.; Damp, J.A.; Greelish, J.P. & Byrne, J.G. (2009). Routine Intraoperative Completion Angiography After Coronary Artery Bypass Grafting and 1-Stop Hybrid Revascularization Results From a Fully Integrated Hybrid Catheterization Laboratory/Operating Room. *Journal of the American College of Cardiology*, Vol.53, No.3, (January 2009), pp. 232–241

4

The 30 Day Complication Rate After Aortic Valve Replacement with a Pericardial Valve in a Mainly Geriatric Population

Wilhelm Mistiaen
Artesis University College Antwerp, Dept of Healthcare Sciences and University of Antwerp, Faculty of Medicine, Antwerp
Belgium

1. Introduction

The stenotic degenerative aortic valve disease is a slowly developing condition. This condition is the result of an active process. Recently, it has been discovered that programmed cell death plays a major role in this progression (1-4). Stenotic degenerative aortic valve disease obstructs the outflow of the left ventricle (LV) and causes a pressure overload, with all its undesirable consequences. Once the disease has become symptomatic, the prognosis without surgical replacement of the valve is dismal: the life expectancy is reduced to 2 or 3 years with occurrence of syncope, angina pectoris and certainly with dyspnea (5). Age, left ventricular dysfunction and neurologic condition played a major role in the denial for AVR (6). Medical treatment and balloon valvotomy (7) do not improve the prognosis. Aortic valve replacement (AVR) is the only way to prolong life and improve its quality. In spite of technical improvements, the procedure involves a major procedure, with all its complications. Moreover, one condition (the valve disease) is replaced by another (the prosthetic valve).

The possible hospital or 30 day complications which can occur after AVR include valve related, cardiac non-valve related and non-cardiac events. Identification of their predictors could lead to an improved referral pattern and, hence to an improved 30 day outcome, provided these predictors are liable to changes.

2. Methods

In one centre for cardiac surgery, 1000 patients who underwent AVR with Carpentier-Edwards cardiac valve, were studied in a retrospective way. The operations were performed between the end of 1986 and the end of 2006. In most patients with degenerative aortic valve disease, coronary artery disease was also present. Hence, patients who received concomitant CABG were also included. Their median age was 75 (71-77) years. The surgical technique remained largely unchanged and was performed through a median sternotomy. After opening the pericardium, the ascending aorta, the vena cava inferior and superior could be accessed for connection to the extracorporeal circulation. The pulmonary artery was ligated temporarily in a gentle way. A vent was placed through the left superior pulmonary vein in order to decompress the left ventricle. Before the extracorporeal circulation was started, the patient was fully heparinized. The patient was cooled to 30° Celsius and the heart was stopped and topically cooled with sludge ice. Systemic blood pressure, central venous pressure and left atrial pressure were continuously monitored. The ascending aorta was opened and cold cardioplegia was instilled within the coronary arteries. In case of severe coronary artery disease, additional cardioplegia was instilled through the coronary sinus. This was repeated after 30 minutes. The calcified aortic valve was inspected and excised. The ring was decalcified if necessary. The interrupted sutures were placed as three separate series through the aortic annulus, and then through the prosthesis in the same order. The valve was lowered into the annulus and the sutures were tied and severed at the desired length. If necessary, the great saphenous vein was harvested by another team for concomitant CABG. The suturing of the bypass on the coronary arteries were performed during the same clamping. The aortotomy was closed with a double running suture and the proximal end of the bypasses were also connected. The internal mammary artery was not often used. The extracorporeal circulation was stopped stepwise and then disconnected. Temporary pacemaker wires were attached to the surface of the ventricles. After thorough hemostasis and placement of drains, the chest cavity was closed. The patient was transferred to the intensive care unit and kept under sedation for 24 hours. In 1996, the anesthesia changed into a "short-track" procedure: the sedation was shortened from one day to 6 hours and extubation was performed as soon as possible thereafter.

The changes is referral pattern were documented by comparison of age and co-morbid conditions in four periods of 5 year (1986-1991; 1992-1996; 1997-2001 and 2002-2006). A chi-square analysis was used as statistical analysis to show significant differences over time.

Twenty five preoperative and five peri-operative factors were screened in two steps. In a first step, the effect on hospital events was studied by an univariate chi-square or a Fisher-exact analysis. In a second step, the significant factors were entered in a multivariate logistic regression analysis in order to identify the predictors.

The results are presented for each risk factor (first column of the table), n/N (second column), p or probability (third column), OR (fourth column) and 95%CI (last column), where N is the number of patients at risk (i.e. having the risk factor) and n the number of these patients who suffered the complication; OR is the odds ratio and 95%CI is the 95% confidence interval.

These factors were defined or dichotomized if appropriate and numbers are given.

Octogenarians	186	
Male gender	530	
COPD (chronic obstructive pulmonary disease)	235	defined on protocol by pneumologist
Impaired renal function	109	plasma creatinine over 1.3 mg%
Previous carcinoma	104	proven by histologic examination and treated with curative intent
Hypertension	654	blood pressure repeatedly over 140/90 mmHg in resting conditions
Diabetes	149	treated by diet, peroral antidiabetics or insulin
Coronary artery disease	631	documented on coronarography
Myocardial infarction	151	documented by ECG, enzymes (during previous admission)

Previous CABG	81	previous admission and operation protocol
Carotid artery disease	238	stenosis of 40% or more on Doppler-duplex
History of TIA/CVA (Transient ischemic attack / cerbrovascular accident)		
	40/68	by history and CT (computer tomography), during previous admission
Left ventricular dysfunction	247	decrease documented by segmental analysis of ventricular wall on echocardiography
LV ejection fraction<50%	155	calculated by data obtained at echocardiography
Atrial fibrillation	197	chronic or paroxysmal, documented by ECG
Ventricular arrhythmias	74	documented by Holter monitoring
Heart failure	216	at least one previous admission for pulmonary edema
NYHA (New York Heart Association) class IV		
	251	by anamnesis at admission for AVR
Need for digitalis	152	by anamnesis at admission for AVR
Conduction defect	270	documented by ECG: of any type and of any degree
First degree AV (atrioventricular) block		
	33	ibid
Previous PaceMaker implant	33	during previous admission
Previous endocarditis	17	documented by bacteriological analysis during previous admission
Need for urgent AVR	25	condition needing AVR at the same day in order for the patient to survive
Cross-clamping>75 min	460	sum of cross clamping time for valve implantation and for additional procedures
Valve size 19	27	sizes ranging from 19 to 27
Concomitant CABG	610	
Mitral ring	13	
Aortoplasty	61	enlargement of reduction of the ascending aorta
Carotid endarterectomy	22	

The adverse events under scrutiny were

- hospital mortality (n=37)
- valve related events
  - endocarditis, documented by clinical signs, echocardiography and blood samples (n=2)
  - thrombo-embolism, with neurological signs (n=25), documented on CT or ischemic events on other locations (n=2)
  - bleeding, evident if external or documented on cerebral CT (n=20)
  - ventricular arrhythmias, documented on ECG (n=37)
- cardiac events not related to the valve
  - congestive heart failure defined by the inability of the heart to maintain an adequate circulation without support of inotropics or assist device (n=36)
  - conduction defects (new or progression of an pre-existing defect), documented on ECG, of any type and of any degree (n=101)

- atrial fibrillation, new or recurrence of a previously paroxysmal atrial fibrillation, documented on ECG (n=381)

- non-cardiac events
  - acute renal function impairment, documented by an increase of plasma creatinine with 0.3 mg% (n=53)
  - pulmonary complications: clinical and radiological signs of atelectasis or respiratory infection or prolonged intubation (n=58).

3. Results

Between the end of 1986 and 1991, 80 patients received a Carpentier-Edwards valve in aortic position. This number was 216 between 1992 - 1996, 345 between 1997 - 2001 and 365 between 2002 and the end of 2006. In our series, the changes in the four 5-year periods showed a significant increase in time for

- patients over 80 (from 6,3% to 25,5%),
- diabetes: 6.5% to 22.7%;
- COPD: 6.5% to 36.4%;
- renal function impairment: 0.9% to 17.7%;
- carotid artery disease: 2.5% to 40.1%;
- preoperative period of congestive heart failure: 12,5% to 28.3%;
- previously performed CABG: 1.3% to 11.3%;

All increases were highly significant ($p<0.001$). Only for the need of digitalis, a significant decrease was observed: from 39.7% to 9.4% ($p<0.001$). These results show that patients referred for AVR became older and have more co-morbidity. The reduction of use of digitalis could be due to the introduction of ACE inhibitors, angiotensin receptor, renin and beta blocking agents.

The hospital results showed a completely different pattern. Only for non-cardiac complications, a significant increase ($p=0.001$) has been found over time, from about 20% in the first two five-year periods to about 30% in the last two five-year periods. Mortality and major cardiovascular complications rates such as ventricular arrhythmias, bleeding, congestive heart failure and thromboembolism all remained well below 5% throughout these observation periods, without a noteworthy increase. Atrial fibrillation remained between 30 and 40%, without an increase over time.

Although patients referred for AVR became older and sicker, 30-day postoperative survival seemed not affected. Therefore, age and the presence of co-morbid conditions do not necessarily represent formal contra-indications for AVR. Nevertheless, an increase of non-cardiac postoperative complications with concomitant increase in length of stay and use of economic resources could be expected if older and sicker patients are operated upon.

Hospital or 30 day mortality

Significant preoperative factors for mortality in an unvariate analysis were:

$P<0.001$:	need for urgent surgery, age over 80, decreased left ventricular function,
$P<0.01$:	renal function impairment, LVEF below 50%, previous AMI, previous heart failure, need for digitalis,
$P<0.05$:	diabetes, chronic or paroxysmal atrial fibrillation,

The other risk factors had no significant effect. NYHA functional class II had a protective effect ($p<0.001$) for mortality.

Multivariate analysis showed following results

Factor	**n/N**	**p**	**OR**	**95%CI**
Urgent AVR	7/25	<0.001	9.0	2.8-28.7
Digitalis	12/152	0.002	3.5	1.6-7.7
Age > 80	17/186	0.005	3.1	1.4-6.6

Mortality in the hospital phase was the most important outcome. It varied between 1.5% (8) and 24% (9). These differences were due to large differences in patient characteristics such as age and co-morbid conditions. With a time span of almost 20 year between the first and the last publication, improvement in surgical techniques and peri-operative care could also be responsible for these differences in mortality.
In most series, the hospital mortality was below 10%. In series where the mortality was over 10%, several risk factors were usually present. Independent predictors for hospital mortality were identified and confirmed that specific co-morbid conditions increased the early postoperative risk.
Most of these factors could be related to the left ventricle and hence to the patient. An emergency need for AVR (i.e. to operate on the same day as the admission in order for the patient to survive) has been identified as the most important predictor, with a increase of mortality of 10 times (10). This has been confirmed in other series (11,12). This indicated to an exhaustion of all compensatory mechanisms to maintain an adequate circulation. A need for urgent AVR has also been identified as a predictor for early postoperative congestive heart failure, which is a highly lethal condition (13). A high preoperative functional class NYHA IV (14,15) and a low-flow low-gradient problem also could be related to a protracted burden, and hence a decreased left ventricular function. Coronary artery disease, previous and the need for concomitant CABG (9,11,12,15) as well as a previous myocardial infarction (10,11) and previous CABG (12) could add to a decrease in left ventricular function.
Valvular factors such as severity of valvular disease and the type and size of valve prosthesis implanted also had an effect (15,16). The effect of non-cardiac factors such as diabetes (15) and renal disease (11,12,17) was also observed. Remarkably, the effect of age over 80 (9,12,18,19), although important, was less compared to the effect of need for urgent surgery on mortality(10).

Thromboembolic events

TE events were one of the most important and devastating events after AVR, especially if permanent neurological deficit was present. One also has to keep in mind that many TE events go unnoticed. In one small series, MRI after cardiac surgery could document silent events in 6 of 34 patients, which is rather high (20). We found this clinically evident thromboembolism in 27 of 1000 patients. In 25 cases, this was neurological. An univariate analysis identified a decreased left ventricular function (p<0.01) as sole risk factor.
This risk factor was confirmed in a multivariate analysis, which showed an ejection fraction below 50% as an independent predictor (11/247 patients), with p=0.027, an odds ratio of 2.5 with a 95% confidence interval between 1.1-5.7.
Some studies reported on the predictors for thromboembolism after AVR on long-term and none reported on such events on short-term. The short-term thromboembolic events, however, have their importance since these are a predictor for future events (21). A preoperative CVA seemed to have a comparable significance (21-24) for long-term events.

A low ejection fraction also has been identified as predictor (24). Congestive heart failure and a dilated ventricle are known risk factors for thromboembolism. Damage to the ventricular wall as well as an abnormal flow of blood (and possible stasis) can promote intra-ventricular thrombosis and hence embolization. If the LVEF is below 30%, life-long anticoagulation is required (25).

Age also has been identified as an independent predictor (23-27). The age distribution of any given patient population should be made known to appreciate fully the effect of this factor. Age might be related, however to co-morbid conditions such as diabetes and atheromatosis of the aorta and the cerebral vessels (23,24).

Carotid artery disease could be a matter for debate. In some series (23,24), it was identified as a predictor for thromboembolism, in other series, this was not (21). A Doppler-duplex investigation is a reliable tool for the detection of lesions and is routinely performed in some institutions. It cannot, however, detect atheromatosis of the intracranial vessels.

A long ECC time (24) might indicate to coronary artery disease (28) and hence, to the need for an associated procedure, which mostly is a CABG. This could confirm atheromatous vessels as a possible source for thromboembolic events. These cannot be considered entirely as valve related. A "smoking gun", however, is often not found. And CABG itself has never been identified as a predictor for thromboembolism.

AF could also be a matter for debate: it is certainly a risk factor for thromboembolic events. However, it is also an indication for anticoagulation, which might cloud the effect of AF. In some series, AF was identified as a predictor (28), in others not (21,24).

It is by no means certain that risk factors for long-term thromboembolic events could be used to predict the occurrence of such events on short term. The latter, however, have their prognostic significance. Moreover, all these predictors indicate that the sources of thromboembolic events are multiple. Hence thromboembolism cannot be considered as entirely valve related (21,29), but also as patient related.

To prevent thromboembolism after AVR with a biological prosthesis, anticoagulant medication is given for three months after implantation, after which it can be replaced by acetyl salicylic acid, with good results (21), unless anticoagulants are indicated for another reason. An RCT to support this strategy does not exist (25), but the general idea is that vitamin K antagonists protect against early thromboembolism while re-endothelialization of the stent and the sutures is not yet complete. For mechanical heart valves, a life-long anticoagulant treatment is necessary. The target level for INR is determined by the valve position (for aortic this is lower than for mitral) and by the type of mechanical heart valves. Older types such as cage ball devices are more thrombogenic and require deeper anticoagulation. A strict classification for thrombogenicity is not available. There are too many patient related factors involved (25).

Bleeding events

Univariate analysis revealed three factors with a significant effect. This was confirmed by a multivariate analysis. The use of vitamin K antagonists could not be included since almost all patients received this medication for three months after operation. The three predictors were:

Factor	n/N	p	OR	95%CI
Concomitant CABG	17/610	0.046	3.6	1.0-12.5
COPD	8/235	0.051	2.6	1.0-6.6
Aortoplasty	4/61	0.058	3.5	1.0-12.6

Bleeding events could be considered as the other side of the coin of anticoagulation with vitamin K antagonists. Effective protection against thromboembolism holds the risk for bleeding. A continuous balance should be made. The INR does not only depend on the dose of vitamin K antagonists, but also on the adsorption of vitamin K by the mucosa of the colon and on its processing by the liver. No other reports concerning predictors for early bleeding after valve replacement appeared. Current results indicated that early bleeding seems related to the procedure and is different compared to bleeding events at long term, which is probably more related to anticoagulation. Nevertheless, other factors such as age and increased cardiothoracic index were identified as predictors for bleeding during long-term follow-up (26). Fragility in elderly might be an important reason. In other series, no predictors or risk factors could be identified (30,31).

Prosthetic valve endocarditis

The number of patients with early prosthetic valve endocarditis was low, hence no risk factors or predictors (such as preoperative endocarditis) could be identified in our series. Literature data only described long-term events.
The linearized rate for long-term prosthetic valve endocarditis was low and mostly under 1% per patient year (26,27,32-39). The most event free rates after 5 to 25 year were well over 90%. This was true for mechanical heart valves (35,40,41) as well as for the different stented (30,42) and stentless tissue valves (27,36,43) as for homografts (8). No risk factors could be identified, although a previous endocarditis could arouse some suspicion. Prosthetic valve endocarditis carried a high risk for mortality, especially if Staphylococcus aureus has been detected (44). These micro-organisms often lead to ring abscesses and prosthetic paravalvular leak. The occurrence of congestive heart failure with prosthetic valve endocarditis has been the main indication for re-operation (45).

Congestive heart failure

Univariate analysis identified following risk factors:

$P<0.001$:	Need for urgent surgery, chronic or paroxysmal atrial fibrillation
$P<0.01$:	Age over 80, decreased left ventricular function, previous infarction
$P<0.05$:	COPD, LVEF below 50%, preoperative heart failure, need for digitalis

NYHA class II had a protective effect ($p<0.001$)

Multivariate analysis showed following results

Factor	n/N	p	OR	95%CI
Urgent AVR	7/25	<0.001	10.5	3.6-30.8
Atrial fibr.	16/197	0.001	3.5	1.7-7.4
EF<50%	10/155	0.055	2.1	1.0-4.4

In-hospital congestive heart failure after AVR is a highly lethal complication (13,46). Hospital heart failure occurred in 2.6% of the patients in an earlier series (13), with need for urgent AVR as the sole independent predictor. This pointed to an exhaustion of all compensatory mechanisms to maintain an adequate circulation and this observation should reason not to postpone AVR, once it has become symptomatic. In another study, the level of B-type natri-uretic peptide was also identified as a predictor (46). Apoptosis or programmed cell death of cardiomyocytes could be an important event in these patients (47). Atrial fibrillation could lead to a decreased ventricular filling and cardiac output since the atrial contraction is lost. In an earlier series, this was also the case in long-term heart failure (13).

Early congestive heart failure should be distinguished from long-term heart failure: the latter was diastolic in nature and has some other risk factors such as conduction defects and coronary artery disease. An impaired relaxation occurred since after regression of the muscle mass, this fibrosis persists for a longer time. This stiffened the LV wall (48). The LVEF remained often normal. Hence, this could be labeled as a "diastolic" form of CHF (13). Concurrent conduction defects thereby could lead to perfusion defects and wall motion abnormalities, even in absence of coronary artery disease (49). Biventricular pacing often could correct this condition (50,51). Coronary artery disease could lead to ischemic loss of myocardial contractility, adding to the left ventricular function. Concomitant CABG, however was not identified as a predictor for postoperative CHF (13).

A small valve size has not been identified as a predictor for long-term heart failure in a previous series (13), neither in the current series for short-term heart failure. Hence, in patients with a small aortic root, it seemed not necessary to enlarge the root or to implant a stentless valve, which requires a more demanding technique, provided the LVF is normal.

However, it becomes important in patients with a low ejection fraction. When, in such patients, a small valve size leads to an even moderate prosthesis-patient mismatch, this might result in heart failure and an increased mortality (52).

Atrial fibrillation

Atrial fibrillation and other non-sinusal rhythms occurs in 20% of the postoperative patients (32). In other series, this was 40% or more (53,54). The definition and the diagnostic method for AF have also an effect on its incidence (54,55). Postoperative AF has not been considered as innocent: it could lead to other complications and an increased stay in the hospital. With atrial fibrillation, there was a higher incidence of postoperative mortality (54) heart failure, renal function impairment, infection and neurologic events (53).

Univariate analysis showed following risk factors

$P<0.01$:	Previous PTCA
$P<0.05$:	LVEF below 50%

In a multivariate analysis, previous PTCA was the only independent predictor ($p=0.006$; odds ratio 2.7; 95% confidence interval 1.3-5.4)

The risk factors for postoperative AF in other series were a history of paroxysmal atrial fibrillation, a large left atrium, a prolonged P wave, heart failure, high age, low ejection fraction and left ventricular hypertrophy (55-57). The effect of age, however remained a matter for debate: atrial fibrillation did not occur more frequently in octogenarians after AVR (27).

It seems that postoperative atrial fibrillation was preventable, at least in part. Pacing could half the frequency of this event (53). Timely and adequate treatment could increase the speed of postoperative rehabilitation and reduce the stay within the hospital (55).

Conduction defects

An univariate analysis showed as risk factors:

$P<0.001$:	preoperative heart failure
$P<0.01$:	carotid artery disease, concomitant CABG
$P<0.05$:	NYHA functional class IV

An AV block grade 1 showed a trend. A large valve size (27 mm) had no effect.

A multivariate analysis showed following results:

Factor	n/N	p	OR	95%CI
Preoperative heart failure	32/215	0.001	3.0	1.7-5.4
Concomitant CABG	69/610	0.007	2.0	1.2-4.2
NYHA class IV	23/249	0.039	1.9	1.0-3.4
AV Block grade 1	7/37	0.078	2.4	1.0-5.7

Conduction defects such as complete atrio-ventricular block, and hence permanent pacemaker implantation, occurred in almost 10% of the patients who underwent AVR (58). The occurrence of all new conduction defects is reported to be 15% (59). Other reports state a lower incidence for permanent pacemaker implantation, since not all conduction defects need this treatment. Sometimes, a new conduction defects could be reversible (58). Development of a new conduction defects resulted to an increased need for monitoring and hence a longer hospital stay (60)

The main predictor for permanent pace maker implantation in other series were preoperative conduction defects (58,61-63). Other predictors were female gender, annular calcification, bicuspid aortic valve, hypertension, myocardial infarction, electrolyte imbalance and prolonged cross-clamping time (60,64,65). Aortic regurgitation might also play a role since this condition usually required implantation of larger valves (58).

Preoperative changes in the conduction system might be degenerative and due to older age, to ischemia and mechanical factors, due to an increased left ventricular pressure (58).

Some factors such as a calcified annulus could lead to trauma of the conduction system during surgery. The link with a congenitally bicuspid aortic valve is less clear. Hypertension could lead to calcification but also to increased septal left ventricular hypertrophy, which makes the conduction system more difficult to protect during cross-clamping (60). Other traumas of the conduction system could be due to impingement by the prosthetic valve or by suturing (58).

Development of a new conduction defects such as left bundle branch block in the postoperative period was a marker for future adverse events, such as sudden death (59), which illustrates the importance of these defects.

Non cardiac hospital complications

Pulmonary complications occurred in 58/1000 patients after AVR (66).

Univariate analysis showed following risk factors

$P=0.001$:	postoperative heart failure
$P<0.01$:	preoperative PM implantation
$P<0.05$:	COPD

Multivariate analysis identified following predictors:

Factor	n/N	p	OR	95%CI
Pacemaker implant	7/33	0.002	4.4	1.8 - 11.2
COPD	21/235	0.073	1.7	0.95 - 3.1
Heart failure	7/34	0.001	4.7	1.8 - 11.9

Respiratory complications after AVR are common (9,66,67) but few reports appeared concerning their predictors. Their rate depends largely on the criteria used (need for prolonged ventilation, respiratory failure, pulmonary infection).

The basic mechanisms of these complications involved a lack of deep inspiration due to postoperative pain, with a shallow breathing pattern, a prolonged recumbent positioning, a temporary diaphragmatic dysfunction and an impaired mucociliary clearance with a decrease in cough effectiveness, increases the risks associated with retained pulmonary secretions and bronchial obstruction (68). Atelectasis, infection and prolonged stay within the intensive care unit could be the result of such obstruction (69,70).

The use of an extracorporeal circulation during cardiac operations certainly has side effects on the respiratory system, due to inflammation (71,72). With greater hemodilution this effect could increase resulting pulmonary edema and pneumonia, especially when endothelial cells are injured (73). Pulmonary edema was also a hallmark of postoperative heart failure, which has been identified as a clear risk factor for postoperative pulmonary complications.

Chronic obstructive pulmonary disease could worsen the production of mucus, thereby increasing the risk for atelectasis and infection. Early postoperative heart failure, and hence pulmonary edema increase the need for ventilator support and prolong the stay on ICU. This also could make the patient more vulnerable for postoperative pulmonary problems (66).

In 58 of 1000 patients, we observed renal function impairment after AVR (17). Renal and cardiovascular disease could be linked in two ways. On the one hand, renal function impairment, even if this modest, has been an established element in the risk profile for atheromatosis (74,75). On the other hand, renal function impairment could also be the result of atheromatosis and has certainly been observed after major cardiovascular surgery such as AVR. Postoperative decrease of the renal function has been considered a serious complication with an increased mortality rate.

The risk factors in an univariate analysis for this complication were

Preop. renal impairment	22/108	29/890	<0.001
Age > 80	22/186	31/814	<0.001
Preop. atrial fibrillation	22/197	29/803	<0.001
Preop. pulmonary oedema	22/216	31/781	0.001
Preop. conduction defect	24/270	28/721	0.002
Diabetes	15/149	37/851	0.006
Preop. myocardial infarction	15/151	36/849	0.006
Postop. heart failure	6/34	47/966	0.007
CCT >75 min. (complete procedure)	29/460	7/275	0.015
Previously performed CABG	9/81	42/916	0.018
concomitant CABG	39/610	14/390	0.031
LV ejection fraction<0.50	13/155	31/723	0.033
Previous TIA/CVA	10/108	41/892	0.035

A multivariate analysis revealed following predictors

Factor	p	OR	95%CI
Preop. renal impairment	<0.001	5.5	2.9 - 10.4
Preop. atrial fibrillation	0.010	2.3	1.2 - 4.2
Age > 80	0.014	2.2	1.2 - 4.1
Myocardial infarction	0.022	2.2	1.1 - 4.4

Age over 80 has been associated with an increase in atheromatosis and myocardial infarction is certainly a marker for it. If atheromatosis also affects the renal arteries, a postoperative decrease in renal function could be expected (17).

Endothelial dysfunction of patients with CAVS could be a link with renal function impairment. This could help explaining the observed association between preoperative AF and postoperative renal complications. There are, however, several confounding factors (76,77).

Other risk factors were hypertension, peripheral arterial disease, bypass time over 70 minutes, severe angina an non-elective surgery (67,78).

Three difficulties could arise by comparing different series. First, the definition of previous renal function impairment as well as of postoperative decrease in renal function varied between series. In one series, a level of 2.0 mg/dl was used (78), in another 1.4 mg/dl (17). This could account for differences in results. The second difficulty has been the estimation of renal function: plasma creatinine , as a routine clinical procedure is not sufficient as estimate for glomerular filtration rate. Hence, its results should be interpreted cautiously. The estimation of glomerular filtration rate requires a 24-h urine collection, which is liable to errors. Third, defining a worsening of renal function by an increase of plasma creatinine (79) also had its difficulties: in patients with a plasma creatinine between 1 and 2 mg and hence, a moderate degree in renal function impairment, an additional increase with 0.3% could mean a serious additional renal damage. In patients with higher initial plasma creatinine , such an increase does not mean necessarily a major change in renal function: the slope of the relation between glomerular filtration rate and plasma creatinine is much less compared to the area with low initial plasma creatinine.

The extracorporeal circulation could have a damaging effect on the glomeruli, especially if the kidney already has been injured. Mechanisms inflicting renal damage are non-pulsatile perfusion, renal hypoperfusion, hypothermia, and increased levels of circulating catecholamines, cytokines, enzymes, free radicals and free hemoglobin (80). Keeping the cross-clamp time as short as possible or installing a minimal ECC could be helpful (81,82).

In spite of increasing age and co-morbid conditions in patients referred for AVR, the increase in hospital complications seemed to be limited to non-cardiac complications, which have a lower fatality rate than cardiovascular complications (83). The occurrence of renal and pulmonary postoperative events should be taken into account, however, if one chooses to operate older and sicker patients with symptomatic aortic valve disease.

4. Discussion and conclusions

Postoperative mortality and valve related complications received much attention in most patients series. Recently, other cardiac complications such as heart failure, conduction defects and atrial fibrillation were also scrutinized. Univariate analysis as screening and subsequent multivariate analysis as identification of risk factors for each event could be helpful patient selection and, more importantly, improve postoperative results if these risk factors are liable for alteration.

Mortality and congestive heart failure, which was identified as the most lethal cardiac complication, were clearly patient related. One might expect a reduction in these events if patients are referred early, once aortic valve degeneration has become symptomatic. This could avoid the appearance of a major risk factor, i.e. the need for urgent valve replacement. This is the clear consequence of a protracted pressure overload on the left ventricle by the diseased aortic valve and the ultimate marker for advanced heart valve disease.

Thromboembolism and bleeding are typically considered as valve related events. The former, however, could also be related to patient factors, while the latter could also be related to the procedure. Both events could have a significance as risk factor for long-term recurrence.

Occurrence of early postoperative conduction defects and of atrial fibrillation could also be considered as markers of advanced valvular heart disease, since some of their risk factors might be the result of protracted pressure overload on the left ventricle. Hence, these events could be seen as patient related.

Non-cardiac complications could clearly be related to co-morbid conditions. These, however are not always liable to alterations. Hence, the peri- and postoperative care should be tailored for each patient. It has also become obvious that age over 80 is not a formal contraindication for AVR. Nevertheless, elderly usually have considerable co-morbidity. The EUROscore, which was developed for CABG patients overestimates the risk for hospital mortality considerably. Low ejection fraction, chronic pulmonary obstructive disease and peripheral artery disease have been identified as predictors, although (84). Pulmonary function after median sternotomy is reduced in a substantial way, probably by several mechanisms such as chest wall restriction, decreased movement of the diaphragm and impairment of diffusion across the alveolar membrane (85).

It seemed worthwhile, therefore, to explore some alternative techniques in valve surgery which could reduce the postoperative risk. These could be 1) minimal surgical access, 2) minimal extracorporeal circulation and 3) transcatheter aortic valve implantation.

The first alternative, minimal surgical access by ministernotomy (85-88) and anterolateral minithoracotomy (89-91) could expose the surgical field adequately. Possible indications could be obesity, chronic obstructive pulmonary disease (86) and previous chest irratiation or CABG with patent left internal mammary artery (91).

Some advantages have been described such as an economic benefit, improved cosmetic result, decrease in postoperative morbidity, length of stay, pain, blood loss and transfusion (86-90,92). Cross clamping time had increased, however (88). Two randomized trials have appeared, which compared minimal and conventional AVR. The first one, was very small and included 20 patients for every group (88). The second one excluded patients with obesity and pulmonary disease (85), in spite of previously mentioned indications (86). Pain and blood loss were less, but there was no less need for transfusion. No other benefits such as a decrease in renal or pulmonary complications or differences in postoperative pulmonary functions could be documented (85,88,93). Results in high risk patients were considered as excellent in a recent review, but randomized controlled trials comparing minimal with conventional AVR are needed (94).

The second approach involves the changes in extracorporeal circulation devices. The use of an extracorporeal circulation during AVR has the risks of hemodilution and of an inflammatory response, which could be reduced by an minimal extracorporeal circulation or MECC. This MECC is a closed system with a centrifugal pump, an oxygenator without a venous and cardiotomy reservoir. The patient functions as the venous reservoir (95). This reduces the contact of blood with artificial surfaces and with air. The risk for hemolysis and the need for blood transfusions also decreases (96). With MECC, there is less increase in C-reactive protein, troponin I level, and better preservation of platelets and renal function. Stroke and cerebral injury were also less. The improved biocompatibility of MECC is of special advantage in high risk patients (age over 65, renal and pulmonary dysfunction). The use of a minimal ECC involves a learning curve, however (82).

More recently, TAVI or transcatheter aortic valve implantation, either through an artery or through the cardiac apex has been developed as third alternative. In patients deemed unfit for conventional AVR, TAVI was compared to balloon valvotomy through a randomized controlled (PARTNER) trial. Mortality (30-day and one-year) from any cause and repeat hospitalization as well as occurrence of cardiac symptoms (higher NYHA functional class) were significantly reduced after TAVI. Major strokes, bleeding events and major vascular events occurred more often, however. Balloon valvotomy did not alter the course of aortic valve disease. Paravalvular leaks after TAVI were usually mild and did not worsen after one year. Postprocedural stroke was troublesome, but might be reduced by developing smaller delivering devices. These results cannot be extrapolated to patients in whom conventional AVR is an option (7). The trans-apical approach for TAVI is a feasible alternative in high risk elderly patients with symptomatic aortic valve disease and peripheral artery disease. There is no need for sternotomy or extracorporeal circulation. No post-procedural stroke was observed, probably due to the avoidance of an atheromatous aortic arch. Presence of preoperative respiratory dysfunction proved to be a risk. The procedural success rate was high. Compared to a control group of patients who underwent conventional AVR (by propensity score analysis), 30-day and one-year survival superior for trans-apical TAVI, but this difference was not significant (97).

To document the superiority of either of these minimal approaches, RCT on sufficiently large scale are needed. For ministernotomy and minithoracotomy, these are feasible, but still lacking. For TAVI, it is currently unethical for patients to subject patients to the still unknown long-term results of TAVI if these are deemed fit for conventional AVR. Conventional AVR still can be considered as the standard therapy for degenerative aortic valve disease, with very predictable results, even in the elderly and patients with co-morbid condition.

5. References

[1] Somers P, Knaapen M, Kockx M, Van Cauwelaert P, Bortier H, Mistiaen W. Histological evaluation of autophagic cell death in calcified aortic valve stenosis. J Heart Valve Dis 2006;15:43-48

[2] Somers P, Knaapen MWM, Mistiaen W. Histolopathology of calcific aortic valve stenosis. Acta Cardiologica 2006; 61(5):557-562.

[3] Mistiaen W, Somers P, Knaapen MWM, Kockx MM. Autophagy as Mechanism for Cell death in Degenerative Aortic Valve Disease: an underestimated phenomenon in cardiovascular disease. Autophagy 2006;2:221-223.

[4] Mistiaen W, Knaapen M. Evaluation of cell death markers in severe calcified aortic valves. Methods In Enzymology 2009, 453:365-378.

[5] Carabello BA, Paulus WJ. Aortic stenosis. Lancet 2009; 373: 956–66.

[6] Iung B, Cacier A, Baron G, Messika-Zitoun D, Delahaye F, Tornos P, Gohlke C, Boersma E, Ravaud P, Vahanian A. Decision-making in elderly patients with severe aortic stenosis: why are so many denied surgery? European Heart Journal 2005;26:2714–2720.

[7] Leon MB, Smith CR, Mack M, et al for the PARTNTER trial investigators. Transcatheter Aortic-Valve Implantation for Aortic Stenosis in Patients Who Cannot Undergo Surgery New England J Med 2010;363:1597-1607.

[8] Hickey E, Langley SM, Allemby-Smith O, Livesey SA, Monro JL. Subcoronary allograft aortic valve replacement: parametric risk-hazard outcome analysis to a minimum of 20 years. Ann Thorac Surg 2007;84:1564-1570.

[9] Kolh P, Lahaye L, Gerard P, Limet R. Aortic valve replacement in the octogenarians: perioperative outcome and clinical follow-up. European Journal of Cardio-thoracic Surgery 1999;16: 68-73.

[10] Mistiaen W, Van Cauwelaert Ph, Muylaert Ph, Wuyts Fl, Harrisson F, Bortier H. Risk factors and survival after aortic valve replacement in octogenarians. J Heart Valve Dis. 2004;13:538-544.

[11] Edwards FH, Peterson ED, Coombs LP, DeLong LR, Jamieson WRE, Shroyer ALW, Grover FL. Prediction of Operative Mortality After Valve Replacement Surgery. J Am Coll Cardiol 2001;37:885-892.

[12] Florath I, Rosendahl UP, Mortasawi A, Bauer SF, Dalladaku F, Ennker IC, Ennker JC.Current Determinants of Operative Mortality in 1400 Patients Requiring Aortic Valve Replacement. Ann Thorac Surg 2003;76:75-83.

[13] Mistiaen W, Van Cauwelaert Ph, Muylaert Ph, Wuyts F, Bortier H. Risk factors for congestive heart failure after aortic valve replacement with a Carpentier-Edwards pericardial prosthesis in the elderly. J. Heart Valve Dis 2005;14:774-779.

[14] Jamieson WRE, Burr LH, Miyagishima RT, Janusz MT, Fradet GJ, Ling H, Lichtenstein SV. Re-operation for bioprosthetic aortic structural failure - risk assessment. European Journal of Cardio-thoracic Surgery 2003;24:873-878.

[15] Alsoufi B, Karamlou T, Slater M, Shen I, Ungerleider R, Ravichandran P. Results of concomitant aorta valve replacement and coronary artery bypass grafting in the VA population. J Heart Valve Dis 2006;15:12-18.

[16] Connolly HM, Oh JK, Schaff HV, Roger VL, Osborn SL, Hodge DO, Tajik AJ. Severe Aortic Stenosis With Low Transvalvular Gradient and Severe Left Ventricular Dysfunction Result of Aortic Valve Replacement in 52 Patients. Circulation. 2000;101:1940-1946.

[17] Mistiaen W, Van Cauwelaert P, Muylaert P, De Worm E. 1000 pericardial valves in aortic position: risk factors for postoperative acute renal function impairment in elderly. J Cardiovasc Surg 2009;50(2):233-237.

[18] Kirsch M, Guesnier L, LeBesnerais P, Hillion ML, Debauchez M, Seguin J, Loisance DY. Cardiac Operations in Octogenarians: Perioperative Risk Factors for Death and Impaired Autonomy. Ann Thorac Surg 1998;66:60-67.

[19] Maillet JM, Somme D, Hennel E, Lessana A, Saint-Jean O, Brodaty D. Frailty after aortic valve replacement (AVR) in octogenarians. Archives of Gerontology and Geriatrics 2009;48:391-396.

[20] Floyd TF, Shah PN, Price CC, Harris F, Ratcliffe SJ, Acker MA, Bavaria JE, Rahmouni H, Kuersten B, Wiegers S, McGarvey ML, Woo JY, Pochettino AA, Melhem RE. Clinically Silent Cerebral Ischemic Events After Cardiac Surgery: Their Incidence, Regional Vascular Occurrence, and Procedural Dependence. Ann Thorac Surg 2006;81:2160-2166.

[21] Mistiaen W, Van Cauwelaert Ph, Muylaert Ph, Sys SU, Harrisson F, Bortier H. Thromboembolism after aortic valve replacement in elderly with a Carpentier-Edwards perimount TM bioprosthesis. J Thorac Cardiovasc Surg. 2004;127:1166-1170.

[22] Minami K, Zittermann A, Schulte-Eistrup S, Koertke H, Körfer R. Mitroflow Synergy Prostheses for Aortic Valve Replacement: 19 Years Experience With 1,516 Patients. Ann Thorac Surg 2005;80:1699 -705.

[23] Gulbins H, Florath I, Ennker J. Cerebrovascular Events After Stentless Aortic Valve Replacement During a 9-Year Follow-Up Period. Ann Thorac Surg 2008;86:769-773.

[24] Filsoufi F, Rahmanian PB, Castillo JG, Bronster D, Adams DH. Incidence, Imaging Analysis, and Early and Late Outcomes of Stroke After Cardiac Valve Operation. Am J Cardiol 2008;101:1472-1478.

[25] Butchart EG, Gohlke C, Antunes MJ, Tornos P, De Caterina R, Cormier B, Prendergast B, Iung B, Bjornstadt H, Leport C, Hall RJC, Vahanian A. Recommendations for the management of patients after heart valve surgery. Eur Heart J 2005;26:2463-2471.

[26] Lund O, Nielsen SL, Arildsen H, Ilkjaer LB, Pilegaard HK. Standard Aortic St. Jude Valve at 18 Years: Performance Profile and Determinants of Outcome. Ann Thorac Surg 2000;69:1459-1465.

[27] Ennker J, Dalladaku F, Rosendahl U, Ennker IC, Mauser M, Florath I. The Stentless Freestyle Bioprosthesis: Impact of Age Over 80 Years on Quality of Life, Perioperative, and Mid-Term Outcome. J Card Surg 2006;21:379-385.

[28] Ruel M, Masters RG, Rubens FD, Bédard PJ, Pipe AL, Goldstein WG, Hendry PJ, Mesana TG. Late Incidence and Determinants of Stroke After Aortic and Mitral Valve Replacement. Ann Thorac Surg 2004;78:77-84.

[29] Horstkotte D, Lengyel M, Mistiaen WP, Völler H, Reibis R, Bogunovic N, Faber L, Hering D, Piper C, on behalf of the Working Group 'Infection, Thrombosis, Embolism and Bleeding' of the Society of Heart Valve Disease. Recommendations for Post-Discharge Patient Follow Up after Cardiac Valve Interventions: A Position Paper. The Journal of Heart Valve Disease 2007;16:575-589.

[30] Rizzoli G, Bottio T, Thiene G, Toscano G, Casarotto D. Long-term durability of the Hancock II porcine Bioprosthesis. J Thorac Cardiovasc Surg 2003;126:66-74.

[31] Sundt TM, Zehr KJ, Dearani JA, Daly RC, Mullany CJ, McGregor CGA, Puga FJ, Orszulak TA, Schaff HV. Is early anticoagulation with warfarin necessary after bioprosthetic aortic valve replacement? J Thorac Cardiovasc Surg 2005;129:1024-31.

[32] Aupart MR, Mirza A, Meurisse YA, Sirinelli AL, Neville PH, Marchand MA. Perimount pericardial bioprosthesis for aortic calcified stenosis: 18-year experience with 1,133 patients. J Heart Valve Dis 2006;15:768-775.

[33] Baudet EM, Puel V, McBride JT, Grimaud JP, Roques F, Clerc F, Roques X, Laborde N, Miller DC. Long-term results of valve replacement with the St Jude Medical prosthesis. J Thorac Cardiovasc Surg 1995;109:858-870.

[34] Burdon TE, Miller DC, Oyer PE, Mitchell RS, Stinson EB, Starnes VA, Shumway NE. Durability of porcine valves at 15 years in a representative North-American patient population. J Thorac Cardiovasc Surg 1992;103:238-252.

[35] Baykut D, Grize L, Schindler C, Keil AS, Bernet F, Zerkowski HR. Eleven-Year Single-Center Experience with the ATS Open Pivot Bileaflet Heart Valve. Ann Thorac Surg 2006;82:847–52.

[36] David TE, Feindel CM, Bos J, Ivanov J, Armstrong S. Aortic valve replacement with Toronto SPV bioprosthesis: Optimal patient survival but suboptimal valve durability. J Thorac Cardiovasc Surg 2008;135:19-24.

[37] Emery RW, Erickson CA, Arom KV, Northrup WF III, Kersten TE, Von Rueden TJ, Lillehei TL, Nicoloff DM. Replacement of the Aortic Valve in Patients Under 50 Years of Age: Long-Term Follow-Up of the St. Jude Medical Prosthesis. Ann Thorac Surg 2003;75:1815-1819.

[38] Goldsmith I, Lip GYH, Patel RL. Evaluation of the Sorin Bicarbon Bileaflet Valve in 488 Patients (519 Prostheses). Am J Cardiol 1999;83:1069–1074

[39] Li HH, Hahn J, Urbanski P, Torka M, Grunkemeier GL, Hacker RW. Intermediate-Term Results With 1,019 Carbomedics Aortic Valves. Ann Thorac Surg 2001;71:1181-1188.

[40] Carrier M, Pellerin M, Perrault LP, Pagé P, Hébert Y, Cartier R, Dyrda I, Pelletier LC. Aortic Valve Replacement With Mechanical and Biologic Prostheses in Middle-Aged Patients. Ann Thorac Surg 2001;71:S253-S256.

[41] Borman JB, De Riberolles C. Sorin Bicarbone bileaflet valve: a 10-year experience. Eur J Cardio-thorac Surg 2003;23:86-92.

[42] Neville PH, Aupart MR, Diemont FF, Sirinelli AL, Lemoine EM, Marchand MA. Carpentier-Edwards Pericardial Bioprosthesis in Aortic or Mitral Position: A 12-Year Experience. Ann Thorac Surg 1998;66:S143-S147.

[43] Butany J, Zhou T, Leong SW, Cunningham KS, Thangaroopan M, Jeggatheeswaran A, Feindel C, David TE. Inflammation and infection in nine surgically explanted Medtronic Freestyle ® stentless aortic valves. Cardiovascular Pathology 2007;16:258-267.

[44] Chirouze C, Cabell CH, Fowler VG Jr., Khayat N, Olaison L, Miro JM, Habib G, Abrutyn E, Eykyn S, Corey GR, Selton-Suty C, Hoen B, and the International Collaboration on Endocarditis Study Group. Prognostic Factors in 61 Cases of *Staphylococcus aureus* Prosthetic Valve Infective Endocarditis from the International Collaboration on Endocarditis Merged Database. Clinical Infectious Diseases 2004; 38:1323-1327.

[45] Habib G, Tribouilloy C, Thuny F, Giorgi R, Brahim A, Amazouz M, Remadi J¨P, Nadji G, Casalta JP, Coviaux F, Avierinos JF, Lescure X, Riberi A, Weiller PJ, Metras D, Raoult D. Prosthetic valve endocarditis: who needs surgery? A multicentre study of 104 cases. Heart 2005;91:954-959.

[46] Nozohoor S, Nilsson J, Lührs C, Roijer A, Algotsson L, Sjögren J. B-Type Natriuretic Peptide as a Predictor of Postoperative Heart Failure After Aortic Valve Replacement. Journal of Cardiothoracic and Vascular Anesthesia 2009;23:161-165.

[47] Gaudino M, Anselmi A, Abbat A, Galiuto L, Luciani M, Glieca F, Possati G. Myocardial apoptosis predicts postoperative course after aortic valve replacement in patients with severe left ventricular hypertrophy. J Heart Valve Dis 2007;16:344-348.

[48] Villari B, Sossalla S, Ciampi Q, Petruzziello B, Turina J, Schneider J, Turina M, Hess OM. Persistent diastolic dysfunction alte after valve replacement in severe aortic regurgitation. Circulation 2009;120:2386-2392.

[49] Bavelaar Croon CD, Wahba FF, Van Hecke MV. Perfusion and functional abnormalities outside the septal region in patients with left bundle branch block assessed with gated SPECT. Q J Nucl Med 2001;45:108-114.

[50] Blanc JJ, Etienne Y, Gilard M. Evaluation of different ventricular pacing sites in patients with severe heart failure: Results of an acute hemodynamic study. Circulation 1997;96:3273-3277.

[51] Sciagra R, Giaccardi M, Porciani MC. Myocardial perfusion imaging using gated SPECT in heart failure patients undergoing cardiac resynchronization therapy. J Nucl Med 2004;45:164-168.

[52] Ruel M, Al-Faleh H, Kulik A, Chan KL, Mesana TG, Burwash IG. Prosthesis–patient mismatch after aortic valve replacement predominantly affects patients with preexisting left ventricular dysfunction: Effect on survival, freedom from heart

failure, and left ventricular mass regression. J Thorac Cardiovasc Surg 2006;131:1036-1044.

[53] Greenberg MD, Katz NM, Iuliano, S, Tempesta BJ, Solomon AJ . Atrial Pacing for the Prevention of Atrial Fibrillation After Cardiovascular Surgery. J Am Coll Cardiol 2000;35:1416-1422.

[54] Mariscalco G, Engström KG. Atrial fibrillation after cardiac surgery: Risk factors and their temporal relationship in prophylactic drug strategy decision. International Journal of Cardiology 2008;129:354-362.

[55] Banach M, Goch A, Misztal M, Rysz J, Jaszewski R, Goch JH. Predictors of paroxysmal atrial fibrillation in patients undergoing aortic valve replacement. J Thorac Cardiovasc Surg 2007;134:1569-76

[56] Baranowska E, Baranowki R, Michalek P, Hoffman P, Rywik T, Rawczylska-Englert I. Prediction of paroxysmal atrial fibrillation after aortic valve replacement in patients with aortic stenosis: identification of potential risk factors. J Heart Valve Dis 2003;12:136-141.

[57] Hayashida N, Shojima T, Yokokura Y, Hori H, Yoshikawa K, Tomoeda H, Aoyagi S. P-Wave Signal-Averaged Electrocardiogram for Predicting Atrial Arrhythmia After Cardiac Surgery. Ann Thorac Surg 2005;79:859-864.

[58] Dawkins S, Hobson AR, Kalra PR, Tang ATM, Monro JL, Dawkins KD. Permanent Pacemaker Implantation After Isolated Aortic Valve Replacement: Incidence, Indications, and Predictors. Ann Thorac Surg 2008;85:108-112.

[59] El-Khally Z, Thibault B, Staniloae C, Theroux P, Dubuc M, Roy D, Guerra P, Macle L, Talajic M. Prognostic Significance of Newly Acquired Bundle Branch Block After Aortic Valve Replacement. Am J Cardiol 2004;94:1008-1011.

[60] Erdogan HB, Kayalar N, Ardal H, Omeroglu SN, Kirali K, Guler M, Akinci E, Yakut C. Risk Factors for Requirement of Permanent Pacemaker Implantation After Aortic Valve Replacement. J Card Surg 2006;21:211-215.

[61] Koplan BA, Stevenson WG, Epstein LM, Aranki SF, Maisel WH. Development and Validation of a Simple Risk Score to Predict the Need for Permanent Pacing After Cardiac Valve Surgery. J Am Coll Cardiol 2003;41:795- 801

[62] Huynh H, Dalloul G, Ghanbari H, Burke P, David M, Daccarett, Machado C, David S. Permanent Pacemaker Implantation Following Aortic Valve Replacement: Current Prevalence and Clinical Predictors. PACE 2009; 32:1520–1525.

[63] Merin O, Ilan M, Oren A, Fink M, Deeb M, Bitran D, Silberman S. Permanent Pacemaker Implantation Following Cardiac Surgery: Indications and Long-Term Follow-Up. PACE 2009; 32:7-12.

[64] Lewis JW Jr., Webb CR, Pickard SD, Lehman J, Jacobsen G. The increased need for a permananet pacemaker after reoperative cardiac surgery. J Thorac Cardiovasc Surg 1998;116:74-81.

[65] Limongelli G, Ducceschi V, D'Andrea A, Renzulli A, Sarubbi B, De Feo M, Cerasuolo F, Calabrò R, Cotrufo M. Risk factors for pacemaker implantation following aortic valve replacement: a single centre experience. Heart 2003;89:901-904.

[66] Mistiaen W, Vissers D. Risk factors for postoperative pulmonary complications after aortic valve replacement within the hospital: an observational study. Austr J Physiotherapy 2008; 54:119-124.

[67] Weerasinghe A, Yusuf M, Athanasiou T, Wood A, Magee P, Uppal R. Role of Transvalvular Gradient in Outcome From Valve Replacement for Aortic Stenosis. Ann Thorac Surg 2004;77:1266-1271.
[68] Overend TJ, Anderson CM, Lucy SD, Bhatia C, Jonsson BI, Timmermans C. The effect of incentive spirometry on postoperative pulmonary complications: a systematic review. Chest 2001;120:971-978.
[69] Lawrence VA, Hilsenbeck SG, Mulrow CD, Dhande R, Sapp J, Page CP. Incidence and hospital stay for cardiac and pulmonary complications after abdominal surgery. Journal of General Internal Medicine 1995;10:671-678.
[70] Johnson LG, McMahan MJ. Postoperative factors contributing to prolonged length of stay in cardiac surgery patients. Dimensions in Critical Care Nursing 1997;16:243-250.
[71] Wynne R, Botti M. Postoperative pulmonary dysfunction in adults after cardiac surgery with cardiopulmonary bypass. clinical significance and implications for practice. Am J Crit Care 2004;13:384-393.
[72] Staton GW, Williams WH, Mahoney EM, Hu J, Chu H, Duke PG, Puskas JD. Pulmonary outcomes of off-pump vs on-pump coronary artery bypass surgery in a randomized trial. Chest 2005;127:892-901.
[73] Habib RH, Zacharias A, Schwann TA, Riordan CJ, Durham SJ, Shah A. Effects of obesity and small body size on operative and long-term outcomes of coronary artery bypass surgery: a propensity-matched analysis. Ann Thorac Surg 2005:1976–86.
[74] Dellegrottaglie S, Saran R, Gillespie B, Zhang X, Chung S, Finkelstein F, et al. Prevalence and predictors of cardiovascular calcium in chronic kidney disease (from the prospective longitudinal RRI-CKD Study). Am J Cardiol 2006;98:571–576.
[75] Qunibi WY. Cardiovascular calcification in nondialyzed patients with chronic kidney disease. Seminars in dialysis 2007;20(2):134-138.
[76] Albahrani MJ, Swaminathan M, Phillips-Bute B, Smith PK, Newman MF, Mathew JP. Postcardiac surgery complications: Association of acute renal dysfunction and atrial fibrillation. Anest Analg 2003;96(3):637-643.
[77] Ngo DTM, Heresztyn T, Mishra K, Marwick TH, Horowitz JD. Aortic stenosis is associated with elevated plasma levels of asymmetric dimethylarginine (ADMA). Nitric Oxide 2007;16:197-201.
[78] Gaudino M, Luciani N, Giungi S, Caradonna E, Nasso G, Schiavello R. Different profiles of patients who require dialysis after cardiac surgery. Ann Thorac Surg 2005;79:825–30.
[79] Cowie MR, Komajda M, Murray-Thomas T, Underwood J, Ticho B on behalf of the POSH Investigators. Prevalence and impact of worsening renal function in patients hospitalized with decompensated heart failure: results of the prospective outcomes study in heart failure (POSH). Eur Heart J 2006;27:1216–1222.
[80] Sajja LR, Mannam G, Chakravarthi MR, Sompalli S, Naidu SK, Somaraju B. Coronary artery bypass grafting with or without cardiopulmonary bypass in patients with preoperative non–dialysis dependent renal insufficiency: A randomized study. J Thorac Cardiovasc Surg 2007;133(2):378-388.
[81] Vaquette B, Corbineau H, Laurent M, Lelong B, Langanay T, de Place C. Valve replacement in patients with critical aortic stenosis and depressed left ventricular

function: predictors of operative risk, left ventricular function recovery, and long term outcome. Heart 2005;91:1324-1329

[82] Remadi JP, Rakotoarivello Z, Marticho P, Trojette F, Benamar A, Poulain H. Aortic valve replacement with the minimal extracorporeal circulation (Jostra MECC System) versus standard cardiopulmonary bypass: A randomized prospective trial. J Thorac Cardiovasc Surg 2004;128:436-441.

[83] Mistiaen W, Van Cauwelaert P, Muylaert P, De Worm E. 1000 Carpentier-Edwards pericardial valves in aortic position: what changed in the last 20 years and what are the effects on hospital complications. J Heart Valve Dis 2007;16:417-422.

[84] Grossi EA, Schwartz CF, Yu PJ, Jorde UP, Crooke GA, Grau JB, Ribakove GH, Baumann FG, Ursumanno P, Culliford AT, Colvin SB, Galloway AC, High-Risk Aortic Valve Replacement: Are the Outcomes as Bad as Predicted? Ann Thorac Surg 2008;85:102-107.

[85] Calderon J, Richebe P, Guibaud JP, Coiffic A, Branchard O, Asselineau J, Janvier G. Prospective Randomized Study of Early Pulmonary Evaluation of Patients Scheduled for Aortic Valve Surgery Performed by Ministernotomy or Total Median Sternotomy. J Cardiothorac Vasc Anesth 2009;23:795-801.

[86] De Amicis V, Ascione R, lannelli G, Di Tommaso L, Monaco M, Spampinato N. Aortic Valve Replacement through a Minimally Invasive Approach. Tex Heart Inst J 1997;24:353-355.

[87] Nair RU, Sharpe DAC. Minimally Invasive Reversed Z Sternotomy for Aortic Valve Replacement. Ann Thorac Surg 1998;65:1165-1166.

[88] Aris A, Camara ML, Montiel J, Delgado LJ, Galan J, Litvan H. Ministernotomy Versus Median Sternotomy for Aortic Valve Replacement: A Prospective, Randomized Study. Ann Thorac Surg 1999;67:1583-1588.

[89] Santana O, Reyna J, Grana R, Buendia M, Lamas GA, Lamelas J. Outcomes of Minimally Invasive Valve Surgery Versus Standard Sternotomy in Obese Patients Undergoing Isolated Valve Surgery. Ann Thorac Surg 2011;91:406-410.

[90] Plass A, Scheffel H, Alkadhi H, Kaufmann P, Genoni M, Falk V, Grünenfelder J. Aortic Valve Replacement Through a Minimally Invasive Approach: Preoperative Planning, Surgical Technique, and Outcome. Ann Thorac Surg 2009;88:1851-1856.

[91] Benetti F, Rizzardi JL, Concetti C, Bergese M, Zappetti A. Minimally aortic valve surgery avoiding sternotomy. Eur J Cardio-thorac Surg 1999;16(Suppl.2):S84-S85.

[92] Korach A, Shemin RJ, Hunter CT, Bao Y, Shapira OM. Minimally invasive versus conventional aortic valve replacement: a 10-year experience. J Cardiovasc Surg 2010;51:417-421.

[93] El Bardissi AW, Shekar P, Couper GS, Cohn LH. Minimally invasive aortic valve replacement in octogenarian, high-risk, transcatheter aortic valve implantation candidates. J Thorac Cardiovasc Surg 2011;141:328-335.

[94] Schmitto JD, Mohr FW, Cohn LH. Minimally invasive aortic valve replacement: how does this perform in high-risk patients? Curr Opin Cardiol 2011;26:118-122.

[95] Frietman PAV, Waanders FGJ, van Boven WJ, de Jong M, van Dongen E, A New Challenge for Mini-Extracorporeal Circulation: Closing Atrial Septal Defects. J Cardiothorac Vasc Anesth 2005;19:656-658.

[96] Nydegger U. Transfusion dependency in cardiac surgery - update 2006. Swiss Med Weekly 2006; 136:781-788.

[97] Walther T, Schuler G, Borger MA, Kempfert J, Seeburger J, Ruckert R, Ender J, Linke A, Scholz M, Falk V1, Mohr FW. Transapical aortic valve implantation in 100 consecutive patients: comparison to propensity-matched conventional aortic valve replacement. Eur Heart J 2010;31;1398-1403.

5

Application of a Novel Venous Cannula for En-Bloc Removal of Undesirable Intravascular Material

Albert K. Chin, Lishan Aklog, Brian J. deGuzman and Michael Glennon
Vortex Medical, Inc.
USA

1. Introduction

Venous occlusive disease encompasses a variety of clinical entities that range the spectrum from being catastrophic and life threatening, such as massive pulmonary embolism, to disease states that may have an occult presentation, such as inferior vena cava occlusion. Other examples of veno-occlusive disease states include deep venous thrombosis and right atrial masses. When venous occlusion is characterized by an overwhelming volume of offending material, clinical therapy may be a significant challenge. This chapter examines the historical background of therapy directed at venous occlusion, and outlines a simplified technique for addressing the occurrence of major undesirable intravascular material.

2. Etiology and incidence

The majority of undesirable material presenting in the major venous circulation have their origins in the lower extremity veins. Deep venous thrombosis has an estimated annual incidence of over 2 million cases in the United States (Hirsh & Hoak, 1996), and accounts for approximately 600,000 hospitalizations per year (Schreiber, 2010). The genesis of venous thrombosis continues to be aptly characterized by the observations of Virchow in 1856 (Virchow, 1998, as cited in Lopez et al., 2004), who is credited with associating the triad of (1) venous stasis, (2) endothelial injury and (3) hypercoagulability with the formation of intravascular clot. The incidence of pulmonary embolism is closely tied to the occurrence of deep venous thrombosis, so much so that the complex of deep venous thrombosis and pulmonary embolism is defined by the term "venous thromboembolism". It is estimated that approximately 50% of patients with deep venous thrombosis have detectable pulmonary emboli (Hirsh, 1996). Lower extremity deep venous thrombosis in the distal vessels, e.g. calf vein thrombosis, has commonly been held to be relatively benign, and mostly asymptomatic; however, some studies have shown that propagation of calf vein clot above the popliteal level occurs in approximately 15% of patients (Lohr et al., 1991). Upon propagation to the popliteal vein, the risk of measurable pulmonary embolism increases to approximately 40% (Kakkar et al., 1969, as cited in Hirsch & Hoak, 1996).

Risk factors for venous thromboembolism are associated with conditions that alter elements of Virchow's triad. These include increasing age, surgery, trauma, hospital or nursing home confinement, malignancy, paralytic neurologic disease, presence of an indwelling venous catheter or pacing lead, varicose veins, previous superficial vein thrombosis, pregnancy, and oral contraceptive use (Heit, 2002). The recurrence rate for patients with a single episode of venous thromboembolism is approximately thirty percent over ten years.

The incidence of pulmonary embolism in the U.S. is estimated to be 1.35 million cases per year (Banovac et al., 2010). Predicted outcomes for patients with pulmonary embolism vary greatly with the hemodynamic stability of the patient upon presentation. Patients with a systolic arterial blood pressure below 90 mm Hg are deemed to have massive pulmonary embolism, while patients with a systolic pressure equal to or above 90 mm Hg are categorized as having non-massive pulmonary embolism. In the International Cooperative Pulmonary Embolism Registry involving 2,342 patients, the vast majority (95.5%) had non-massive pulmonary embolism, while 4.5% had massive pulmonary embolism. Patients with massive pulmonary embolism had a 90 day mortality of 52.4%, compared with a 90 day mortality of 14.7% in patients with non-massive pulmonary embolism (Kucher et al., 2006). In hospital mortality for patients with pulmonary embolism rose from 8.1% in clinically stable patients to 25% in unstable patients, and increased to 65% in patients requiring cardiopulmonary resuscitation, in a separate study of 1,001 patients (Kasper et al., 1997).

Inferior vena cava thrombosis is also associated with deep venous thrombosis, although to a lesser extent than the tie between deep venous thrombosis and pulmonary embolism. The frequency of IVC thrombosis in patients with deep venous thrombosis is estimated to be between 4 - 15% (Fernandez & Geehan, 2008). Other causes of inferior vena cava thrombosis include malignancy, trauma, surgery, abdominal aortic aneurysm, and indwelling venous catheters. In one series, carcinoma of the kidney was the most common cause of IVC thrombosis, accounting for 31% of cases presenting over a 23 year period (Siqueira-Filho et al., 1976). The actual incidence of inferior vena cava thrombosis is difficult to cite, due to the variability of its presentation. It is estimated that in patients with IVC thrombosis, over one-half remain asymptomatic until their initial presentation with pulmonary embolism. Iatrogenic causes of inferior vena cava thrombosis are also significant. IVC thrombosis maybe a complication of vena cava filter placement, in the treatment of or prophylaxis for pulmonary embolism. The occurrence of IVC thrombosis was 2.7% in a 26 year review of 1731 patients implanted with 1765 vena cava filters (Athanasoulis et al., 2000). Vena cava thrombosis may also be caused by indwelling intravascular devices such as pacemaker leads, parenteral nutrition catheters, or hemodialysis catheters (Krug & Zerbe, 1980; Mulvihill & Fonkalsrud, 1984; Gouge et al., 1988).

Masses presenting in the cardiac portion of the venous circulation are relatively rare. Most of such masses are primary atrial myxomas. A study of 33108 consecutive cardiac surgical patients found an incidence of right atrial myxoma to be 0.036%; this incidence represents less than 10% of all atrial myxomas, as most atrial myxomas are left sided. Thrombus formation on the tumor surface or dislodged tumor fragments may cause pulmonary embolism. Thrombus originating in the iliofemoral system or the inferior vena cava may propagate into the right atrium (Khurana & Tak, 2004). Once clot presents in the right atrium, the prognosis is poor without active thrombectomy. A review of the literature involving twenty patients with right atrial thrombus found that the condition was uniformly fatal without treatment, while a 50% mortality rate was observed when either anticoagulation or thrombolytic therapy was administered. When surgical extraction was performed, the mortality rate was reduced to 14% (Armstrong et al., 1985).

3. Therapeutic history

3.1 Medical therapy

Medical treatment of venous thromboembolism was instituted in 1960 with the first randomized clinical trial evaluating the efficacy of anticoagulation in patients with pulmonary embolism (Barrett & Jordan, 1960). Anticoagulation therapy does not resolve existent thrombus, but prevents its propagation, and significantly reduces the mortality rate of pulmonary embolism. Untreated pulmonary embolism carries a mortality rate of approximately 30%; this is reduced to approximately 8% when anticoagulation is instituted (Banovac et al., 2010). The typical therapeutic approach involves intravenous infusion of unfractionated or low molecular weight heparin, followed by oral anticoagulation with warfarin , which is continued for a period of several months. It has been suggested that little benefit is gained by extending anticoagulation therapy from three to six months in venous thromboembolism patients (Campbell et al., 2007).

Fibrinolytic agents provide active dissolution of clot; they were introduced into clinical treatment of venous thromboembolic disease in the 1970s (Tibbutt et al., 1974). Streptokinase, urokinase, and recombinant tissue plasminogen activator (rTPA) are compounds available for fibrinolytic therapy. All three agents convert plasminogen to plasmin, with subsequent enzymatic degradation of fibrin clot. Studies on the efficacy of the three available fibrinolytic agents demonstrate no difference in clot resolution after twenty-four hours (Almoosa, 2002). The positive effect of thrombolytic agents is partially offset by their potential for major bleeding complications, including intracerebral hemorrhage. The risk of hemorrhage during fibrinolytic therapy varies between 6 - 20% (Harris & Meek, 2005). A meta-analysis of nine randomized, controlled clinical trials comparing anticoagulation alone to anticoagulation plus thrombolysis demonstrated no difference in overall mortality between the two treatment regimes in non-selected patients with acute pulmonary embolism (Thabut, G. et al., 2002). Therefore, fibrinolytic therapy is indicated for patients with massive pulmonary embolism characterized by hypotension, or potentially for normotensive pulmonary embolism patients demonstrating right heart dysfunction, as this subgroup of patients has been associated with a higher risk of mortality in previous studies (Goldhaber, 1993, as cited in Harris & Meeks, 2005). Fibrinolytic agents may be delivered intravenously, or selectively into the pulmonary artery at the site of occlusion. A prospective, multi-center trial comparing intrapulmonary fibrinolytic infusion with intravenous fibrinolytic administration found no significant benefit with intrapulmonary catheter therapy (Verstraete et al., 1988). Instead, a prolonged intravenous thrombolytic infusion over seven hours appeared to yield a superior benefit to a single infusion over two hours. Direct insertion of an infusion catheter into the substrate of the embolus has been suggested as a more efficacious method of fibrinolytic delivery. Insufficient clinical data is available at this time to establish superiority of intra-embolic infusion over intrapulmonary or intravenous fibrinolysis.

3.2 Surgical therapy

Patients with massive venous thromboembolism and particularly those with contraindications to thrombolytic therapy are candidates for surgical thrombectomy and embolectomy. Pulmonary embolectomy is a substantial procedure, necessitating a median sternotomy and cardiopulmonary bypass, but without cardioplegic arrest. An arteriotomy in the main pulmonary artery is performed to allow instrumental extraction of thrombus under direct vision, in an en bloc fashion, if possible. In one surgical series of 29 consecutive patients, surgical pulmonary embolectomy was successful in all cases, and the resultant survival rate at one month was 89% (Aklog et al., 2002). A review of 1,300 total patients undergoing operative pulmonary embolectomy in 46 reported series from 1961 to 2005 demonstrated an average mortalityof 30% (Stein et al., 2007). Due to its degree of invasiveness, surgical embolectomy is generally reserved as the last therapeutic option.

3.3 Catheter therapy

Instrumentation for surgical embolectomy dates back to 1963, with the introduction of the Fogarty embolectomy balloon catheter (Fogarty, 1963). The venous thrombectomy version of the Fogarty balloon is a 6F or 8F catheter with inflated balloon sizes up to 19 mm in diameter. The venous thrombectomy catheter is primarily applied to patients with deep venous thrombosis. It incorporates a flexible distal tip to facilitate catheter passage through venous valves. Procedures are performed in the operating theater, with surgical access used to gain vascular control during the thrombectomy process.

A variety of devices have been devised for a percutaneous approach to thrombectomy. Greenfield developed a suction tip catheter for pulmonary embolectomy in 1971 (Greenfield et al., 1971). The catheter was previously available in the form of a 10F steerable catheter with either a 5 mm or a 7 mm diameter cupped tip. Percutaneous entry was performed in either the femoral or jugular vein, and embolectomy conducted under fluoroscopic control. Vacuum was established by means of a syringe to aspirate a portion of the embolus into the cup, whereupon sustained vacuum was maintained as the catheter was withdrawn to remove the clot. Multiple passes of the suction cup catheter were applied until improvements in the pulmonary artery pressure and cardiac output denoted a successful clinical result. A series of 46 patients undergoing Greenfield suction pulmonary embolectomy between 1970 to 1992 demonstrated an overall success rate of 76%, with a one month survival rate of 70% (Greenfield et al., 1993). Conventional straight catheter sheaths may be employed for percutaneous embolectomy. An approach termed the "Meyerovitz technique" applies vacuum via a connected 60 cc syringe to a readily available 8F or 9F coronary guiding catheter without distal side holes, advanced through a 10F introducer sheath (Goldhaber, 1998). However, limited volumes of clot are extracted, due to the small caliber of the guiding catheters used.

Multiple catheter designs address venous thromboembolism via clot fragmentation. Peripheral angioplasty balloon catheters have been applied to restore patency in intraluminal occlusion. Dilatation of thrombus in large caliber vessels may result in significant distal embolization; therefore, balloon angioplasty may be combined with wallstent placement to decrease recurrent embolism resulting from dislodgement of balloon dilated endoluminal thrombus. Another approach to fragmentation therapy utilizes manual rotation of a pigtail catheter to disrupt clot, with concomitant site specific thrombolytic injection to augment the mechanical therapy (Schmitz-Rode et al., 1998). The 5F pigtail catheter is ensheathed in a coaxial 5.5F introducer sheath. This device seeks to recanalize an occluded vessel, without retrieval of disrupted segments. Treated patients are subjected to distal embolization that may potentially be clinically significant. Another specialized catheter fragmentation device devised by Amplatz applies high speed rotation of a distal impeller on a 7F catheter to draw clot towards the impeller, resulting in disintegration of thrombus into tiny particles. Micro thrombi generated by this system are not removed from the circulation. The smaller clot fragments generated by the Amplatz impeller is an improvement over pigtail embolectomy; however, the presence of circulating micro-hemolytic fragments may be of concern, particularly if a substantial volume of debris is generated. Clot fragmentation coupled with embolic removal has a theoretic edge over fragmentation alone. An 11F Aspirex device integrating high-speed rotation of a distally situated spiral with vacuum capability is undergoing clinical trials to evaluate its effectiveness in pulmonary arteries between 6 mm and 14 mm in diameter (Kuchar, 2007). This device combination of mechanical thrombolysis with vacuum removal addresses organized thrombus and seeks the removal of fragmentation byproducts.

Another approach to clot fragmentation is catheter rheolysis. This class of therapeutic catheter utilizes a multi-lumen catheter with separate injection and retrieval ports. High pressure fluid infusion through one or more injection ports serve to fragment thrombus upon contact. Infusion through the injection port or ports create a Venturi effect, establishing a pressure differential between the injection and retrieval ports that create a backflow through the retrieval lumen for removal of thrombus fragments and infused fluid. Rheolytic catheters are sized in the 6F to 7F range, and are not designed to be used in vessels greater than 12 mm in diameter (Kuchar, 2007). Their application in massive pulmonary embolism has been described in small clinical series, with resultant limited effectiveness (Siablis, 2005, Chiam, 2005, Zeni, 2003, and Koning, 1997, as cited in Kuchar, 2007).

3.4 En Bloc removal of undesirable intravascular material

A simplified approach to the en bloc removal of undesirable intravascular material is proposed. One of the authors noticed that during surgical embolectomy, it is often possible to perform en bloc removal of a large mass of organized thrombus, when a venous drainage cannula inserted into the main pulmonary artery gains purchase of the tail of the clot. The flow rate established by the cardiopulmonary bypass pump generates significant vacuum that in some cases may pull a thrombotic cast of the pulmonary vasculature into the extracorporeal circulation, where it is trapped by the in-line filter. In other cases, the large caliber of the main pulmonary artery and the subsequent girth of the embolus prevent its introduction into the venous outflow cannula; however, it may be grasped by the cannula tip and extracted via the pulmonary arteriotomy. The mechanics of thrombectomy gained as a result of the open surgical experience suggested a possible technique of percutaneous venous extraction. An extracorporeal circuit may be established containing a large bore outflow line, a centrifugal pump, an in-line filter, and an inflow line. The distal end of the venous outflow cannula is fitted with a balloon-activated funnel tip that expands to the luminal diameter of the occluded vessel. The venous outflow cannula is advanced into proximity of the obstructing venous material, while the venous inflow cannula is inserted into a separate venous entry site. Activation of the centrifugal pump creates a uni-directional flow that serves two functions: One, it creates a vacuum at the funnel drainage side to extract undesirable intravascular material; and two it performs simultaneous reinfusion of filtered blood volume to maintain circulatory homeostasis. The extracorporeal circuit is placed percutaneously or via femoral venous cutdown. The technique establishes a venous to venous bypass circulation without oxygenation, powered by a compact centrifugal pump generating a flow rate up to 5 liters per minute. The sizes of both outflow and inflow venous cannulae are maximized, to accommodate the large girth of the pulmonary vasculature. Whereas previous suction thrombectomy devices extracted clot in piecemeal fashion with multiple catheter insertions and removals, due to their limited bore, the extracorporeal veno-venous system strives for en bloc extraction, with intraluminal passage of clot in the venous cannulae.

3.4.1 Instrumentation and technique

Elements of the funnel drainage cannula and extracorporeal circuit used to extract occluding venous material are shown in Figure 1. The funnel cannula (AngioVac® Cannula, Vortex Medical Inc., Norwell, MA) contains a 22F body with distal fingers that are balloon expandable to generate a maximal funnel diameter of 48F. The funnel drainage cannula is connected to ½ inch polyvinyl chloride tubing that leads to the in-line filter with a 90 cc capacity. The centrifugal pump is downstream of the filter, and connected to the reinfusion cannula, completing the extracorporeal circuit. In preparation for establishment of extracorporeal bypass, a 10,000 unit bolus of intravenous heparin is administered to the patient, and a constant intravenous infusion of approximately 1,000 units per hour continued to maintain the patient's activated clotting time (ACT) at 300 seconds. If the ACT is maintained at 300 or above, use of a heparin coated bypass circuit is unnecessary. Prior to use, the circuit is primed with normal saline, yielding a closed system that accomplishes vacuum extraction, filtering and reinfusion in concurrent fashion. With use of the Rotaflow centrifugal pump (MAQUET Cardiovascular, Wayne, New Jersey), priming of the circuit requires approximately 500 cc of saline. In use, venous access is established via the femoral or jugular vein, and an angiographic catheter advanced to the site of the occlusion. If extraction of pulmonary emboli in a branch vessel is anticipated, cannulation of the target vessel is performed using a 5F to 8F pigtail catheter (Andrews, 2004), and an 0.038" guidewire left in position. A 26F introducer sheath (Gore® DrySeal Sheath, W.L. Gore & Associates, Inc., Medical Products Division, Flagstaff, AZ) is inserted in the femoral or jugular venous access site and the drainage cannula fitted with its internal tapered dilator is advanced over the emplaced 0.038" guidewire to position the funnel tip approximately 10 cm proximal to the occlusion. The dilator is removed from the drainage cannula, and the balloon inflated with saline to a pressure of 1 atmosphere to expand the collecting funnel. The centrifugal pump is activated prior to advancement of the funnel cannula towards the occlusion. The rotational speed of the pump is increased in increments of 500 ml/minute until thrombus extraction occurs. Flow rate indicated on the pump generally increases as the speed is increased. A sudden drop to zero flow may be a signal that a large mass has become seated in the funnel. Pump velocity is maintained, and as the mass is compressed and extracted through the cannula, flow will be re-established. If the diameter and density of a mass of dislodged organized thrombus prevents its passage through the venous drainage cannula, the cannula may be removed from the body and its lumen cleared externally. Following suction embolectomy, a completion venogram or pulmonary arteriogram is performed via the drainage cannula to evaluate the completeness of thrombus extraction.

3.4.2 Functional mechanics of En Bloc intravascular extraction

Intravascular extraction with the funnel cannula is a flow directed process, with the centrifugal pump generating sufficient flow to perform suction embolectomy at one end of the circuit and vascular reinfusion at the opposite end of the circuit. The balloon situated at the funnel portion of the drainage cannula not only serves to expand the funnel for vessel wall apposition and removal of intravascular material, but also provides inflow regulation during the extraction procedure (Figure 2). Modulation of antegrade venous flow assists the

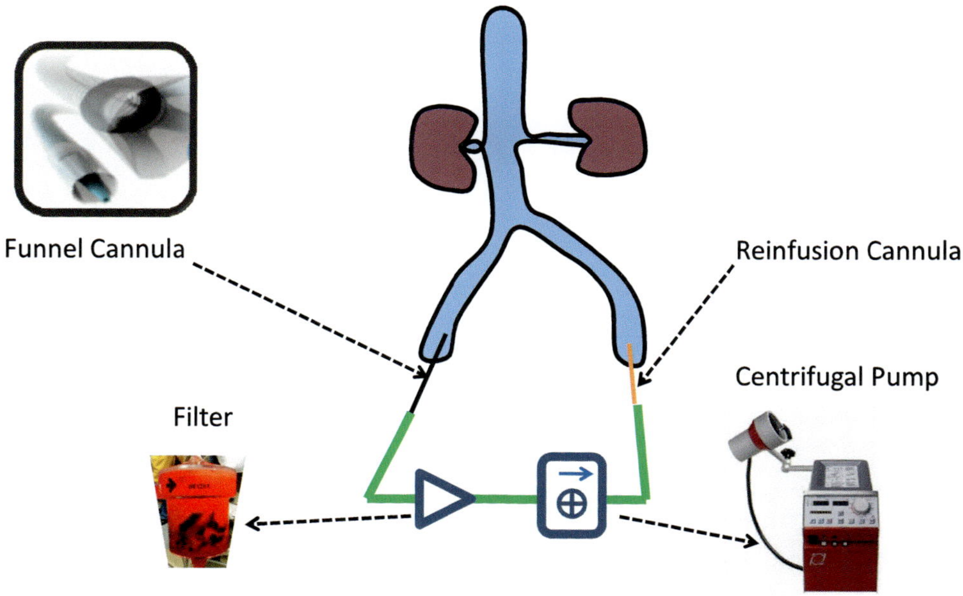

Fig. 1. Elements of the funnel drainage cannula and extracorporeal circuit

centrifugal pump in generating the necessary retrograde flow to initiate movement of the thrombotic material and its subsequent excursion the length of the drainage cannula. The degree of collateralization in the native circulation facilitates intravascular extraction, as it preserves the potential for retrograde flow at the treatment site. If retrograde flow at the occlusion site is diminished or removed, intravascular extraction may be inhibited. In order to delineate the significance of retrograde flow on the dynamics of en bloc extraction, a flow model was constructed to allow empirical evaluation of the vacuum extraction process.

3.4.3 Material and methods

Branched, tapering vinyl tubing was connected with fittings in a configuration that mimics the morphology of the pulmonary vasculature, and a valve was placed immediately distal to the site of embolic extraction (Figure 3). Saline was heated to 37 degrees Celsius and continuously circulated through the circuit by means of an impeller pump and a peristaltic pump in series, at a flow rate of 5.0 L/minute. Organized thrombus was modeled using calf liver sectioned into15 mm x 80 mm strips. Calf liver was used to model thrombus, as its density is similar to the density of mammalian clot (Nahimyak, 2006 amd Baraislas. 2007), and it lacks the propensity for disintegration in a mechanical flow model. With the thrombus model placed in the vascular circuit in a position equivalent to the main pulmonary artery, the valve proximal to the thrombus model was adjusted to three different positions: (1) completely closed position, (2) completely open position, and (3) partially closed position. The separation distance at thrombus model capture, centrifugal pump speed at capture, and flow rate generated in the funnel drainage cannula at capture were measured.

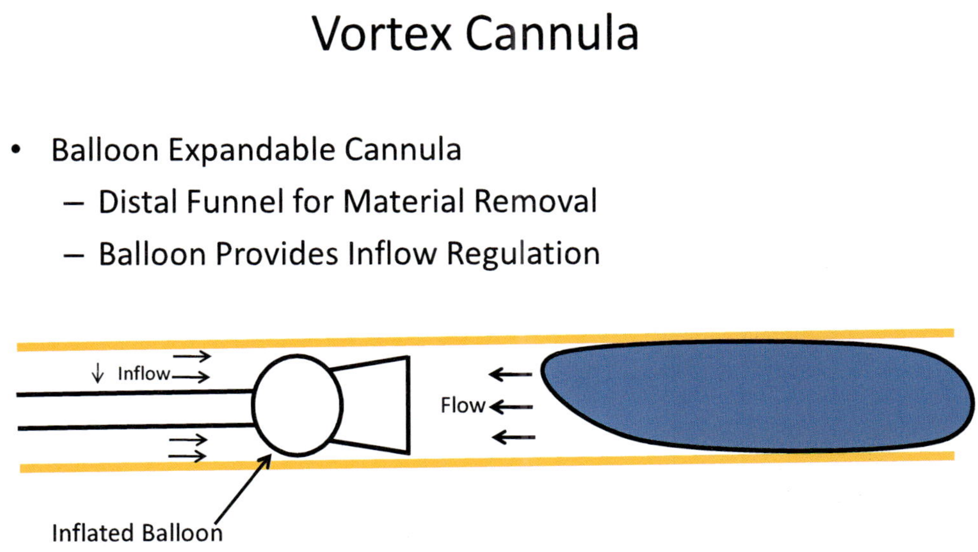

Fig. 2. Flow dynamics of the funnel drainage cannula

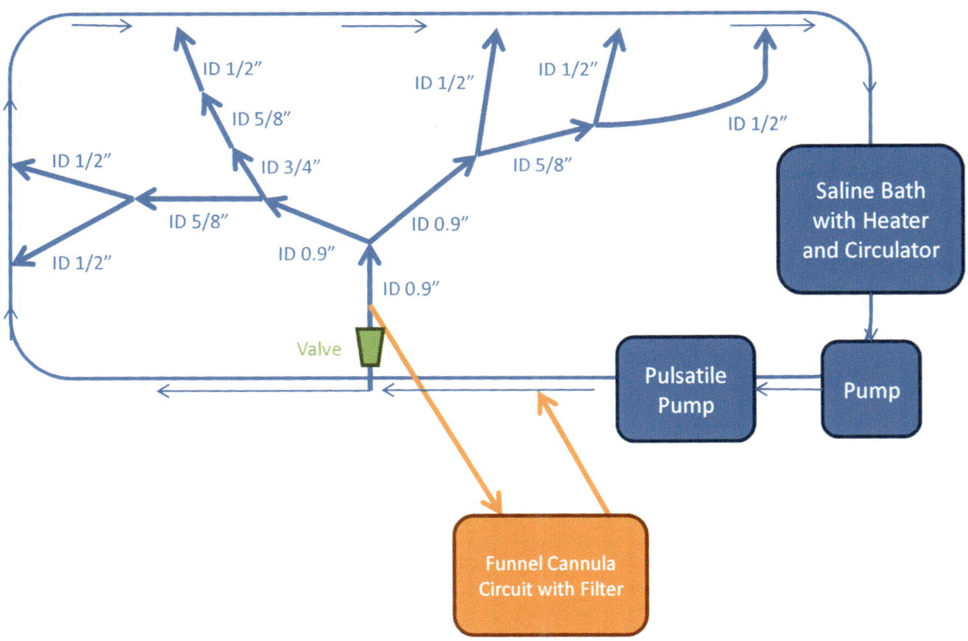

Fig. 3. Test fixture to evaluate the mechanics of the vacuum extraction process

3.4.4 Results

At a separation distance of 11 cm between the tip of the funnel and the clot model, no movement of the clot was noted with the valve closed completely, at all pump flow rates increased to a maximum of 6 liters per minute. Advancement of the funnel cannula to the proximity of the clot model, at 5 cm of separation, allowed extraction at 4.6 liters per minute of pump flow rate. With the valve completely open, allowing ample backflow, the clot model was extracted at a separation distance of 11 cm with a pump flow rate of 2.5 liters per minute. When the valve was 80% closed, clot extraction did not occur at 11 cm; however, removal was observed at 5 cm of separation distance at a pump flow rate of 6 liters per minute.

3.4.5 Clinical experience

Between December 2009 and May 2011, a total of 49 patients underwent removal of undesirable intravascular material using the funnel-tipped venous drainage cannula under extracorporeal veno-venous bypass. Procedures were conducted both in the fluoroscopy suite, and in the surgical theater under C-arm guidance. Veno-occlusive states addressed by these procedures included the following: (1) A retained segment of fibrin sheath from a pacemaker lead was extracted from the right atrium of a patient. (2) Vegetation was removed from the tricuspid valve of a patient who developed endocarditis from an indwelling line. (3) Thrombus and tumor was removed from a patient with an inferior vena cava occlusion due to a retroperitoneal malignancy. (4) A saddle embolus was removed from a patient with pulmonary embolism. (5) Organized and soft thrombus was removed from a patient presenting with bilateral iliofemoral and inferior vena cava occlusion. IVC thrombosis and pulmonary embolism accounted for the majority of the procedures, 43% and 29%, respectively. Seven patients had right atrial thrombus removed via suction embolectomy; in four of these patients, the thrombus extended up into the superior vena cava, and cannulation of the the SVC was required to remove the occluding clot. Four patients had vegetative endocarditic masses removed from their right atria. Several representative procedures may be detailed as follows:

Example 1:

A 63 year old female presented with severe bilateral lower extremity edema, bordering on phlegmasia cerulean dolens. She had an inferior vena cava filter placed two weeks previously for deep venous thrombosis, and her history is also significant for a recent neurosurgical procedure. The patient's situation was additionally complicated by a documented history of heparin induced thrombocytopenia. A venogram demonstrated complete IVC thrombosis extending proximal to the IVC filter and involving both iliofemoral systems distally (Figure 4).

Thrombolytic therapy was contraindicated in this patient, due to the recent neurosurgical procedure and the history of heparin induced cytopenia. Rheolytic thrombectomy, applied in an attempt to recanalize the vena cava and distal venous circulation, was unsuccessful. The patient was brought back to the fluoroscopy suite, where the suction funnel cannula was inserted through a 26F introducer sheath via a percutaneous right femoral vein entry site. Upon establishment of flow via the centrifugal pump, a large amount of fresh and organized thrombus was retrieved in the filter. The suction cannula was advanced into the vena cava, as well as the contralateral iliac vein. Two full filter canisters of occluding material, totaling 180 cc in volume, was removed from the patient (Figure 5). In addition, the

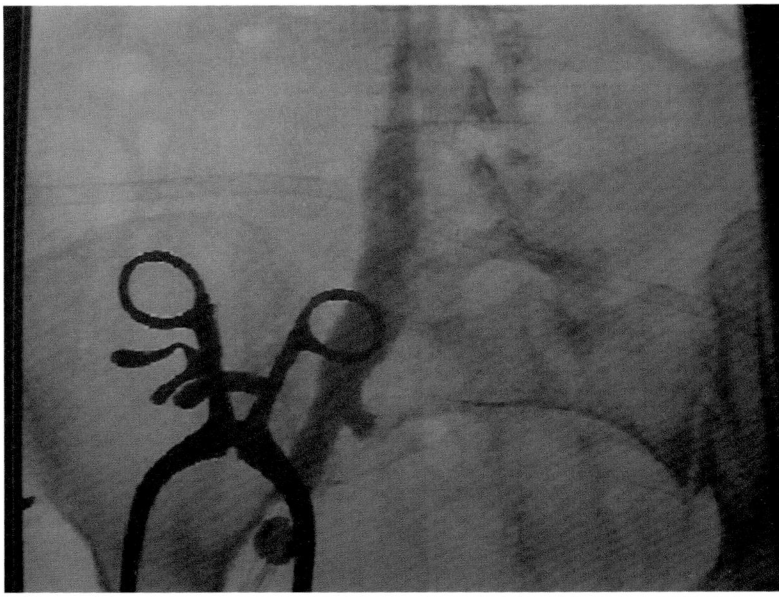

Fig. 4. Venogram depicting complete IVC thrombosis

previously placed IVC filter was removed through the central lumen of the suction cannula, while the extracorporeal circulation was maintained to prevent distal embolization from occurring during vena caval filter retrieval. Upon completion of the embolectomy procedure, a new IVC filter was placed. The post-extraction venogram showed a widely patent IVC and iliofemoral vasculature (Figure 6). The patient remained stable throughout the procedure. The procedure was conducted under administration of intravenous Bivalirudin (Angiomax®, The Medicines Company, Parsippany, NJ), due to the patient history of heparin induced thrombocytopenia.

Example 2:

A 40kg 23 year old female on renal dialysis via an indwelling right subclavian catheter, with a history of end stage renal disease and a failed renal transplant, presented with chest pain. She was found to have an embolus in a distal lobar branch of the left pulmonary artery, and an echocardiogram and CT scan revealed a fluttering clot at the distal tip of the subclavian catheter, and a 3 cm sessile mass on the free wall of the right atrium (Figure 7). Suction embolectomy was performed under general anesthesia in the operating room under echocardiographic guidance. Due to the small stature of the patient and subsequent limited caliber of her vasculature, the left and right femoral veins were exposed via open groin incisions. The 22F funnel cannula was introduced directly into the right femoral venotomy, and a 17F cannula placed into the left femoral vein for reinfusion. The funnel cannula was advanced into the right atrium and positioned in proximity to the subclavian catheter. Flow was initiated with the centrifugal pump, and chronic thrombotic material trapped by the filter. The subclavian dialysis catheter was removed, and the cannula advanced into the superior vena cava while circulating flow was maintained. A large amount of organized thrombus was noted in the filter (Figure 8). The echocardiogram showed removal of all

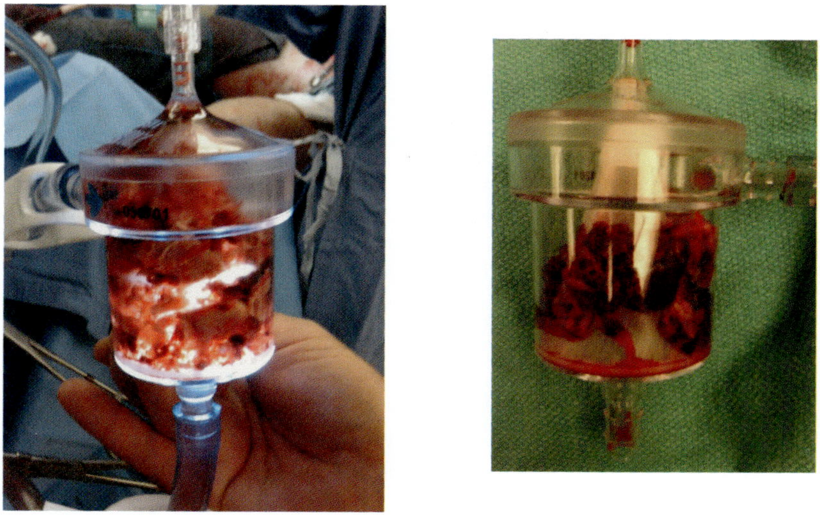

Fig. 5. Thrombotic material captured in two filters

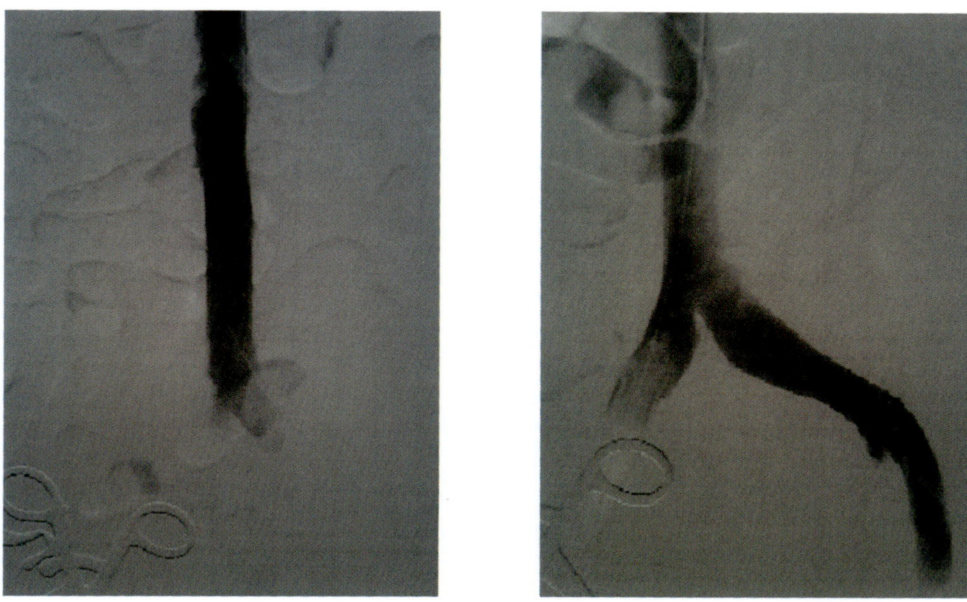

Fig. 6. Completion venogram demonstrating recanalization of the IVC and iliac veins

mobile thrombus, and a patent proximal superior vena cava (Figure 9). The sessile mass remained attached to the wall of the right atrium; no additional attempts were made to detach this immobile mass. A new dialysis catheter was placed, and the patient was discharged from the hospital under anticoagulation.

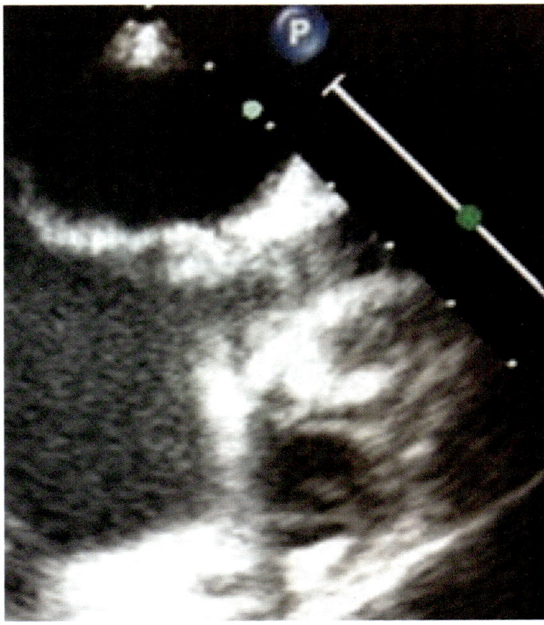

Fig. 7. Echocardiogram depicting mobile thrombus and sessile mass in the right atrium

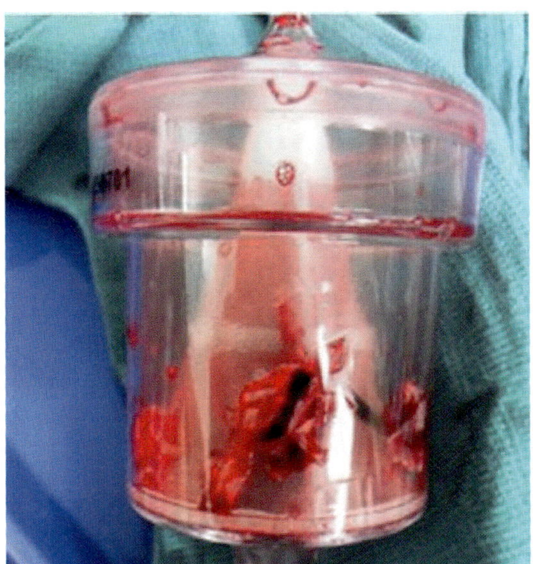

Fig. 8. Organized thrombus extracted from right atrium and superior vena cava

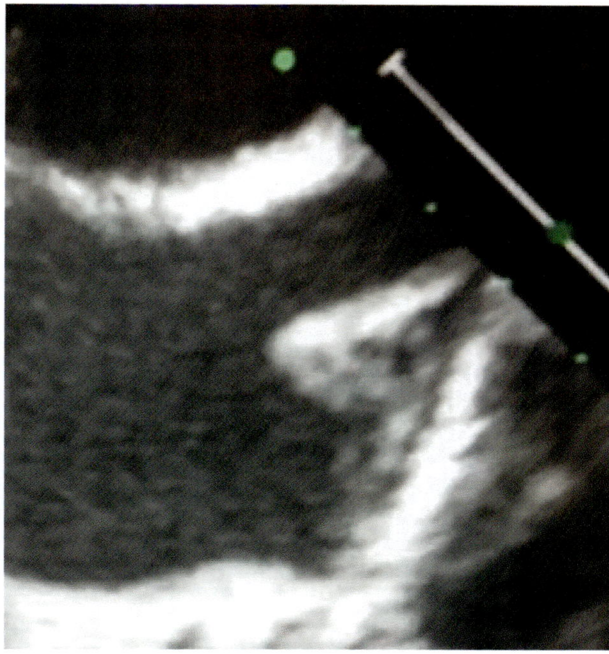

Fig. 9. Post extraction echocardiogram depicting absence of mobile thrombus

3.4.6 Clinical results

Of the 49 total patients in this series, 27 patients were male, and 22 female. The average age of the male patients was 53 years with a range between 27 and 88 years, and the average age of the female patients was 51 years, with a range between 19 and 82 years. Twelve of the procedures were performed in a totally percutaneous manner, while thirty-seven procedures were performed via surgical exposure of the femoral veins. Success of an extraction procedure is defined as removal of occluding material, fluoroscopic or echocardiographic evidence of venous patency, and stabilization of patient hemodynamic parameters. Forty of the forty-nine procedures resulted in removal of intravascular material for an 80% overall success rate. In 9 cases, minimal or no material was removed. In one case, spontaneous fragmentation and distal embolization of the thrombus occurred prior to initiation of the suction embolectomy procedure. One perioperative death occurred in a hemodialysis patient with a right atrial mass and an inferior vena cava occlusion. Hemothorax from a suspected guidewire perforation of the right atrium was noted during the procedure. The patient was brought to the operating room, and surgical exploration found a substantial fibrotic mass encasing the right atrium and inferior vena cava, preventing cannulation for cardiopulmonary bypass. The patient survived the surgery, but succumbed within 48 hours in the intensive care unit. No hemolysis or thrombocytopenia was observed in any of the patients in this study, and the patients' hematocrit values remained stable post procedure.

3.4.7 Discussion

The propensity for clot to propagate as well as to organize renders treatment of thromboembolic disease difficult. Anticoagulation addresses further propagation of thrombus; however, once a patient presents with a significant mass of clot, vascular recanalization becomes a formidable task. Complete occlusions in major or great venous vessels tend to be unresponsive to thrombolytic therapy, as circulating thrombolytic agents are unable to access the inner mass of a substantial body of clot that typifies massive pulmonary embolism or total vena cava occlusion. Thrombolytic dissolution occurs at the periphery of the occlusion, proceeding progressively inwards with time. Hemodynamic instability may curtail the opportunity window for therapeutic intervention, and immediate bulk extraction of occlusive material is warranted. Percutaneous interventional devices utilizing mechanical or rheolytic fragmentation of clot increase the rate of thrombolysis. Dissolution is a function of the amount of interaction achieved by the device with the clot. Higher surface contact area between the active components of the device and resident clot yields greater thrombolytic activity. Presently available percutaneous devices are limited by their size relative to clot in the great vessels. The luminal cross-sectional area of a 7F catheter is equal to 3 mm^2, which encompasses 0.5% of the surface area of a 30 mm diameter inferior vena cava or pulmonary artery with a luminal cross-sectional area of 615 mm^2. This means that a 7F catheter approaching an occluding thrombus in the vena cava contacts only 0.5% of the cross-sectional area of a clot on a single pass. An impractical number of catheter passes would be required to clear a total occlusion in the great vessels.

The large bore of the funnel cannula facilitates material removal from the great vessels. The large conduit size also minimizes the potential for hemolysis during vacuum extraction. Suction therapy is conducted by a centrifugal pump which generates typical flow rates up to 5 liters per minute via the 22 F cannula. At this flow rate and cannula size, laminar flow is maintained in the extracorporeal circuit, providing atraumatic passage for circulating erythrocytes.

4. Conclusion

Removal of undesirable intravascular material using extracorporeal recirculation with a funnel venous drainage cannula seeks to mimic surgical removal of massive emboli, by maximizing physical contact with the leading edge of the occlusion, and conducting en bloc removal of substantial embolic masses. The significant flow rates (on the order of 4 or 5 liters per minute) established in the drainage cannula while extracting major emboli, are matched by simultaneous reinfusion to maintain hemodynamic stability during the embolectomy process. A funnel cannula tip that matches the size of the occluded vessel and a high circulating flow rate are necessary elements to facilitate embolectomy. Bench top tests indicate that backflow must be present to support the level of pump flow rate that generates vacuum sufficient to remove large masses. In some of the procedures that yielded little or no material extraction, it is possible that a lack of backflow was exhibited due to absent or severely limited retrograde collateralization. Guidewire or angiographic catheter passage through the thrombotic substrate may yield partial recanalization that provides the requisite degree of retrograde flow for successful embolic removal. Another cause of unsuccessful extraction may be an advanced degree of fibrotic attachment associated with aged thrombus that is not amenable to vacuum dislodgment. Further clinical experience will delineate additional associated techniques and define best patient selection criteria for optimal application of vacuum extraction with the funnel cannula. The experience to date generates a sense of optimism that suction embolectomy with associated extracorporeal recirculation has potential as a functional therapeutic component in the battle against thromboembolic disease. Continued research into this and other approaches is certainly warranted.

5. References

Aklog, L., Williams, C., Byrne, J., & Goldhaber, S. (2002). Acute pulmonary embolectomy: A contemporary approach. *Circulation*, 105, (March 2002), pp. (1416-1419)

Almoosa, K. (2002). Is thrombolytic therapy effective for pulmonary embolism? *Am Fam Physician*, 65, (March 2002), pp. (1097-1102)

Andrews, R. (2004). Contrast peripheral phlebography and pulmonary angiography for diagnosis of thromboembolism. *Circulation*, 109[Suppl I], (March 2004), pp. (I-22-I-27)

Armstrong, W., Feigenbaum, H., & Dillon, J. (1985). Echocardiographic detection of right atrial thromboembolism. *Chest*, 87(6), (June 1985), pp. (801-806)

Athanasoulis, C., Kaufman, J., Halpern, E., Waltman, A., Geller, S., & Fan, C. (2000). Inferior vena caval filters: Review of a 26-year single-center clinical experience. (2000). *Radiology*, 216, (July 2000), pp. (54-66)

Banovac, F., Buckley D., Kuo, W., Lough D., Martin L., Millward S. Clark T., Kundu S., Rajan D., Sacks D., & Cardella J. (2010). Reporting standards for endovascular treatment of pulmonary embolism. *J Vasc Interv Radiol*, 21(1), (January 2010), pp. (44-53)

Barauskas, R., Gulbinas, A., & Baraskas, G. (2007). Investigation of radiofrequency ablation process in liver tissue by finite element modeling and experiment. *Medicina (Kaunas)*, 43(4), (April 2007), pp. (310-325)

Barritt, D., & Jordan, S. (1960). Anticoagulant drugs in the treatment of pulmonary embolism: a controlled trial. *Lancet*, 275 (7138), (June 1960), pp. (1309-1312)

Campbell, I., Bentley, D., Prescott, R., Rouytledge, P., Shetty H., & Williamson, I. (2007). Anticoagulation for three verasus six months in patients with deep vein thrombosis or pulmonary embolism, or both: randomized trial. *BMJ*, 334(7595), (March 2007), pp. (674-671)

Fernandez, L., & Geehan, D. (2008). Inferior vena cava thrombosis. In: *eMedicine General Surgery*, April 19, 2011, Available from http://emedicine.medscape.com/article/191103-print

Fogarty, T., Cranley, J., Krause, R., Strasser, E, & Hafner, C. (1963). A method for extraction of arterial emboli and thrombi. *Surg Gynecol Obstet*, 116, (February 1963), pp. (241-244)

Goldhaber, S. (1998). Integration of catheter thrombectomy into our armamentarium to treat acute pulmonary embolism. *Chest*, 114, (November 1998), pp. (1237-1238)

Gouge, S., Paulson, W., & Moore J. (1988). Inferior vena cava thrombosis due to an indwelling hemodialysis catheter. *Am J Kidney Dis*, 11(6), (June 1988), pp. (515-518)

Greenfield, L., Bruce, T., & Nichols, N. (1971). Transvenous pulmonary embolectomy by catheter device. *Ann Surg*, 174(6), (December 1971), pp. (881-886)

Greenfield, L., Proctor, M., Williams, D., & Wakefield, T. (1993). Long-term experience with transvenous catheter pulmonary embolectomy. *J Vasc Surg*, 18(3), (September 1993), pp. (450-458)

Harris, T., & Meek, S. (2005). When should we thrombolyse patients with pulmonary embolism? A systematic review of the literature. *Emerg Med J*, 22(11), (November 2005), pp. (766-771)

Heit, J. (2002) Venous thromboembolism epidemiology: implications for prevention and management. *Semin Thromb Hemost*, 28(Suppl 2),(June 2002), pp. (3-13)

Hirsh, J., & Hoak, J. (1996). Management of deep vein thrombosis and pulmonary embolism. *Circulation*, 93, (June 1996), pp. (2212-2245)

Kasper, W., Constantinides, S., Geibel, A., Olchewski, M., Heinrich, F., Grosser, K., Rauber, K., Iversen, S., Redecker, M., & Kienast, F. (1997). Management strategies and determinants of outcome in acute major pulmonary embolism: Results of a multicenter registry. *J Am Coll Cardiol*, 30, (November 1997), pp. (1165-1171)

Khurana, A., & Tak, T. (2004). Venous thromboembolic disease presenting as inferior vena cava thrombus extending into the right atrium. *Clinical Medicine & Research*,2(2), (May 2004), pp. (125-127)

Krug, H., & Zerbe, F. (1980). Major venous thrombosis: a complication of transvenous pacemaker electrodes. *Br Heart J*, 44,(August, 1980), pp.(158-61)

Kucher, N., Rossi, E.,De Rosa, M., & Goldhaber, S. (2006). Massive pulmonary embolism. *Circulation*, 113(4), (January 2006), pp. (577-582)

Kuchar, N. (2007). Catheter embolectomy for acute pulmonary embolism. *Chest*, 132, (August 2007), pp. (657-663)

Lohr, J., Kerr T, Lutter, K., Cranley, R., Spirtoff, K, & Cranley, J. (1991). Lower extremity calf thrombosis: To treat or not to treat? *J Vasc Surg*, 14(5), (November 1991), pp. (618-623)

Lopez J., Kearon C., & Lee A. (2004). Deep venous thrombosis. *Proceedings of American Society of Hematology*, San Diego, California, (December 2004), pp. (439 - 464)

Mulvihill, S., & Fonkalsrud E. (1984). Complications of superior versus inferior vena cava occlusion in infants receiving central total parenteral nutrition. *J Pediatr Surg*, 19(6), (December 1984), pp. (752-757)

Nahimyak, V., Yoon, S., & Holland, C. (2006). Acousto-mechanical and thermal properties of clotted blood. *J Acoust Soc Am*, 119(6), (June 2006), pp. (3766-3772)

Schreiber, D. (2010). Deep venous thrombosis and thrombophlebitis. In: *eMedicine Emergency Medicine*, March 27, 2011, Available from:
http://emedicine.medscape.com/article/1911303-overview

Siqueira-Filho, A., Kottke, B., & Miller W. (1976). Primary inferior vena cava thrombosis. *Arch Intern Med*,136(7), (July 1976), pp. (799-802)

Schmitz-Rode, T., Jannsens, U., Schild, H., Basche, S., Hanrath, P., & Gunther, R. (1998). Fragmentation of massive pulmonary embolism using a pigtail rotation catheter. Chest, 114, (November 1998), pp. (1427-1436)

Stein, P., Alnas, M., Beemath, A., & Patel, N. (2007). Outcome of pulmonary embolectomy. *Am J Cardiol*, 99(3), (February 2007), pp. (421-423)

Thabut, G., Thabut, D., Myers, R., Bernard-Chabert, B., Marrash-Chahla, R., Mal, H., & Fournier, M. (2002). Thrombolytic therapy of pulmonary embolism. *JACC*, 40(9), (November 2002), pp. (1660-1667)

Tibbutt, D., Davies J., Anderson, J., Fletcher, E., Hamill, J., Holt, J., Thomas, M., Lee, G., Miller G., Sharp, A., & Sutton, G. (1974). Comparison by controlled clinical trial of streptokinase and heparin in treatment of life-threatening pulmonary embolism. *BMJ*, 1, (March 1974), pp. (343-347)

Verstraete, M., Miller, G., Bounameaux, H., Charbonnier, B., Colle, J., Lecorf, G., Marbet, G., Mombaerts, P., & Olsson, C. (1988). Intravenous and intrapulmonary recombinant tissue-type plasminogen activator in the treatment of acute massive pulmonary embolism. *Circulation*, 77(2), (February 1988), pp. (353-360)

6

Conduit Selection for Improved Outcomes in Coronary Artery Bypass Surgery

Zane B. Atkins[1,2,*], Kristine V. Owen[3] and Walter G. Wolfe[1,2]
[1]*Department of Surgery, Veterans Affairs Medical Center Durham, NC*
[2]*Department of Surgery, Duke University Hospital Durham, NC*
[3]*Department of Medicine, Charles George Veterans Affairs Medical Center Asheville, NC*
USA

1. Introduction

Coronary artery bypass grafting (CABG) is one of the most studied operations in medical history, but many of the data forming the basis for clinical decisions in patients with coronary artery disease (CAD) were derived in the 1970s and 1980s, when the procedure and medical therapy were in their relative infancy. Advances in medical therapy (beta adrenergic blockers, thienopyridines, statins, and others), percutaneous coronary interventions (PCI), and surgical techniques have changed the decision making for patients with CAD. In addition, patient populations referred for surgery have changed since the original studies documenting advantages of CABG over other forms of therapy.

Since percutaneous transluminal coronary angioplasty (PTCA) was introduced, significant advances have been made in the percutaneous treatment of CAD. When drug-eluting stents (DES) were introduced in the early 2000s, many predicted the demise of CABG surgery. Enthusiasm for percutaneous treatment of CAD has most recently led to promoting PCI for unprotected left main coronary artery (LMCA) disease, an anatomical state typically reserved for CABG [1-3]. Percutaneous options have indelibly changed the face of CABG surgery and raise questions concerning the "gold standard" of care in coronary revascularization. For instance, recent reports document that patients referred for redo coronary artery surgery have declined, presumably due to the increased enthusiasm, possibly among surgeons themselves, for PCI in this setting [4]. Despite this, few studies have actually compared PCI with CABG. Two notable studies are recently available, both demonstrating advantages for CABG over PCI for left main CAD and/or three-vessel CAD [5, 6].

Concurrently, details pertaining to short-term outcomes of CABG have been questioned. For example, historical saphenous vein graft (SVG) patencies were reported as approximately 50% at 10 years [7]. However, several studies published in the mid-2000s indicate that early-term patencies of aorto-coronary SVG conduits are not as good as the historical figures that are still often quoted [8-10]. While the long-term patency and performance of the left internal mammary artery (LIMA) has not been questioned, the recent poor performance of

* Corresponding Author

SVG, coupled with increasing enthusiasm and demand for DES has lead to the emergence of "hybrid" coronary revascularization, typically consisting of LIMA-to-LAD and PCI of other coronary lesions. [11].

Coronary artery surgery itself has undergone several iterative changes recently. In the 1990s, great enthusiasm existed for the "mid-CAB" (minimally-invasive direct coronary artery bypass) procedure, an approach integral to "hybrid" revascularizations and primarily involving a small left anterior thoracotomy to harvest the LIMA and expose the left anterior descending [LAD] coronary artery. However, outside of the context of hybrid procedures, mid-CAB has had little widespread applicability, particularly since most patients referred for coronary surgery have multivessel disease. Introduction of mid-CAB procedures help usher in the era of off-pump CABG, which was heralded as an approach to reduce the risks associated with on-pump CABG, particularly myocardial dysfunction and cerebrovascular complications [12]. Finally, technology has introduced minimally invasive platforms for performing multi-vessel CABG, most recently the introduction of "totally endoscopic" and robotic CABG surgery [13]. However, it should be noted that these "improved techniques" continue to utilize the same conduit selection and comparative trials with objective evidence are lacking. Since minimally invasive strategies for CABG do not routinely incorporate changes to the operation known to improve short- and long-term results, there appears little reason to suspect that graft patency rates will be improved by less invasive procedures. Rather, one could argue that these alterations in approach to CABG are primarily based on industry involvement, public demands for less invasive procedures, and as marketing strategies by hospital systems.

Are there alternatives to CABG, which could improve long-term outcomes for graft patency and the composite of major adverse coronary events (MACE) particularly when compared with PCI? The answer is a resounding "yes," and it is found in arterial conduits for coronary bypass. CABG with multiple arterial grafts have been shown to have improved graft patency, reduced need for reoperation or reintervention, and prolonged survival compared with patients undergoing CABG with one IMA and SVG [14-17]. For instance, Sabik et al reviewed a 27-year experience at the Cleveland Clinic with regard to need for reintervention after primary CABG and found that the extent of arterial grafting correlated with freedom from subsequent reintervention [18]. Specifically, patients who received two IMA grafts at initial surgery had approximately 10% risk for reintervention at 10 years; those with one IMA had 20% risk; and those with no IMA had approximately 30% risk for reintervention at 10 years [18].

However, the surgical community has not fully utilized these assets despite numerous, compelling data [19-23]. Jones succinctly summarized the decision point facing conventional, open surgery in the face of rapidly advancing technologies, particularly PCI, and the impact on referral trends for surgical intervention: " improve the long-term outcome, lessen resources used, or both." [24]. Therefore, one important philosophic principle regarding use of multiple arterial conduits is that the focus is on the *long-term* results, not the short-term.

The purpose of this chapter is to review the data available for CABG with multiple arterial grafts including bilateral IMA use, radial artery, and other conduits. Finally, we will demonstrate the advantages of multiple arterial grafting and make the argument that this strategy yields superior long-term results compared to any strategy for coronary revascularization based on PCI or CABG with traditional conduit selection.

2. Percutaneous coronary interventions

PCI was introduced in 1977 and has undergone consistent improvements in technologies and approaches, offering a less invasive treatment modality for CAD [25]. With the introduction of DES in 2003, the percentage of CAD patients treated with PCI have increased consistently [26, 27]. However, recent studies evaluating long-term outcomes for DES have revealed increased morbidity and mortality secondary to late stent thrombosis [28-30]. While DES therapy has reduced need for target lesion reintervention [31, 32], there is a strict therapeutic requirement for dual anti-platelet therapy (DAPT). Current DAPT recommendations are for at least one year after DES therapy, but the ideal length of treatment still not yet known [33].

3. Comparing coronary bypass surgery and PCI

Shortly after the emergence of PCI as a reliable and durable therapy for CAD, comparisons between angioplasty and CABG were designed in order to determine the relative advantages of each modality. The BARI (Bypass Angioplasty Revascularization Investigation) trial compared balloon angioplasty with CABG in patients with multivessel CAD and severe angina or inducible coronary ischemia. After 5 and 10 years follow-up, no difference in long-term survival was demonstrated [34, 35]. Similar results were noted in other randomized trials of PTCA versus CABG [36, 37]. It was commonly noted in these trials that reintervention for recurrent angina symptoms was significantly more common for patients treated with an initial strategy of PTCA [BARI, RITA, GABI]. However, on subgroup analysis, survival advantage for CABG was demonstrated among diabetic patients in the BARI trial [35]. Finally, a meta-analysis of 13 randomized controlled trials comparing CABG with PTCA showed improved survival for CABG at 5-8 years in those with multivessel CAD and in diabetic patients [38].

Even as studies comparing PTCA with CABG were enrolling, bare-metal stents (BMS) were introduced, and trials to compare the new technology with CABG emerged. The randomized Stent or Surgery (SoS) trial compared multivessel CAD treatment by CABG or by PCI with BMS [39]. At a median follow-up of 2 years, these data showed reduced rates of coronary reintervention and significantly fewer deaths after CABG. Similar trials comparing CABG and PCI with BMS did not demonstrate a survival advantage for either therapy [40], although diabetic patients appeared to have improved survival after CABG in the Arterial Revascularization Therapies Study (ARTS 1) [41].

The US Food and Drug Administration approved DES therapy in 2003, stimulating another round of comparisons between CABG and PCI with the newer technology. Hannan et al reviewed risk-adjusted data from the NY State Dept of Health comparing patients who underwent CABG or PCI with DES for multivessel CAD over a 15-month period shortly after DES approval [5]. At a mean follow-up of 19 months, CABG patients experienced reduced hazard ratio for death, reduced mortality, reduced death/myocardial infarction composite, and less need for repeat revascularization [5]. However, the data were not acquired in the context of a randomized trial. Finally, the SYNTAX trial, a prospective randomized trial conducted across Europe and the US, compared PCI with DES and CABG in patients with 3-vessel CAD, left main CAD, or both [6]. The primary outcomes were major adverse cardiovascular or cerebrovascular events, and follow-up was provided for 12 months after intervention. The SYNTAX data demonstrated increased rates of MACE in the

PCI group, primarily related to the increased need for repeat intervention. Death and post-procedure MI were not significantly different between the two groups, but there was an increased stroke rate in the CABG group compared with PCI, which is somewhat offset by the fact that surgical patients were not managed with aggressive antiplatelet therapy as compared to the PCI group, and many of the cerebrovascular events occurred outside of the perioperative period. More recently, three-year follow up SYNTAX data were reported confirming advantages of CABG over PCI with regard to MACE. Unlike 12-month data, however, composite safety endpoints were no longer different between the two groups, including a similar stroke rate [42]. The SYNTAX authors concluded that CABG remains the preferred therapy for 3-vessel or left main CAD but recommend longer follow up, as is planned for an additional two years [6].

Despite the favorable data for CABG emanating from carefully designed and conducted randomized trials, rates of CABG referral have decreased consistently since the introduction of PCI with stent technologies [43]. Preference for PCI appears driven by disparate interpretation of PCI-versus-CABG studies, by strong patient preference for less invasive procedures with presumed lower periprocedural risk, and by the promise for faster recovery. As a result, the percentage of patients referred for CABG with previous PCI has increased steadily [44] with higher acuity relative to patients without previous intervention [45]. Additionally, technical details of CABG in current surgical practices are considered more challenging compared with previous eras due to more diffuse CAD, subjectively smaller distal coronary targets, particularly among diabetic patients, and the high incidence of prior PCI [46]. Consequently, contemporary results for CABG following PCI are characterized by worse perioperative outcomes when compared with CABG patients without previous intervention. For example, higher rates of postoperative mortality, MACE, and other perioperative complications following CABG in both diabetic and nondiabetic patients have been observed [47-50]. More importantly, increased mid-term mortality in diabetic patients with prior PCI has been observed after CABG [50], and Rao et al demonstrated increased long-term mortality in patients with prior PCI who subsequently underwent CABG [51].

4. Saphenous vein graft conduits

Reversed saphenous vein grafts (RSVG) have been utilized for CABG since the procedure's inception [52] and remain an important graft conduit option in the present era and in numerous clinical scenarios [53, 54]. Historically, patency rates of RSVG aorto-coronary artery grafts have been observed to be approximately 50-60% at 10 years [7, 55]. However, as previously noted, recent RSVG patency data are less encouraging [8-10]. For example, the PREVENT-IV study evaluated 3,000 patients undergoing CABG with 1-year routine angiographic follow-up. At this early time point, 30% of RSVG conduits were occluded and over 45% had "failed," as defined by ≥ 75% stenosis [10]. Importantly, study patients with vein graft failure had significantly increased rates of perioperative complications including MI, death or MI, or MACE relative to the cohort without vein graft complications [10]. Similar results have been noted elsewhere [56-59]. Additionally, surprisingly poor early-to-mid-term RSVG patency rates have been reported elsewhere. The Portland Endoscopic SVG Harvest Trial demonstrated 69% [8], patency by angiography at 6-months, while the PRAGUE 4 trial showed one-year RSVG patency of 52.5% [9]. The potential impact of poor vein graft performance cannot be overstated as RSVG failure is significant contributor to redo coronary surgery [60]. In addition, early vein graft failure is associated with increased perioperative myocardial infarction [10, 61], which consequently affects survival after CABG [58, 59].

Several potential explanations exist for the recently chronicled poor performance of RSVG as aorto-coronary conduits including early technical errors, endothelial injury, and early thrombosis, which may be related to insufficient biologic reaction to aspirin or inadequate antiplatelet effect of aspirin [62-64]. One important contributor to poor RSVG conduit performance, receiving significant recent attention, may be the practice of harvesting the conduit endoscopically (EVH). This technique was introduced and popularized in the 1990s and has been widely adopted due to increased incisional comfort and patient satisfaction, and decreased wound complications compared to open vein harvesting [65, 66] such that at least 70% of CABG patients undergo EVH based on recent Society of Thoracic Surgeons Database reporting [67]. However, EVH has been associated with increased endothelial injury, which may have significant negative consequences including graft patency and possibly long-term survival [68, 69]. Desai et al recently demonstrated using optical coherence tomography that EVH operators had a steep learning curve with regard to subtle RSVG injuries and that vein grafts with four or more intimal or medial dissections showed significantly worse early patency rates than those with fewer intimal injuries (67% vs. 96%) [70].

In contrast, when RSVGs are harvested using a "no touch" technique, better patency results have been noted. The "no touch" method avoids vein stripping, taking surrounding tissue, and avoids over-distending the vein conduit as it is being prepared for coronary anastomosis [71]. This has also been shown recently to preserve the venous vasa vasorum [72]. Perhaps this helps to explain differences in contemporary SVG patency rates versus those reported historically, which were always done by an open surgical technique. Other predictors of improved vein patency include grafting to the LAD coronary artery versus other target sites, smaller venous conduit size, and larger diameter target coronary artery. In contrast, young age and low EF reduced long-term patency [60]. The type of distal anastomosis (sequential, y- or t-grafts, or other composite grafts) did not affect long-term patency [60]. Based on these data, some suggest SVG from the calf/lower leg since size and possible thickness of the vein is better [60]. Additionally, EVH is more difficult to perform on the lower leg; therefore, programs committed to EVH likely neglect this potentially advantageous conduit.

Current surgical patient cohorts have also been implicated in reduced vein graft patencies. For example, it is generally accepted that contemporary patients referred for surgery are older and more medically complex [73]. For example, many patients referred for CABG are diabetic, a condition that is notorious for more complicated and diffuse CAD [46, 74]. In addition, it has been proposed that venous grafts in elderly may be of inferior quality relative to younger patients [75].

5. General advantages of arterial grafting

Several advantages to arterial grafting have been demonstrated relative to CABG without arterial grafts. Most notably, the LIMA-LAD graft has been shown to be an independent predictor of survival after CABG when compared with patients not receiving LIMA-LAD [76]. In addition, using more than one IMA graft reduces the need for subsequent reintervention and prolongs survival relative to patients receiving only one arterial grafts

[15, 17]. Similarly, Guru et al evaluated the potential benefit of multiple arterial grafting in over 53,000 patients undergoing primary CABG between 1991 and 2001. After propensity matching, patients receiving ≥ 2 arterial grafts had decreased rates of cardiac readmission and reduced incidence of the composite of cardiac readmission, death, and repeat revascularization relative to those with ≤ one arterial grafts [23]. Furthermore, patients receiving ≥ 2 arterial grafts had improved survival compared with patients receiving only one arterial graft [23]. Similar findings were reported by Nasso, et al, who found no differences at 2 years between groups receiving RA, in-situ RIMA, or free RIMA as the 2nd arterial graft, although each of these groups was superior to patients receiving only one arterial graft (LIMA-LAD) with respect to cardiac event-free survival [77]. Zacharias et al also demonstrated advantages of RA grafting as a 2nd arterial conduit on long-term survival when compared to RSVG conduits [14].

In addition, multiple arterial grafts and their arrangements in all coronary distributions have been proven superior to venous grafts with regard to long term patency regardless of the anatomic details of the native coronary and distal anastomosis [55]. These results are particularly applicable in the context of recurrent angina [16, 55, 78]. Finally, perhaps one of the best recent demonstrations of the advantages of arterial grafting over RSVG conduits was provided by Gaudino et al, who studied 60 CAD patients who had previously undergone PCI and developed in-stent restenosis. After undergoing CABG, patients receiving IMA and RA grafts had patency rates of 90% while those undergoing RSVG had patency rates of 50% at a mean follow-up of 52 months [79].

5.1 Total arterial revascularization

Since SVG conduits inevitably fail, particularly late [62], there has been increased enthusiasm for total arterial revascularization for CABG. Total arterial revascularization may obviate the concerns of vein graft failure and has been shown to have good short-term results [80]. However, little evidence is available to suggest that outcomes are improved with "all-arterial" grafting [81]. Zacharias et al have recently demonstrated that patients with multi-vessel CAD undergoing all-arterial grafting had improved 12-year survival compared with matched patients who underwent standard CABG with LIMA-LAD and RSVG to other distal targets [82]. Furthermore, complete coronary revascularization and use of all-arterial grafting strategy was associated with improved 12-year survival [82, Figure].

It has been estimated that all-arterial grafting is possible in 90% of patients using various conduits and their configurations [55], and even patients with advanced age have been shown to benefit from all-arterial revascularization strategies in terms of freedom from recurrent coronary events and improved graft patency [83].

6. Bilateral internal mammary artery conduits

In the 1980s, the LIMA-to-LAD graft was shown to be an independent predictor of improved short- and long-term results when used as a conduit for CABG compared to RSVG-only grafting [76]. Unequivocal advantages of the LIMA-LAD graft include prolonged survival relative to use of RSVG to LAD, reduced rates of recurrent angina, reduced postoperative MI and other ischemic events, and decreased need for coronary reintervention [76, 84]. The superiority of the LIMA in comparison to other CABG conduits

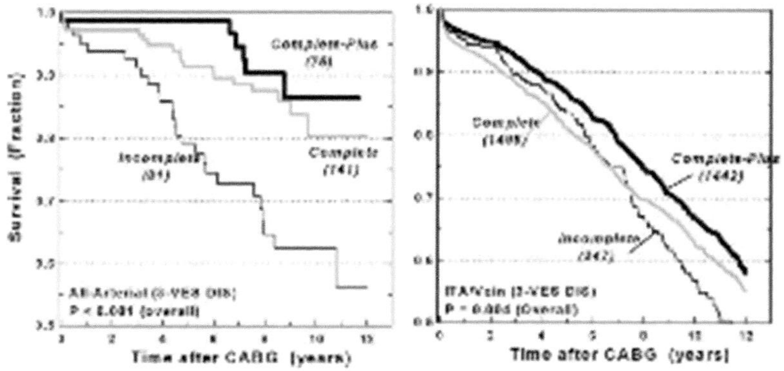

Fig. 1. Effects of completeness of revascularization on 12-year old Kaplan-Meier survival in triple-vessel disease (3-Ves Dis) patients. (Left) All-arterial patients. (Right) Internal thoracic artery/saphenous vein (ITA/Vein) patients. Incomplete - completeness of revascularization index (CRI) less than 1, or 2 grafts; complete CRI equal to 1, or 3 grafts; complete plus - CRI greater than 1, or 4 or more grafts. All p values by log-rannk (Mantel-Cox) test. (CABG - coronary artery bypass graft surgery.)

may be related to its unique freedom from arteriosclerosis and due to the rich run-off bed provided by the LAD coronary and its branches [85]. Since there is no basis for suggesting or concluding that the biological and mechanical properties of the right IMA are different from the LIMA, successes with the LIMA have prompted investigation of the potential benefits of bilateral IMA (BIMA) grafting.

The original description of BIMA for CABG is credited to Kay in 1969 [86]. Since then, multiple centers including our own have investigated the impact of BIMA grafting on long-term results of CABG. Advantages of BIMA have been somewhat difficult to prove definitively without randomized controlled trials in this area, which have not been conducted secondary to cost concerns and administrative requirements associated with studies inherently requiring significant longitudinal follow-up [87]. Instead, investigation and documentation of BIMA benefits have relied on evaluating institutionally maintained observational databases to show differences between the "treatment group" and the "control group" by way of propensity matching [87]. Analysis of these data show improved long-term results for patients receiving BIMA grafting as compared with single IMA grafting. However, survival curves do not separate until several years postoperatively, which has been a consistent finding [15, 88, 89; Figure]. The demonstrated clinical advantages of BIMA grafting strategies include prolonged survival and reduced need for coronary reintervention on the basis of recurrent myocardial ischemia, including freedom from the need for coronary reintervention [15, 88, 90] which hold true for women as well as for men, where it has been demonstrated that use of BIMA had 3-fold improved cardiac-related survival compared with patients who did not receive an IMA graft [91].

Reported rates of BIMA use in CABG range from 4.0% to nearly 50% depending upon several factors including the contributing authors' practice preferences and the particular patient cohort treated [19-22, 92]. However, it has been estimated that up to 80% would be candidates for BIMA grafting [93]. Subjective and potential obstacles to BIMA use include increased surgical times, increased technical challenges, especially related to the positioning

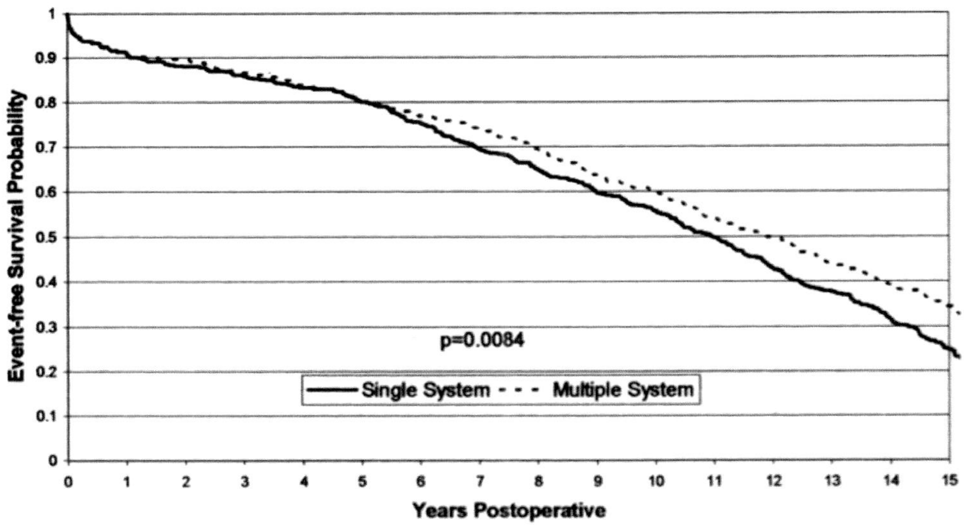

Fig. 2.

of the non-LIMA-to-LAD graft, and increased rates of sternal wound complications relative to patients with one or less IMAs harvested [94]. After 10 years of experience with BIMA CABG, Gansera et al noted increased OR and aortic cross clamp times among BIMA patients compared with single IMA CABG patients. In addition, patients receiving BIMA grafting had higher rates of bleeding requiring postoperative mediastinal reexploration (2.9% vs. 0.6%) along with increased rates of wound complications [95]. However, they also noted that nearly one full additional distal graft was completed when both IMAs were used and, most importantly, BIMA grafting was associated with improved 30-day survival, particularly among diabetic patients, compared with only one IMA graft. [95]. In this same study, a grafting strategy not incorporating 2 IMA conduits was an independent predictor of *perioperative* mortality, directly disputing biases that BIMA grafting is associated with increased perioperative complications [95]. Similarly, Kurlansky et al reviewed their collective experience with more than 4,500 consecutive CABG procedures (2,369 single IMA; 2,215 BIMA) and demonstrated that hospital mortality was significantly reduced among patients undergoing BIMA grafting compared with controls [92].

Nevertheless, selection of patients for BIMA grafting should be performed cautiously, particularly when performing surgery through a standard median sternotomy incision. This is primarily related to the well-demonstrated risk for sternal wound infection after BIMA grafting in patients with diabetes, obesity, and other comorbidities [96-100]. However, BIMA grafting can be performed safely without significant increased risk for sternal wound infection as has been frequently demonstrated [24, 98, 100, 101]. For example, Jones et al reviewed their experience with 500 consecutive patients undergoing BIMA CABG over an 11-year period, excluding only those with proximal coronary stenoses <70% and emergency cases with HD instability. Nevertheless, the reported rates of perioperative complications were low: operative mortality was 1.8%; deep sternal wound infections were 1%; and 1.8% had take back for bleeding. Incredibly, only 2 patients out of the 500 required reoperation for myocardial ischemia in the follow-up period. [24]. Interestingly, however, Jones et al point out that if strict criteria for selecting patients for BIMA grafting had been used, nearly 70% of patients in their series would have been excluded [24].

As noted previously, RSVG conduits for CABG have not been compared directly to DES, but comparisons of BIMA grafting with a strategy primarily employing DES for coronary revascularization do exist [102, 103]. After matching for multiple comorbidities, significantly improved angina, reduced need for reintervention, and improved reintervention-free survival at one year have been observed among patients undergoing BIMA CABG relative to PCI [102]. In a similar study, Locker et al examined BIMA CABG versus PCI in diabetic patients and demonstrated more complete coronary revascularization, improved angina, reduced need for reintervention, and increased cardiovascular event-free survival (80% vs. 30%, $p < 0.001$) in patients undergoing BIMA CABG [103]. More importantly, 6-year survival among patients with left main CAD or 3-vessel CAD was significantly better with BIMA revascularization, providing rare evidence for superiority of multiple arterial grafting strategy relative to PCI [103].

One controversial and often-debated point concerning BIMA CABG relates to the native coronary artery planned as a target for the second (right) IMA. Initial opinion considered best results of BIMA CABG to occur when the RIMA was grafted to the "next most" important coronary bed angiographically, assuming that LIMA to LAD was nearly always performed [104]. Schmidt et al found that multiple left-sided grafts lead to improved survival relative to a cohort of patients in which the RIMA was placed to the right coronary artery distribution along with LIMA-LAD grafting [104]. However, it should be noted that graft patency was quite good in both groups (91.7 % vs. 89.6%), as was survival, and freedom from heart failure, angina and need for reintervention [104]. They argued that maximum long-term benefit from BIMA grafting is realized when the 2nd IMA is placed to the coronary distribution subtending the most amount of viable myocardium, which was most commonly the circumflex artery distribution.

The requirement for the 2nd IMA targeted to the left coronary system has been refuted by other data. Analysis of Cleveland Clinic data shows that benefits of BIMA CABG are similar regardless of the recipient coronary artery for the 2nd IMA graft [89]. Sabik et al found that risk-adjusted and unadjusted outcomes did not differ between a strategy for the 2nd IMA going to the right coronary or the circumflex coronary artery territory, but several important caveats are applicable, particularly with regard to the right coronary artery if the RIMA is to be used as an in situ graft to this coronary distribution. For instance, the distal RCA should be free of disease, and the proximal RCA stenosis should be $\geq 70\%$ in diameter to avoid competitive native coronary flow, which may be detrimental to IMA patency. Finally, distal viable myocardium should be ensured [105]. More recently, Kurlansky et al reviewed their experience in over 2,200 consecutive patients who underwent BIMA grafting. In 2/3 of patients, the 2nd IMA was placed to the left coronary system, while in 1/3 of patients, the 2nd IMA was placed to the right coronary system. Incredibly, 98% of patients had complete coronary revascularization performed with in-situ arterial configurations, that is, avoiding free IMA utilization. At a mean follow-up of nearly 13 years, long-term survival was no different between groups [106, Figure].

Gansera et al recently described their strategy for with BIMA versus single IMA in which the RIMA was usually directed anteriorly and to the left as pedicled conduit for the LAD, while the LIMA was typically directed for revascularization of the lateral wall (circumflex artery distribution) [95]. Importantly, RIMA crossover grafts to the LAD coronary system appear to have patency rates that are not different from LIMA-LAD configurations [107]. In

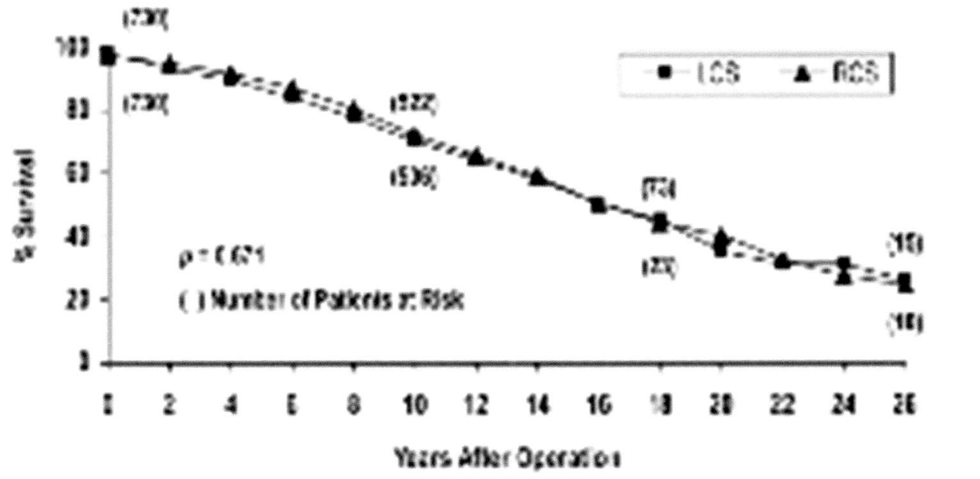

Fig. 3. Actuarial survival of optimally matched patients who underwent coronary artery bypass grafting to the left coronary system (LCS [boxes]) and the right coronary system (RCS [triangles]). Number of patients at risk is in parentheses; results are mean = standard error of the mean.

fact, Chow et al reported that RIMA patency was similar to LIMA patency regardless of the coronary distribution to which the artery was grafted [108]. However, a "crossover" configuration for the RIMA places the RIMA-LAD graft at significant risk for injury during subsequent redo sternotomy (as potentially required for aortic valve replacement or other procedures). Consequently, when performing this procedure, we often apply a protective barrier to the mediastinum prior to sternal closure (Repel-CV, SyntheMed, Inc., Iselin, NJ, USA) and often reapproximate the thymic remnant to protect the RIMA-LAD graft [108].

Therefore, the specific BIMA configuration doesn't seem to affect MACE, graft patency, or morbidity/mortality outcomes [110]. Glineur et al evaluated BIMA grafting with both IMA grafts targeted to the left coronary system in either an in-situ or Y-graft configuration, noting equivalent patencies and other mid-term results. In addition, the T-graft configuration has been shown to be safe and effective in grafting multiple distal coronary targets [111].

Most results with BIMA grafting are improved by harvesting the conduit as a "skeletonized" graft rather than as a pedicled graft, in which the accompanying mammary veins and surrounding chest wall muscle and fascia were mobilized along with the artery. Skeletonized IMA harvesting preserves sternal perfusion relative to pedicled IMA harvesting [112, 113]. As a result, skeletonized IMA harvesting is associated with reduced sternal wound complications and longer IMA graft length, allowing more distal coronary targets to be bypassed [Figure, 92, 98, 100]. Skeletonized IMAs also have increased blood flow through the conduit [114], possible as the result of decreased spasm, since skeletonized IMA is typically accomplished without the need for electrocautery on the chest wall [100, 106, 115].

7. Radial artery

Professor Alain Carpentier is credited with introducing the radial artery (RA) as an alternative conduit for CABG [116], but initial results with the RA were unfavorable, leading Carpentier and others to abandon its use. Subsequently, several RA grafts were empirically observed to be patent at follow-up coronary angiography, leading to the concept's reintroduction in the late 1980s [117]. Since then, the RA has since been widely used and aggressively investigated as a conduit option for CABG due to ease of use, availability in at least 90% of patients, good length allowing reach to any distal target for anastomosis, and it is amenable to concurrent harvesting methods (the IMA, SVG, and RA can be harvested simultaneously) [118]. Depending upon the details of RA grafting, including the target coronary bed and the proximal degree of coronary artery stenosis, long-term RA graft patency approaches 90% and can approximate that of pedicled IMA graft patencies [55, 119, 120].

Since most coronary grafting strategies employing RA grafts do so to evaluate alternatives to SVG conduits, numerous trials comparing RA with SVG for patency and long-term outcomes have been conducted recently [14, 78, 121-123]. In general, these data demonstrate equivalent or improved patency for the RA compared with SVG. One recent randomized controlled trial in the US Veterans Affairs system evaluated RA and SVG as coronary bypass grafts to the "best remaining recipient vessel," with the primary end point of one-year angiographic patency [123]. These data demonstrated equivalent graft patencies for RA compared with SVG, but one-year patency for both groups approached 90% [123]. This is in line with many previous reports on early RA patency, and far exceeds other recent estimations of early graft SVG patency for [8-10]. In contrast, the Radial Artery Versus Saphenous Vein Patency (RSVP) trial compared 5-year graft patency for RA versus SVG when placed to circumflex coronary artery branches that were at least 70% stenotic [121]. These data demonstrated a significantly improved patency for RA grafts (98.3%) relative to SVG grafts (86.4%) [122].

Perhaps the most recognized comparison of RA and SVG is provided by the Radial Artery Patency Study (RAPS), which randomized 561 patients at 13 centers (Canada, New Zealand) to receive a RA graft to the right coronary system or the circumflex coronary system [78]. Saphenous vein grafts were placed to the coronary system not receiving the RA graft, and all patients underwent LIMA-LAD grafting. One-year angiographic follow-up was performed in 440 patients and demonstrated significantly improved patency for RA grafts compared with SVG (91.8% vs. 86.4%, $p = 0.009$). However, angiographic "string sign" was significantly increased in RA grafts compared with SVG (7% vs. 0.9%, $p = 0.001$) [78]. It is unclear as to the long-term significance of this finding; as Carpentier originally noted, others have since reported that patency of the RA graft with a "string sign" may actually improve as the native disease worsens [124]. When patient characteristics and target vessel characteristics were considered in the interpretation of the RAPS data, RA grafts were protective of graft patency by multivariable analysis, while smaller distal targets, less proximal coronary artery stenosis, and diabetes were associated with reduced patency rates for SVG or RA grafts [125]. Graft occlusion was significantly more common among diabetics with SVG (19%) compared with RA grafts in diabetics (12%). In fact, RA grafting conferred even greater protection effect from graft occlusion was among diabetic patients than in the study cohort as a whole [125].

Despite the positive comparisons of RA with SVG patency rates, it has been more difficult to ascribe improved clinical outcomes with RA versus SVG [126]. However, some data suggest that better long-term survival is seen in those receiving RA conduits as compared with SVG (Figure). Zacharias et al evaluated the influence of RA and SVG as a 2nd graft (all patients receiving LIMA-LAD) with regard to survival in 2 groups of 925 matched patients each [14]. 6-year survival was improved in RA patients [14, Figure.].

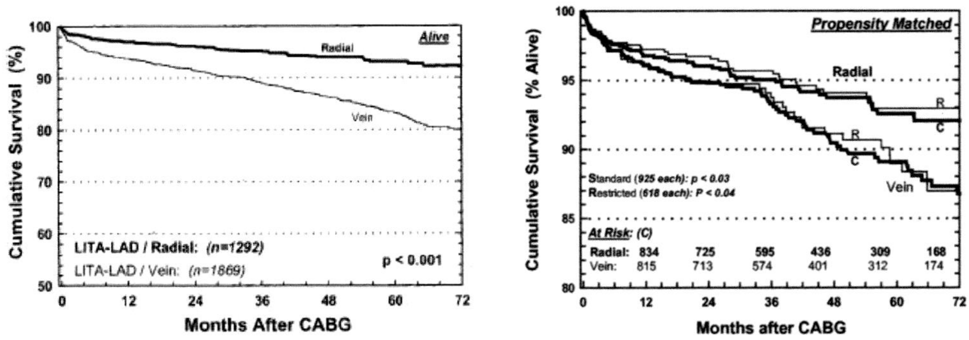

Fig. 4.

Similar data have been reported by Tranbaugh et al, who compared over 800 patients undergoing CABG utilizing LIMA, RA, and SVG with matched patients undergoing CABG with LIMA and SVG only [127]. They showed significantly improved survival in the RA group in addition to improved patency of RA as compared to SVG (81% vs. 47%) in symptomatic patients who subsequently underwent diagnostic angiography after CABG (mean time to repeat catheterization 4.3 years) [127]. Importantly, RA use emerged as independent predictor of survivalat 14 years when the data were assessed by multivariable analysis [127, Figure].

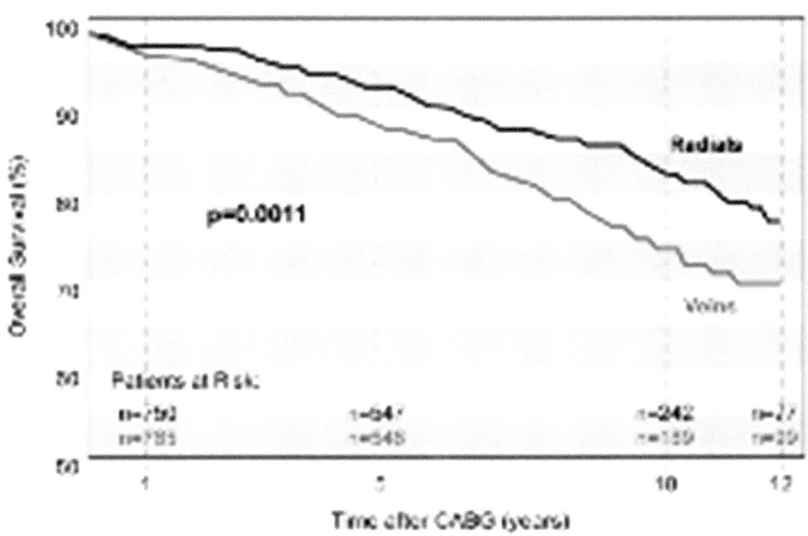

Fig. 5. Comparison of Kaplan-Meier survival for propensity-matched patents (p - 0.0011, log rank test), CABG - coronary artery bypass graft surgery.

Conduct of these well-designed trials incorporating angiographic follow-up of RA grafts has provided a wealth of insight into features important to successful RA grafting. For example, as noted, early graft failures in the form of "string sign" have been noted in randomized trials [78], and several explanations for this are possible. For example, RA grafts appear notoriously susceptible to competitive flow within the native coronary circulation, as may occur when native coronary stenosis is not severe (≤ 70%) [128, 129]. Based on this frequent observation, use of the RA is not recommended as a conduit for CABG unless the native coronary artery stenosis is high grade (≥ 70%). This strategy has been associated with improved patency and reduced "string sign" in the RAPS study [78]. Radial artery graft patency is also dependent upon coronary target location, as has been noted for the RIMA graft [89]. For instance, Maniar et al found that grafts to the right coronary artery were more likely to be occluded compared with those placed to the LAD or to the circumflex coronary artery [129], which has been corroborated by others [130].

Certain inherent, unique characteristics of the RA may also contribute to "string sign" formation [131]. Limb arteries such as the RA are known to be more prone to spasm than somatic (IMA) or splanchnic arteries [132]. One key difference between the IMA and the RA is that the RA is significantly more muscular, leading to increased tendency for spasm requiring prolonged vasodilation [133]. Vasodilation of the harvested RA should begin intraoperatively by exposing the conduit to papaverine or verapamil/nitroglycerin. Verapamil/nitroglycerin may be more effective than papaverine in regards to degree of vasodilation and preservation of endothelial function, which can be a problem with papaverine (especially if injected intraluminally) and with the alpha-blocking agent phenoxybenzamine [118]. Postoperatively, most authors have recommended vasodilation with calcium channel blocking agents or long-acting nitrates for at least one month after surgery.

It is debated as to whether the proximal RA graft anastomosis should be performed to the ascending aorta or as a composite graft to other conduits. In a study of over 1,500 radial artery grafts, Maniar et al found no difference between these two types of grafting strategies [129]. Collins et al, reporting the results of the Radial Artery Versus Saphenous Vein Patency (RSVP) trial, demonstrated superior patency of RA grafts compared with SVG, and all proximal anastomoses were performed to the aorta directly [122]. Jung et al recently demonstrated using postoperative CT angiography that RA patency was better when the proximal anastomosis was made to the aorta and did not use the IMA as RA inflow [134]. However, Desai et al found that at one year, 21% of RA grafts going directly to the aorta had "some degree" of angiographic stenosis, which was significantly less than SVG proximal anastomoses [78].

Testing for appropriateness of RA harvesting to gauge the likelihood of hand ischemia after RA harvesting is recommended. The Modified Allen's Test (MAT) is abnormal in wide ranges (<1% to 27%), often attributed to observer variability [135]. When MAT was compared with Doppler ultrasonography of the thumb artery, MAT was noted to have a sensitivity of 100% and specificity of 97% for thumb ischemia [136]. Various adjuncts to the MAT have been proposed, including pulse oximetry, plethysmography, and Doppler ultrasonography of the hand [136-138]. However, none of these modalities have been proven to add significantly to the diagnostic accuracy of a properly performed MAT, which appears to accurately and safely select patients for RA harvesting.

Harvesting of the RA has been performed traditionally by the open, "no-touch" technique [127]. However, more recently, the trend appears to have shifted toward endoscopic RA harvesting with demonstrated functional and cosmetic advantages [139] and no increase in vasoreactivity or damaged endothelium [140]. However, harvesting the RA as a pedicle with harmonic scalpel appears to be less injurious than using electrocautery for tissue dissection [140]. Patency rates are similar regardless of method of harvesting [142].

8. Summary

Coronary artery bypass grafting remains one of the most frequently performed major operations worldwide. Even in the burgeoning era of percutaneous approaches to coronary heart disease, the indications for CABG continue to be based on relief of angina, prevention of myocardial damage from ischemic complications, and prolonged expected survival in select patients. In order to provide the best results for CABG patients, the surgeon's chief focus should be on improved long-term outcomes. Based on the information available, the best long-term outcomes of CABG are achieved when incorporating a strategy of grafting with arterial conduits.

9. References

[1] Park SJ, Kim YH, Park DW, et al. Randomized trial of stents versus bypass surgery for left main coronary artery disease. N Engl J Med 2011; 364: 1718-27.

[2] Lee MS, Tseng CH, Barker CM, et al. Outcome after surgery and percutaneous intervention for cardiogenic shock and left main disease. Ann Thorac Surg 2008; 86: 29-34.

[3] Babaev A, Frederick PD, Pasta DJ, et al. Trends in management and outcomes of patients with acute myocardial infarction complicated by cardiogenic shock. JAMA 2005; 294: 448-54.

[4] Epstein AJ, Polsky D, Yang F, et al. Coronary revascularization trends in the United States, 2001-2008. JAMA 2011; 305: 1769-76.

[5] Hannan EL, Wu C, Walford G, et al. Drug-eluting stents vs. coronary-artery bypass grafting in multivessel coronary disease. N Engl J Med 2008; 358: 331-41.

[6] Serruys PW, Morice MC, Kappetain AP, et al. Percutaneous coronary intervention versus coronary-artery bypass grafting for severe coronary artery disease. N Engl J Med 2009; 360: 961-72.

[7] Bourassa MG, Campeau L, Lesperance J, Grondin CM. Changes in grafts and coronary arteries after saphenous vein aortocoronary bypass surgery: results at repeat angiography. Circulation 1982; 65: 90-7.

[8] Yun KL, WU Y, Aharonian V, et al. Randomized trial of endoscopic versus open vein harvest for coronary artery bypass grafting: six-month patency rates. J Thorac Cardiovasc Surg 2005; 129: 496-503.

[9] Widimsky P, Straka Z, Stros P,et al. One-year coronary bypass graft patency: a randomized comparison between off-pump and on-pump surgery angiographic results of the PRAGUE-4 trial. Circulation 2004; 110; 3418-23.

[10] Alexander JH, Hafley G, Harrington RA, et al. Efficacy and safety of edifoligide, an E2F transcription factor decoy, for prevention of vein graft failure following coronary artery bypass graft surgery: PREVENT IV: a randomized controlled trial. JAMA 2005; 294: 2446-54.

[11] Vassiliades TA, Douglas JS, Morris DC, et al. Integrated coronary revascularization with drug-eluting stents: immediate and seven-month outcome. J Thorac Cardiovasc Surg 2006; 131: 956-62.

[12] Shroyer AL, Grover FL, Hattler B, et al. On-pump versus off-pump coronary-artery bypass surgery. N Engl J Med 2009; 361: 1827-37.

[13] de Canniere D, Wimmer-Greinecker G, Cichon R, et al. Feasibility, safety, and efficacy of totally endoscopic coronary artery bypass grafting: multicenter European experience. J Thorac Cardovasc Surg 2007; 134: 710-6.
[14] Zacharias A, Habib RH, Schwann TA, Riordan CJ, Durham SJ, Shah A. Improved survival with radial artery versus vein conduits in coronary bypass surgery with left internal thoracic artery to left anterior descending artery grafting. Circulation 2004; 109: 1489-96.
[15] Burfeind WR, Jr., Glower DD, Wechler AS, et al. Single versus multiple internal mammary artery grafting for coronary artery bypass: 15-year follow-up of a clinical practice trial. Circulation 2004; 110: II-27-35.
[16] Cho KR, Kim JS, Choi JS, Kim KB. Serial angiographic follow-up of grafts one year and five years after coronary artery bypass surgery. Eur J Cardiothorac Surg 2006; 29: 511-6.
[17] Nishida H, Tomizawa Y, Endo M, Kurosawa H. Survival benefit of exclusive use of in situ arterial conduits over combined use of arterial and vein grafts for multiple coronary artery bypass grafting. Circulation 2005; 112: I-299 -303.
[18] Sabik JF III, Blackstone EH, Gillinov AM, Smedira NG, Lytle BW. Occurrence and risk factors for reintervention after coronary artery bypass grafing. Circulation 2006; 114 [suppl I]: I-454-60.
[19] Tabata M, Grab JD, Khalpey Z, et al. Prevalence and variability of internal mammary artery graft use in contemporary multivessel coronary artery bypass graft surgery: analysis of the Society of Thoracic Surgeons National Cardiac Database. Circulation 2009; 120: 935-40.
[20] Grover FL, Johnson RR, Marshall G, et al. Impact of mammary grafts on coronary bypass operative mortality and morbidity. Ann Thorac Surg 1994; 57: 559-69.
[21] Galbut DL, Traad EA, Dorman MJ, et al. Seventeen-year experience with bilateral mammary artery grafts. Ann Thorac Surg 1990; 49: 195-201.
[22] Kappetain AP, Dawkins KD, Mohr FW, et al. Current percutaneous intervention and coronary bypass grafting procedures for three-vessel and left main coronary artery disease. Insights from the SYNTAX run-in phase. Eur J Cardio-thorac Surg 2006; 29: 486-91.
[23] Guru V, Fremes SE, Tu JV. How many arterial grafts are enough? A population-based study of midterm outcomes. J Thorac Cardiovasc Surg 2006; 131: 1021-8.
[24] Jones JW, Schmidt SE, Miller R, Nahas C, Beall AC Jr. Suitability and durability of multiple internal thoracic artery coronary artery bypasses. Ann Surg 1997; 225: 785-92.
[25] Gruntzig A. Transluminal dilatation of coronary-artery stenosis. Lancet 1978; 1: 263.
[26] Moses JW, Stone GW, Nikolsky E, et al. Drug-eluting stents in the treatment of intermediate lesions: pooled analysis from four randomized trials. J Am Coll Cardiol 2006; 47: 2164-71.
[27] Tonino PAL, De Bruyne B, Pijls NHJ, et al. Fractional flow reserve versus angiography for guiding percutaneous coronary intervention. N Engl J Med 2009; 360: 213-24.
[28] Pfisterer M, Brunner-La Rocca HP, Buser PT, et al. Late clinical events after clopidogrel discontinuation may limit the benefit of drug-eluting stents: an observational study of drug-eluting verusus bare-metal stents. J Am Coll Cardiol 2006; 48: 2584-91.

[29] Bavry AA, Kumbhani DJ, Helton TJ, Borewk PP, Mood GR, Bhatt DL. Late thrombosis of drug-eluting stents: a meta-analysis of randomized clinical trial. Am J Med 2006; 119: 1056-61.
[30] Eisenstein EL, Anstrom KJ, Kong DF, et al. Clopidogrel use and long-term clinical outcomes after drug-eluting stent implantation. JAMA 2007; 297: 159-68.
[31] Moses JW, Leon MB, Popma JJ, et al. Sirolimus-eluting stents versus standard stents in patients with stenosis in a native coronary artery. N Engl J Med 2003; 349: 1315-23.
[32] Morice MC, Serruys PW, Sousa JE, et al. A randomized comparison of a sirolimus-eluting stent with a standard stent for coronary revascularization. N Engl J Med 2002; 346: 1773-80.
[33] Park SJ, Park DW, Kim YH, et al. Duration of dual antiplatelet therapy after implantation of drug-eluting stents. N Engl J Med 2010; 362: 1374-82.
[34] The BARI Investigators. Comparison of coronary bypass surgery with angioplasty in patients with multivessel disease. N Engl J Med 1996; 335: 217-25.
[35] The BARI Investigators. The final 10-year follow-up results from the BARI randomized trial. J Am Coll Cardiol 2007; 49: 1600-6.
[36] Henderson RA, Pocock SJ, Sharp SJ, et al. Long-term results of RITA-1 trial: clinical and cost comparisons of coronary angioplasty and coronary-artertу bypass grafting. Randomised Intervention Treatment of Angina. Lancet 1998; 352: 1419-25.
[37] Hamm CW, Reimers J, Ischinger T, Rupprecht HJ, Berger J, Bleifeld W. A randomized study of coronary angioplasty compared with bypass surgery in patients with symptomatic multivessel coronary disease. German Angioplasty Bypass Surgery Investigation (GABI). N Engl J Med 1994; 331: 1037-43.
[38] Hoffman SN, TenBrook JA Jr., Wolf MP, Pauker SG, Salem DN, Wong JB. A meta-analysis of randomized controlled trials comparing coronary artery bypass graft with percutaneous transluminal coronary angioplasty: one-to eight-year outcomes. J Am Coll Cardiol 2003; 41: 1293-304.
[39] SoS Investigators. Coronary artery bypass surgery versus percutaneous coronary intervention with stent implantation in patients with multivessel coronary artery disease (Stent or Surgery trial): a randomised control trial. Lancet 2002; 360: 965-70.
[40] Rodriguez AE, Baldi J, Fernandez Pereira C, et al. Five-year follow-up of the Argentine randomized trial of coronary angioplasty with stenting versus coronary bypass surgery in patients with multiple vessel disease (ERACI II). J Am Coll Cardiol 2005; 46: 582-8.
[41] Serruys PW, Ong ATL, van Herwerden LA, et al. Five-year outcomes after coronary stenting versus bypass surgery for the treatment of multivessel disease: the final analysis of the Arterial Revascularization Therapies Study (ARTS) Randomized Trial. J Am Coll Cardiol 2005; 46: 575-81.
[42] Kappetein AP, Feldman TE, Mack MJ, et al. Comparison of coronary bypass surgery with drug-eluting stenting for the treament of left main and/or three-vessel disease: 3-year follow-up of the SYNTAX trial. Eur Heart J 2011; 32: 2125-34.
[43] Ulrich MR, Brock DM, Ziskind AA. Analysis of trends in coronary artery bypass grafting and percutaneous coronary intervention rates in Washington State from 1987 to 2001. Am J Cardiol 2003; 92: 836-9.
[44] Abramov D, Tamariz MG, Fremes SE, et al. Trends in coronary artery bypass surgery results: a recent, 9-year study. Ann Thorac Surg 2000; 70: 84-90.

[45] Eifert S, Mair H, Boulesteix AL, et al. Mid-term outcomes of patients with PCI prior to CABG in comparison to patients with primary CABG. Vasc Health Risk Manag 2010; 6: 495-501.
[46] Zhao DX, Leacche M, Balaguer JM, et al. Routine intraoperative completion angiography after coronary artery bypass grafting and 1-stop hybrid revascularization. J Am Coll Cardiol 2009; 53: 232-41.
[47] Massoudy P, Theilmann M, Lehmann, et al. Impact of prior percutaneous coronary intervention on the outcome of coronary artery bypass surgery: a multicenter analysis. J Thorac Cardiovasc Surg 2009; 137: 840-5.
[48] Theilmann M, Neuhauser M, Knipp S, et al. Prognostic impact of previous percutaneous coronary intervention in patients with diabetes mellitus and triple-vessel disease undergoing coronary artery bypass surgery. J Thorac Cardiovasc Surg 2007; 134: 470-6.
[49] Chocron S, Baillot R, Rouleau JL, et al. Impact of previous percutaneous transluminal coronary angioplasty and/or stenting revascularization on outcomes after surgical revascularization: insights from the imagine study. Eur Heart J 2008; 29: 673-9.
[50] Tran HA, Barnett SD, Hunt SL, Chon A, Ad N. The effect of previous coronary artery stenting on short- and intermediate-term outcome after surgical revascularization in patients with diabetes mellitus. J Thorac Cardiovasc Surg 2009; 138: 316-23.
[51] Rao C Stanbridge RD, Chikwe J, et al. Does previous percutaneous coronary stenting compromise the long-term efficacy of subsequent coronary artery bypass surgery? A microsimulation study. Ann Thorac Surg 2008; 85: 501-7.
[52] Sabiston DC, Jr. The William F. Rienhoff, Jr Lecture: The Coronary Circulation. The Johns Hopkins Medical Journal. 1974; 134: 314.
[53] Dacey LJ, Braxton JH Jr, Kramer RS, et al. Long-term outcomes of endoscopic vein harvesting after coronary artery bypass grafting. Circulation 2011; 123: 147-153.
[54] Atkins BZ, Salomone JP, Subramanian A, Burke R, Vercruysse GA. Management of traumatic coronary artery injuries: advantages of off-pump coronary artery bypass. Eur J Trauma Emerg Surg 2010; 36: 380-4.
[55] Tatoulis J, Buxton BF, Fuller JA. Patencies of 2,127 arterial to coronary conduits over 15 years. Ann Thorac Surg 2004; 77: 93-101.
[56] Rasmussen C, Thiis JJ, Clemmensen P, et al. Significance and management of early graft failure after coronary artery bypass grafting: feasibility and results of acute angiography and re-re-vascularization. Eur J Cardiothorac Surg 1997; 12: 847-52.
[57] FitzGibbon GM, Leach AJ, Keon WJ, Burton JR, Kafka HP. Coronary bypass graft fate. Angiographic study of 1,179 vein grafts early, one year, and five years after operation. J Thorac Cardiovasc Surg 1986; 91: 773-8.
[58] Verrier ED, Shernan SK, Taylor KM, et al. Terminal complement blockade with pexelizumab during coronary artery bypass graft surgery requiring cardiopulmonary bypass: a randomized trial. JAMA 2004; 291: 2319-27.
[59] Yusuf S, Zucker D, Passamani E, et al. Effect of coronary artery bypass graft surgery on survival: overview of 10-year results from randomized trials by the Coronary Artery Bypass Graft Surgery Trialists Colaboration. Lancet 1994; 344: 563-70.
[60] Shah PJ, Gordon I, Fuller J, et al. Factors affecting saphenous vein graft patency: clinical and angiographic study in 1402 symptomatic patients operated on between 1977 and 1999. J Thorac Cardiovasc Surg 2003; 126: 1972-7.

[61] Thielmann M, Massoudy P, Jaeger BR, et al. Emergency re-revascularization with percutaneous coronary intervention, reoperation, or conservative treatment in patients with acute perioperative graft failure following coronary artery bypass surgery. Eur J Cardiothorac Surg 2006; 30: 117-25.

[62] Tector AJ, Schmahl TM, Janson B, et al. The internal mammary artery graft. Its longevity after coronary bypass. JAMA 1981; 246: 2181-3.

[63] Gluckman TJ, McLean RC, Schulman SP, et al. Effects of aspirin responsiveness and platelet reactivity on early vein graft thrombosis after coronary artery bypass graft surgery. J Am Coll Cardiol 2011; 57: 1069-77.

[64] Rousou LJ, Taylor KB, Lu XG, et al. Saphenous vein conduits harvested by endoscopic technique exhibit structural and functional damage. Ann Thorac Surg 2009; 87: 62-70.

[65] Hayward TZ III, Hey LA, Newman LL, et al. Endoscopic vein versus open saphenous vein harvest: the effect on postoperative outcomes. Ann Thorac Surg 1999; 68: 2107-10.

[66] Felisky CD, Paull DL, Hill ME, et al. Endoscopic greater saphenous vein harvesting reduces the morbidity of coronary artery bypass surgery. Am J Surg 2002; 183: 576-9.

[67] Shahian DM, O'Brien SM, Filardo G, et al. The Society of Thoracic Surgeons 2008 cardiac surgery risk models, part 1: coronary artery bypass grafting surgery. Ann Thorac Surg 2009; 88: S2-22.

[68] Zenati MA, Shroyer AL, Collins JF, et al. Impact of endoscopic versus open saphenous vein harvest technique on late coronary artery bypass grafting patient outcomes in the ROOBY (Randomized On/Off Bypass) Trial. J Thorac Cardiovasc Surg 2011; 141: 338-44.

[69] Lopes RD, Hafley GE, Allen KB, et al. Endoscopic versus open vein-grafting harvesting in coronary-artery bypass surgery. NEJM 2009; 16: 235-44.

[70] Desai P, Kiani S, Thiruvanthan N, et al. Impact of the learning curve for endoscopic vein harvest on conduit quality and early graft patency. Ann Thorac Surg 2011; 91: 1385-91.

[71] Souza DS, Johansson B, Bojo L, et al. Harvesting the saphenous vein with surrounding tissue for CABG provides long-term patency comparable to the left internal thoracic artery: results of a randomized longitudinal trial. J Thorac Cardiovasc Surg 2006; 132: 373-8.

[72] Dreifaldt M, Souza DS, Loesch A, et al. The "no-touch" harvesting technique for vein grafts in coronary artery bypass surgery preserves an intact vasa vasorum. J Thorac Cardiovasc Surg. 2011; 141: 145-50.

[73] Shroyer ALW, Coombs LP, Peterson ED, et al. The Society of Thoracic Surgeons: 30-day operative mortality and morbidity risk models. Ann Thorac Surg 2003; 75: 1856-65.

[74] Flaherty JD, Davidson CJ. Diabetes and coronary revascularization. JAMA 2005; 293: 1501-8.

[75] Muneretto C, Bisleri G, Negri A, et al. Total arterial myocardial revascularization with composite grafts improves results of coronary surgery in elderly: a prospective randomized comparison with conventional coronary artery bypass surgery. Circulation 2003; 108: II-29-33.

[76] Loop FD, Lytle BW, Cosgrove DM, et al. Influence of the internal-mammary-artery graft on 10-year survival and other cardiac events. N Engl J Med 1986; 314: 1-6.
[77] Nasso G, Coppola R, Bonifazi R, et al. Arterial revascularization in primary coronary artery bypass grafting: direct comparison of 4 strategies-results of the Stand-in-Y Mammary Study. J Thorac Cardiovas Surg 2009; 137: 1093-1100.
[78] Desai ND, Cohen EA, Naylor CD, Fremes SE. A randomized comparison of radial-artery and saphenous-vein coronary bypass grafts. N Engl J Med 2004; 351: 2302-9.
[79] Gaudino M, Cellini C, Pragliola C, et al. Arterial versus venous bypass grafts in patients with in-stent restenosis. Circluation 2005; 112 [suppl I]: I-265-9.
[80] Tatoulis J, Buxton BF, Fuller JA, Royce AG. Total arterial coronary revascularization: techniques and results in 3,220 patients. Ann Thorac Surg 1999; 68: 2093-9.
[81] Tector AJ, McDonald ML, Kress DC, et al. Purely internal thoracic artery grafts: outcomes. Ann Thorac Surg 2001; 72: 450-5.
[82] Zacharias A, Schwann TA, Riordan CJ, Durham SJ, Shah AS, Habib RH. Late results of conventional versus all-arterial revascularization based on internal thoracic and radial artery grafting. Ann Thorac Surg 2009; 87: 19-26.
[83] Muneretto C, Bisleri G, Negri A, et al. Total arterial myocardial revascularization with composite grafts improves results of coronary surgery in elderly: a prospective randomized comparison with conventional coronary artery bypass surgery. Circulation 2003; 108 [suppl II]: II-29-33.
[84] Cameron A, Davis KB, Green G, Schaff HV. Coronary bypass surgery with internal-thoracic-artery grafts—effects on survival over a 15-year period. N Engl J Med 1996; 334: 216-19.
[85] Barner HB, Standeven JW, Reese J. Twelve-year experience with internal mammary artery for coronary artery bypass. J Thorac Cardiovasc Surg 1985; 90: 668-75.
[86] Kay EB. Internal mammary artery grafting. Letter to the editor. J Thorac Cardiovasc Surg 1987; 94: 312.
[87] Rankin JS, Harrell FE Jr. Measuring the therapeutic efficacy of coronary revascularization: implications for future management. J Thorac Cardiovasc Surg 2006; 131: 944-8.
[88] Lytle BW, Blackstone EH, Sabik JF, Houghtaling P, Loop FD, Cosgrove DM. The effect of bilateral internal internal thoracic artery grafting on survival during 20 postoperative years. Ann Thorac Surg 2004; 78: 2005-14.
[89] Sabik JF III, Stockins A, Nowicki ER, Blackstone EH, Houghtaling PL, Lytle BW, Loop FD. Does the location of the second internal thoracic artery graft influence outcome of coronary artery bypass grafting? Circulation 2008; 118 [suppl 1]: S210-5.
[90] Lytle BW, Blackstone EH, Loop FD, et al. Two internal thoracic artery grafts are better than one. J Thorac Cardiovasc Surg 1999; 117: 855-72.
[91] Gansera B, Gillrath G, Lieber M, Angelis I, Schmidtler F, Kemkes BM. Are men treated better than women? Outcome of male versus female patients after CABG using bilateral internal thoracic arteries. Thorac Cardiovasc Surg 2004; 52: 261-7.
[92] Kurlansky PA, Traad EA, Dorman MJ, et al. Thirty-year follow-up defines survival benefit for second internal mammary artery in propensity-matched groups. Ann Thorac Surg 2010; 90: 101-8.
[93] Green GE, Sosa JA, Cameron A. Prospective study of feasibility of routine use of multiple internal mammary artery anastomoses. J Cardiovasc Surg 1989; 30: 643-7.

[94] Borger MA, Cohen G, Buth KJ, et al. Multiple arterial grafts. Radial versus right internal thoracic arteries. Circulation 1998; 98 (suppl II): II7 – 14.

[95] Gansera B, Schmidtler F, Gillrath G, et al. Does bilateral ITA grafting increase perioperative complications? Outcome of 4,462 patients with bilateral versus 4,202 patients with single ITA bypass. Eur J Cardiothorac Surg 2006; 30: 318-23.

[96] Saso S, James D, Vecht JA, et al. Effect of skeletonization of the internal thoracic artery for coronary revascularization on incidence of sternal wound infection. Ann Thorac Surg 2010; 89: 661-70.

[97] Toumpoulis IK, Anagnostopoulos CE, Derose JJ jr, Swistel DG. The impact of deep sternal wound infection on long-term survival after coronary artery bypass grafting. Chest 2005; 127: 464-71.

[98] Pevni D, Mohr R, Lev-Run O, et al. Influence of bilateral skeletonized harvesting on occurrence of deep sternal wound infection in 1,000 consecutive patients undergoing bilateral internal thoracic artery grafting. Ann Surg 2003; 237: 277-80.

[99] Diez C, Koch, D, Kuss O, Silber RE, Friedrich I, Boergermann J. Risk factors for mediastinitis after cardiac surgery-a retrospective analysis of 1700 patients. J Cardiothorac Surg 2007; 2: 23.

[100] Pevni D, Uretzky G, Mohr A, et al. Routine use of bilateral skeletonized internal thoracic artery grafting: long-term results. Circulation 2008; 118: 705-12.

[101] Momin AU, Deshpande R, Potts J, et al. Incidence of sternal infection in diabetic patients undergoing bilateral internal thoracic artery grafting. Ann Thorac Surg 2005; 80: 1765-72.

[102] Herz I, Moshkovitz Y, Loberman D, et al. Dru-eluting stents versus bilateral internal thoracic grafting for multivessel coronary disease. Ann Thorac Surg 2005; 80: 2086-90.

[103] Locker C, Mohr R, Lev-Ran O, et al. Comparison of bilateral thoracic artery grafting with percutaneous coronary interventions in diabetic patients. Ann Thorac Surg 2004; 78: 471-5.

[104] Schmidt SE, Jones JW, Thornby JI, Miller CC 3rd, Beall AC Jr. Improved survival with multiple left-sided bilateral internal thoracic artery grafts. Ann Thorac Surg 1997; 64: 9-14.

[105] Sabik JF III; Lytle BW, Blackstone EH, Khan M, Houghtaling PL, Cosgrove DM. Does competitive flow reduce internal thoracic artery graft patency? Ann Thorac Surg 2003; 76: 1490-6.

[106] Kurlansky PA, Traad EA, Dorman MJ, Galbut DL, Zucker M, Ebra G. Location of the second internal mammary artery graft does not influence outcome of coronary artery bypass grafting. Ann Thorac Surg 2011; 91: 1378-84.

[107] Dion R, Etienne PY, Verhelst R, et al. Bilateral mammary grafting. Eur J Cardiothorac Surg 1993; 7: 287-94.

[108] Chow MS, Sim E, Orszulak TA, Schaff HV. Patency of internal thoracic artery grafts: comparison of right versus left and importance of vessel grafted. Circulation 1994; 90: II:129-32.

[109] Lodge AJ, Wells WJ, Backer CL, et al. A novel resorbable film reduces postoperative adhesions after infant cardiac surgery. Ann Thorac Surg 2008; 86: 614-21.

[110] Glineur D, Hanet C, Poncelet A. Comparison of bilateral internal thoracic artery revascularization using in-situ or Y graft configurations: a prospective randomized

clinical, functional, and angiographic midterm evaluation. Circulation 2008; 118: S216-21.

[111] El Nakadi B, Choghari C, Joris M. Complete myocardial revascularization with bilateral internal thoracic artery T-graft. Ann Thorac Surg 2000; 69: 498-500.

[112] Lorbergoym M, Medalion B, Bder O, Lockman J, Cohen N, Schachner A, Cohen AJ. 99mTc-MDP bone SPECT for the evaluation of sternal ischaemia following internal mammary artery dissection. Nucl Med Commun 2002; 23: 47-52.

[113] Knobloch K, Lichtenberg A, Pichlmaier M, Mertsching H, Krug A, Klima U, Haverich A. Microcirculation of the sternum following harvesting of the left internal mammary artery. Thorac Cardiovasc Surg 2003; 51: 255-9.

[114] Mannacio V, Di Tommaso L, De Amicis V, Stassano P, Vosa C. Randomized flow capacity comparison of skeletonized and pedicled left internal mammary artery. Ann Thorac Surg 2011; 91: 24-30.

[115] Gurevitch J, Kramer A, Locker C, et al. Technical aspects of double-skeletonized internal mammary artery grafting. Ann Thorac Surg 2000; 69: 841-6.

[116] Carpentier A, Guermonprez JL, Deloche A, Frechette C, DuBost C. The aorto to coronary radial artery bypass graft. A technique avoiding pathological changes in grafts. Ann Thorac Surg 1973; 16: 111-21.

[117] Acar C, Jebara VA, Portoghese M, et al. Revival of the radial artery for coronary artery bypass grafting. Ann Thorac Surg 1992; 54: 652-60.

[118] Attaran S, John L, El-Gamel A. Clinical and potential use of pharmacological agents to reduce radial artery spasm in coronary artery surgery. Ann Thorac Surg 2008; 85: 1483-9.

[119] Cameron J, Trivedi S, Stafford G, Bett JHN. Five-year angiographic patency of radial artery bypass grafts. Circulation 2004; 110 [suppl II]: II-23-6.

[120] Tatoulis J, Buxton BF, Fuller JA, et al. Long-term patency of 1108 radial arterial-coronary angiograms over 10 years. Ann Thorac Surg 2009; 88: 23-9.

[121] Cameron J, Trivedi S, Stafford G, Bett JHN. Five-year angiographic patency of radial artery bypass grafts. Circulation 2004; 110 [suppl II]; II-23 – 6.

[122] Collins P, Webb CM, Chong CF, Moat NE. Radial artery versus saphenous vein patency randomized trial: five-year angiographic follow-up. Circulation 2008; 117: 2859-64.

[123] Goldman S, Sethi GK, Holman W, et al. Radial artery grafts vs. saphenous vein grafts in coronary artery bypass surgery: a randomized trial. JAMA 2011; 305: 167-74.

[124] Possati G, Gaudino M, Alessandrini F, et al. Midterm clinical and angiographic results of radial artery grafts used for myocardial revascularization. J Thorac Cardiovasc Surg 1998; 116: 1015-21.

[125] Desai ND, Naylor CD, Kiss A, et al. Impact of patient and target-vessel characteristics on arterial and venous bypass graft patency: insight from a randomized trial. Circulation 2007; 115: 684-91.

[126] Hayward PAR, Hare, DL, Gordon I, Buxton BF. Effect of radial artery or saphenous vein conduit for the second graft on 6-year clinical outcome after coronary artery bypass grafting. Results of a randomized trial. Eur J Cardiothorac Surg 2008; 34: 113-7.

[127] Tranbaugh RF, Dimitrova KR, Friedmann P, et al. Radial artery conduits improve long-term survival after coronary artery bypass grafting. Ann Thorac Surg 2010; 90: 1165-72.

[128] Hashimoto H, Isshiki T, Ikari Y, et al. Effects of competitive blood flow on arterial graft patency and diameter. J Thorac Cardiovasc Surg 1996; 111: 399-407.

[129] Maniar HS, Sundt TM, Barner HB, et al. Effect of target stenosis and location on radial artery graft patency. J Thorac Cardiovasc Surg 2002; 123: 45-52.

[130] Achouh P, Boutekadjirt R, Toledano D, et al. Long-term (5- to 20-year) patency of the radial artery for coronary bypass grafting. J Thorac Cardiovasc Surg 2010; 140: 73-9

[131] Parolari A, Rubini P, Alamanni F, et al. The radial artery: which place in coronary operation? Ann Thorac Surg 2000; 69: 1288-94.

[132] He GW. Arterial grafts for coronary artery bypass grafting: biological characteristics, functional classification and clinical choice. Ann Thorac Surg 1999; 67: 277-84.

[133] Pevni D, Mohr R, Lev-Ran O, et al. Technical aspects of composite arterial grafting with double skeletonized internal thoracic arteries. Chest 2003; 123: 1348-54.

[134] Jung SH, Song H, Choo SJ, et al. Comparison of radial artery patency according to proximal anastomotic site: direct aorta to radial artery anastomosis is superior to radial artery composite grafting. J Thorac Cardiovasc Surg 2009; 138: 76-83.

[135] Brzezinski M, Luisetti T, London MJ. Radial artery cannulation: a comprehensive review of recent anatomic and physiologic investigations. Anesth Analg 2009; 109: 1763-81.

[136] Ruengsakulrach P, Brooks M, Hare D, Gordon I, Buxton B. Preoperative assessment of hand circulation by means of Doppler ultrasonography and the modified Allen's test. J Thorac Cardiovasc Surg 2001; 121: 526-31.

[137] Johnson WH II, Cromartie RS III, Arrants JE, Wuamett JD, Holt JB. Simplified method for candidate selection for radial artery harvesting. Ann Thorac Surg 1998; 65: 1167.

[138] Fuhrman TM, Pippin WD, Talmage LA, Reilley TE. Evaluation of collateral circulation of the hand. J Clin Monit 1992; 8: 28-32.

[139] Navia JL, Brozzi N, Chiu J, et al. Endoscopic versus open radial artery harvesting for coronary artery bypass grafting. Scand Cardiovasc J 2011 May 16 (Epub ahead of print).

[140] Shapira OM, Eskenazi BR, Anter E, et al. Endoscopic versus conventional radial artery harvest for coronary artery bypass grafting: functional and histologic assessment of the conduit. J Thorac Cardiovasc Surg 2006; 131: 388-94.

[141] Brazio PS, Laird PC, Xu C, et al. Harmonic scalpel versus electrocautery with hemoclips for harvest of radial artery conduits: reduced risk of spasm and intimal injury on optical coherence tomography. J Thorac Cardiovasc Surg 2008; 136: 1302-8.

[142] Bleiziffer S, Hettich I, Eisenhauer B, et al. Patency rates of endoscopically harvested radial arteries one year after coronary artery bypass grafting. J Thorac Cardiovasc Surg 2007; 134: 649-56.

7

Current Evidence of On-Pump Versus Off-Pump Coronary Artery By-Pass Surgery

Kim Houlind
Dept. of Vascular Surgery,
Kolding Sygehus - Little Belt Hospital
Denmark

1. Introduction

Conventional coronary artery by-pass grafting (CCABG) performed using cardioplegic arrest and cardiopulmonary by-pass is a very well documented treatment for ischemic heart disease. The operation often relieves chest pain and it improves survival for patients with triple- vessel disease and left main coronary artery disease.
Since it was introduced in the late 1960´es, CCABG has become one of the most commonly performed operations. In 2007, an estimated 408.000 surgical coronary revascularizations were performed in the United States alone (1)
Given the ageing populations in large parts of the world, CCABG is also increasingly being offered to elderly patients and to patients with co-morbidities. As a consequence, a significant number of operated patients suffer major or minor complications. Concerns have been raised that the use of cardiopulmonary by-pass (CPB) could cause neuro-cognitive dysfunction. Also, CPB has been linked to myocardial, renal and pulmonary damage. Several mechanisms have been suggested: Manipulation of the aorta during cannulation and clamping may cause dislodgment and embolization of atherosclerotic deposits, cardiac arrest may induce myocardial damage, and the long-lasting and repeated contact of blood with the non-biological surfaces of filters and tubing of the heart- lung- machine induce mechanical wearing of the formed elements and biochemical over-activation of the immune- and coagulation systems
Development of the Off-pump Coronary Artery By-pass (OPCAB) technique has been driven by concerns of these possible side-effects from CPB. On the other hand, concerns have been raised about whether the quality of anastomoses constructed "on the beating heart" - i.e. without cardiopulmonary by-pass and cardioplegic arrest – would be as good as that of the anastomoses performed during CCABG. The question remains controversial. Best estimates of the proportion of surgical coronary revascularizations performed as OPCAB in the United States is around 25%. Some surgical centres perform almost all coronary by-pass operations off-pump, while others hardly or never use this technique. Tradition and economy dictate that OPCAB is the preferred method in some parts of the developing world. In the beginning of the OPCAB-experience, evidence was limited to small, published series by individual surgeons (2-3). Although seemingly providing good results, these observations were hampered by the lack of a control group. Later studies from databases were difficult to interpret because the original intention-to-treat was not

recorded. This may have caused high-risk patients to be moved from one treatment group to the other (4-5).

From the late 1990ies to 2002 a significant technical development in stabilizing equipment led to a fast rise in the number of OPCAB procedures. From 2002 results from the first randomized studies failed to show a clear benefit and interest has cooled somewhat. A significant number of randomized studies have been conducted comparing very different end-points after OPCAB and CCABG. This chapter aims to review the results of these studies to assess the comparative effectiveness and safety of the two techniques.

2. Methods

Searching MEDLINE and Cochrane library using the terms » *OPCAB* «, » *off-pump* «, » *offpump* « OR »MIDCAB«, limited to English language june 23rd, 2010, provided 4788 abstracts that were read manually to find randomized, controlled trials. Two-hundred and twenty nine papers were retrieved and read before 90 papers, reporting results from 61 individual randomized, controlled trials, were identified.

3. Results

3.1 Effectiveness

Long term survival

The comparative long-term survival of OPCAB and CCABG is not well evaluated. The longest follow-up is in the OCTOPUS-study (6). Five years postoperatively 130/142 OPCAB-patients and 130/139 CCABG patients were alive (p=ns). Other studies with up to twelve months follow-up also failed to show any difference (7-13). Due to the relatively low risk of mortality associated with either operation, however, the statistical strength to detect any difference is not present in any of these studies.

The largest randomized study, the ROOBY-trial (14) showed a trend towards higher mortality in the OPCAB group at one year follow-up (4.1% vs. 2.9%, p=0.15) and a significant difference in cardiac deaths only (2.7% vs. 1.3%, p=0.03). On the other hand, another study with a mean 3.8 years follow-up of 300 patients showed a trend in the opposite direction with 5 deaths in the OPCAB-group and 10 in the CCABG-group (15).

Graft patency

Even with the use of contemporary cardiac stabilizers and intracoronary shunts, OPCAB remains more technically challenging than CCABG. Difficulties with positioning the heart may cause the surgeon to graft a less favourable part of the coronary artery. Performing the anastomosis is more difficult and may lead to stenosis at the anastomosis site. Furthermore, the coagulability of blood is increased after OPCAB compared to CCABG (16-20). Hence, a serious concern when introducing the OPCAB technique has been whether the number and quality of the grafts would be equivalent to what could be achieved using CPB.

In the vast majority of randomized, controlled trials, the OPCAB-patients tended to receive a lower number of grafts than the patients operated using CPB. In the largest studies and in a meta-analysis this difference was statistically significant (13-14, 21, 22) with a mean difference of 0.1-0.3 grafts. Several studies compared the number of grafts compared to a preoperative plan. In most of these studies, no difference was found (8-9,12, 14, 23), a few studies showed a difference in favour of CCABG, and one study found a difference in favour of OPCAB (24). In this study, however, the absolute number of grafts was 0.2 lower in the OPCAB-group.

Allmost all of the earlier studies showed a trend towards poorer graft patency in OPCAB patients. A single, smaller study found this difference to be statistically significant (25). Also, the proportion of patent grafts in the largest study, the ROOBY-trial, was 82.6% in the OPCAB group and 87.8% in the CCABG group ($p<0.01$) (14). This difference, however, did not result in a higher number of myocardial infarctions in the OPCAB group.

In studies performed by few, dedicated OPCAB surgeons, the difference in number of grafts was very small and not statistically significant (12, 24). The study by Khan (25), the SMART study (14), and the Best Bypass Surgery Study (26) differentiated the findings and found a higher proportion of occluded grafts at right and circumflex territories and fewer occlusions in the LAD territory. Lingaas et al only found differences in graft patency between OPCAB and CCABG to be significantly different when comparing vein grafts as opposed to internal mammary artery grafts (10).

Recurrent or persistent chest pain

An important parameter is freedom from chest pain. In the Octopus trial (6, 24), 89.0% experienced freedom from chest pain in the OPCAB group compared to 89.3% in the CCABG-group (p=ns). At five years follow-up, these numbers were down to 82.3% and 87.7%, respectively (p=ns). At one year follow-up, ergometer testing was performed in 81% of the patients. It was found to be negative in 79.8% of CCABG patients and 83.1% of OPCAB patients (p=ns). In the SMART-study, chest pain was present at one-year follow-up in 0% of CCABG and 3% of OPCAB patients, respectively (p=ns) (12). In a separate publication, using a specific questionnaire on chest pain in the 400 patients involved in the BHACAS1 and BHACAS2-studies, no difference was found after a median follow-up of three years (27).

Reintervention

Given the lower number of patent grafts in the OPCAB groups, a greater need for coronary re-intervention might be expected. Only few of the published trials have had long enough follow-up for this question to be evaluated. In the BHACAS-1 study, three percent of both OPCAB and CCABG patients had had a reintervention - either percutaneous or surgical - within a median three years follow-up (7). The longest follow-up, which was published by the Octopus trialists, reported 7.7% of OPCAB-patients and 5% of CCABG patients to have undergone reintervention after five years (6). In the ROOBY-trial, the proportion undergoing reintervention was 4.6% in the OPCAB group and 3.4% in the CCABG group at one year follow-up. Neither individual studies nor metanalyses found thiese differences to be statistically significant (21, 26).

Quality of life

A number of studies compare self-reported, health related quality of life after OPCAB and CCABG. Medical Outcomes Study-Short Form 36 (MOS SF-36) is the most commonly used tool. In this questionnaire eight scales cover physical, mental, and social well-being (28). One study found a significantly higher score among CCABG-patients in one of the eight scales ("Role emotional") in contrast to another study who favoured OPCAB patients in the dimension "Social Relationships", using another questionnaire (29,30). In general, few significant inter-group differences have been found, given the multiple tests being performed.

On the other hand, a significant increase in self-reported, health related quality of life is invariably found in both groups comparing preoperative and postoperative status (24, 27, 31).

3.2 Safety

Periperative mortality

Most of the randomized trials have included either consecutive patients or patients with low perioperative risk due to young age, few comorbidities, and need for relatively few grafts. The expected operative mortality for this group of patients is too low for any of the randomized trials to have sufficient statistical strength to detect a difference between treatment groups. This is also true for metaanalyses of randomized trials.
Among the larger non-randomized studies, Cleveland et al. analyzed data from the Society of Thoracic Surgeons (STS) database (4). They included operations performed in 1998 and 1999 in 126 centers with experience in OPCAB surgery. A total of 118.140 CCABG and 11.717 OPCAB procedures were included. The risk adjusted mortality in this comparison was 2.94% in the CCABG group and 2.32% in the OPCAB group ($p < 0.0001$). Magee and co-workers compared the results of 6.466 CCABG and 1.983 OPCAB procedures in two American centres in 1998-2000 (5). In spite of a significantly higher preoperative morbidity in the OPCAB-group, mortality in the OPCAB group was 1.8% against 3.5% in the CCABG-group ($p = 0.002$). However, these comparisons were not performed according to the principle of intention–to-treat. This is a significant drawback, since patients who were converted to CCABG during the operation after initially attempting to perform OPCAB are analyzed as belonging to the CCABG group. Hence, the complications of the most complicated OPCAB-procedures were exported to the CCABG-group.
It is worth noting that one of the few randomized studies that specifically included high-risk patients who received an acute operation, found a significantly higher mortality in the CCABG group than in the OPCAB group (7.7% vs. 1.6%, $p=0.04$) (32). However, this study exclusively included patients who only needed grafting the LAD territory, which would be expected to favour OPCAB.

3.3 Other cardiac complications

Myocardial damage

None of the randomized studies or meta-analyses has documented any significant difference in the incidence of clinical peri-operative myocardial infarction. However, many randomized studies provide evidence of a lower, subclinical release of biochemical markers of myocardial damage among patient operated using OPCAB (12, 25, 32-42). This tendency is very robust across the different studies, and it is even preset in a study that showed a significantly higher proportion of graft occlusions in the OPCAB group (25). These differences are ascribed to ischemia and reperfusion with cardioplegia. Apart from creatinine-kinase type B (CK-MB) and Troponine T, also atrial natriuretic peptide and heart type fatty-acid binding protein tend to exhibit a higher raise after CCABG than after OPCAB (36). All of these differences, are, however in an order of magnitude smaller than what has so far been considered clinically relevant. By detailed measurement of left ventricular ejection fraction between groups, no inter-group differences were found (42). On the other hand, the long term follow-up of the OCTOPUS-study showed that the patients with the highest release of CK-MB had the highest risk of experiencing a clinical myocardial infarction during the following year (43). A number of confounding issues may, however, be relevant.

In a study of myocardial biopsies, it was found that the concentration of reduced glutathion recovered more rapidly in CCABG than OPCAB patients (38). For the OPCAB-operations, a proximal snare was used for occlusion of the vessel while performing the anastomosis. This finding suggests that cardioplegia is better tolerated than occlusion. Still, a higher increase in CK-MB was found in the CCABG-group. Together, these findings suggest that the myocardium in the territory of the occluded vessel suffers more from occlusion but a less profound damage to the entire myocardium is caused by ischemia and reperfusion. Which of these two situations pose the largest threat to heart function is not clear. Gadolinium contrast enhanced magnetic resonance perfusion imaging, reflecting permanent damage to the myocardium, failed to detect a difference between treatment groups despite a higher release of Troponine- I in the CCABG-group (39). On this background, it was speculated whether some of the Troponine leak represented protein release from non-structurally bound cytosolic pools, rather than true myocardial necrosis. In another study, micro-dialysis was used to sample myocardial interstitial fluid during and after surgery (44). More abnormal values were found during CCABG than during OPCAB. It was not stated in the paper whether samples were taken within or outside the area of the temporally occluded vessel during OPCAB.

Atrial fibrillation

In the BHACAS-1 study, Heart rate and rhythm were continuously monitored for 72 postoperative hours. The incidence of postoperative atrial fibrillation was found to be 45% among CCABG patients as compared to 8% among patients operated with OPCAB ($p<0.001$) (45). A large number of later studies, including the BHACAS-2 study, have confirmed this tendency but with a much smaller difference between groups. The tendency is statistically significant in some of these studies and in meta-analyses (21).

Postoperative inotropic support and low cardiac output syndrome

Need for inotropic drugs after the operation may reflect either transient or permanent heart failure. Several, larger studies do not report this end-point (13-14), but among the ones that do, there is a trend towards a higher incidence in patients operated using cardiopulmonary by-pass. A meta-analysis of 16 studies including 1655 patients found a need for inotropic support postoperatively in 23.6% of CCABG and 15.1% of OPCAB patients ($p=0.04$)(21). Other studies report the incidence of "low cardiac output syndrome", defined as need for intra-aortic balloon pump, need for inotropic drugs or pressor drugs. One of the larger studies reports a significant difference (12), while others do not (13, 46).

3.4 Neurological complications

Stroke

Theoretically, the use of cardiopulmonary by-pass may cause stroke by a number of different mechanisms. These include the manipulation of the ascending aorta for cannulation and clamping, gaseous or particulate emboli formed in the by-pass circuit, and accidental interruption of flow.

Also, post-operative atrial fibrillation may cause strokes in spite of adequate antithrombotic treatment. For these reasons, an important argument for favouring OPCAB has been the intention to reduce the rate of peri-operative strokes.

In low risk patients, the risk of suffering a peri-operative stroke is between 1 and 1.5%. Hence, none of the individual, randomized, controlled trials have had the statistical strength to prove a difference. A single meta-analysis only just managed to show a significant difference (47), but other analyses, comprising just as many or more trials and patients, failed to prove OPCAB superior (21). Therefore, until the time of the publication of the ROOBY-trial (14), evidence was ambiguous. In the ROOBY trial, however, the trend was opposite that of most earlier studies with 1.3% strokes in the OPCAB-group and 0.7% in the CCABG-group (p=0.28). In view of the large volume of this trial compared to all the other trials, it can no longer be stated that there is a clear trend in favour of OPCAB to reduce the rate of peri-operative strokes in younger, low-risk patients. It is, however, worth noting, that the OPCAB technique is still being developed in order to reduce stroke rate. An increasing number of surgeons favour a "no-touch-aorta" technique, placing proximal anastomoses end-to-side in a mammary artery graft rather than on the aorta itself. In addition, some centers aim to reduce the risk of embolisation due to atrial fibrillation by ligating the left atrial appendage. Excellent results have been produced, but not tested in randomized trials.

Neurocognitive dysfunction

Several randomized trials have used neuro-psychological or neuro-cognitive tests to detect perioperative cerebral damage lesser than overt stroke. In some of these studies, early postoperative testing favoured OPCAB (48-49) while others found no significant difference (50-53). Zamvar and coworkers, only including patients with triple-vessel disease, performed a battery of neuro-cognitive tests one week and ten weeks postoperatively, comparing with pre-operative test results. At both occasions, they found a significantly higher degree of neuro-cognitive dysfunction in CCABG-patients than in OPCAB-patients (54).

In the Octopus trial (6, 41, 49), a significant difference in favour of OPCAB was found after three months but not after one year nor after five years of follow-up. At five years follow-up, a more than fifty per cent decline in scores at neuro-cognitive testing was found in both groups, illustrating the fact that patients with ischemic heart disease in general have an increased risk of neurocognitive decline. A similar decline has been documented after three years in a non- surgical control group (55).

Surrogate end-points of brain damage are often used in randomized trials comparing OPCAB with CCABG. These include release of the S-100 peptide and detection of High Intensity Transcranial Doppler Signals (HITS) as well as changes in serum concentrations of different hormones.

When S-100 is detected in peripheral blood, it is seen as a marker of damage to, and increased permeability of, the blood-brain barrier. There is good evidence from randomized controlled trials that the increase of S-100 is higher after CCABG than after OPCAB (48, 51, 56). In two out of three studies these increases are compared to the results of postoperative, neurocognitive tests, but none of the studies showed any correlation between S-100 levels and neurocognitive function. In one of the studies one patient suffered a major stroke resulting in paralysis of an arm and a leg without a major increase in blood concentrations of S-100. Hence, the clinical significance of relase of S-100 is uncertain.

Characteristic high-intensity signals - HITS - can be detected by trans-cranial measurement of Doppler signals from the medial cerebral artery. The amount of HITS increase during manipulation of the aorta, especially during cannulation, clamping, and declamping. A lower number of HITS are observed at the beginning of cardiopulmonary by-pass. It is not clear, to what extent HITS represent particulate emboli being released from vessel walls, tubes or filters and what proportion of HITS are being generated by gaseous microemboli and turbulence. Several studies have demonstrated a larger amount of HITS in patients undergoing CCABG than in patients undergoing OPCAB (48, 53). One study showed a correlation between the number of HITS detected in the CCABG-group and the results of one out of three neurocognitive tests. This correlation, however, according to a figure in the publication, relies heavily on the results from one patient (48). No correlation was found with the results of any of the other two tests nor, in the OPCAB group, between the number of HITS and the results of any of the three tests. In a larger study, a lower neuro-cognitive score was found at discharge from hospital in patients who had undergone CCABG compared to patients operated with OPCAB-tecghnique (53). This difference was not found at six weeks and six months follow-up and no correlation was found between number of HITS and postoperative cognitive function.

To summarize, there is strong evidence of more HITS when performing CCABG than OPCAB. There is, however, no evidence that these HITS represent emboli or that they have any significance with regard to early or late postoperative cognitive dysfunction.

In another study, cerebral SPECT-scans revealed more evidence of microemboli after CCABG than after OPCAB (50). However, like in the case of HITS and S-100 release, this finding could not be shown to correlate with the performance of patients in neuro-cognitive tests.

One study suggests that changes in neuro-cognitive function and tendency to mental depression after both CCABG and OPCAB are related to disturbance of the circadian rhytms of cortisol and melatonine release (57). These disturbances are, though, also susceptible to other factors and they occur after both types of procedures. The clinical significance of this finding is not clear.

3.5 Renal function

Transient or permanent renal impairment are well known complications to cardiac surgery (58). This risk has be attributed to the systemic, inflammatory response, hypoperfusion of the kidneys during operation and, possibly, the non-pulsatile nature of flow during cardiopulmonary by-pass (59).

Clinically significant, new onset renal failure - defined either as need for dialysis or by increase in biochemical markers to pathological levels - occur at a rate of approximately 1-2 per cent of the low-risk patients typically included in randomized, controlled trials. None of these studies have, therefore, had the statistical strength to detect a difference in the incidence of this end-point between patients operated with OPCAB or CCABG. Even in a large meta-analysis by Cheng et al (21) showing an odds ratio of 0.58 in favour of OPCAB the confidence limits were too wide to allow statistical significance.

On the other hand, when comparing biochemical markers of sub-clinical renal damage, evidence from several clinical trials is in favour of OPCAB (11, 60-61). This difference is clear whether glomerular or tubular damage is compared (60). In one study, the difference between creatinine clearance after CCABG compared to OPCAB was especially high in patients with diabetes, hypertension and heart failure (11). In one trial, comparing patients operated using pulsatile flow in the cardiopulmonary by-pass circuit, no difference in postoperative renal function was found between patients operated with OPCAB and CCABG. This finding seems to confirm the theory that non-pulsatile flow contributes to the subclinical renal impairment often seen after cardiac surgery using cardiopulmonary by-pass (61).

3.6 Lung function

During cardiopulmonary by-pass, ventilation is commonly stopped to prevent the motion of the lungs interfering with surgery. During the early postoperative period patients who have

undergone cardiac surgery are prone to develop atelectasis. Theoretically, this may be prevented by OPCAB where the lungs are continuously ventilated.
Most of the authors addressing this question, found that postoperative ventilation times were longer for patients who underwent CCABG than for those who underwent OPCAB. There is good evidence from a meta-analysis for a lower incidence of chest infections and shorter postoperative need for ventilator assistance after OPCAB (21), although one study of low-risk patients contradicts this finding (23). Most of these studies may be biased by the fact that the staff members deciding the time when the patients should be weaned from the ventilator were not blinded with regard to the type of operation that had been performed. On the other hand, evidence is strengthened by the fact that the one study in which the staff was indeed blinded also found a shorter postoperative need of ventilation in the OPCAB group (12).
In two trials, patients with chronic obstructive pulmonary disease were studied specifically. In one of these studies, a significantly higher postoperative decrease in lung function was found among post-CCABG patients (62). In the other study, a shorter time to extubation and shorter stay in intensive care unit was found among OPCAB patients (63). Also, in a study of patients with recent myocardial infarction, a shorter ventilation time was documented for OPCAB-patients compared to CCABG-patients (32).
It has been suggested, that the mechanism behind impaired lung function after CCABG was changes in alveolar gas exchange as a result of increased interstitial oedema. This effect has, however, been specifically addressed by several studies finding that this effect is comparable in OPCAB and CCABG-patients and most significant during the first few postoperative hours (23, 42, 64-65).In a randomized comparison of patients with single- and double-vessel disease, a significantly higher veno-arterial shunting was found after cardio-pulmonary by-pass (23). It is still unknown whether this result can be generalized to patients with triple vessel disease where the OPCAB-technique is complicated by the need to manipulate the heart.

3.7 Gastro-intestinal complications

There is evidence from a single, large, randomized trial that the risk of gastro-intestinal complications - including ischaemic bowel, hepatic failure, gastric bleeding, perforated duodenal ulcer, acute cholecystitis, and acute pancreatitis - is higher after CCABG than after OPCAB (66). This study, however, excluded patients needing grafts to the circumflex territory. This selection can be expected to favour OPCAB. Other, larger, randomized trials either do not find this difference or do not report this endpoint (6-7, 12-14).

3.8 Inflammatory response

A generalized inflammatory response is activated by any sort of surgery, but is aggravated by cardio-pulmonary by-pass. The blood–air interface and the contact between the blood and the artificial surfaces of the CPB circuit play important roles. Cooling and heating as well as ischemia and reperfusion of the myocardium are other factors that tend to activate a systemic inflammatory response.
The inflammatory response includes both humoral and cellular elements. Randomized comparisons between CCABG and OPCAB shows the CCABG patients to have increased serum-levels of a multitude of different substances including tumor necrosis factor-alpha, interleukins 6 and 8, selectin, c-reactive protein, intracellular adhesion molecule – 1, and vascular endothelial growth factor (39,67-72). Also, the expression of a scavenger molecule on monocytes is significantly higher in "on-pump" patients (73). It has been proposed that

this inflammatory over-activation can be harmful and lead to organ failure and infections. No definitive coupling has, however been made in coronary artery by-pass patients between inflammatory markers and clinical outcome.
Similarly, oxidative stress is known to be higher in patients undergoing cardiopulmonary by-pass. Theoretically, this may cause tissue damage, but no practical clinical consequence has been proven in patients (74).

3.9 Blood loss and coagulation

Transfusions have been shown to be associated with substantial incremental increases in risks of mortality and morbidity for patients undergoing cardiac surgery. There is good evidence from a number of large, randomized trials that blood loss and need for transfusions is lower after OPCAB than after CCABG (7,15, 24, 45, 74-76). This finding is often explained by the activation and subsequent deactivation of platelets and humoral coagulation factors by the non-biological surfaces of the cardiopulmonary by-pass circuit. The alpha granules of the platelets are being depleted and the platelet count is reduced by dilution. Also fibrinolytic cascades are activated.
Some characteristics of the study protocols may, however, influence these results. Typically, different protocols for heparinization and reversion with protamine are used for the study groups, increasing bleeding tendency in the CCABG-groups. In addition, some studies apply a fixed value of haematocrit as an indication for transfusion. Because of dilution caused by the priming volume of the cardiopulmonary by-pass circuit this will increase the risk of transfusion in the CCABG-group compared to the OPCAB-group, even if this dilution were better treated using diuretics.

3.10 Cost-effectiveness

Some of the clinical trials have covered heath economic analyses up to twelve months after surgery. All these studies find OPCAB to be less costly while providing a similar gain of Quality Adjusted Life Years (12-13, 24, 29, 50). As an example, the Octopus study (24) found costs of OPCAB to be $13.069 versus $14.908 ($P<0,01$) at one year follow up for a one year QALY of 0,83 in the CCABG group versus 0,82 in the OPCAB group. Long term data on health economics are not available.

4. Summary

In conclusion, this review of currently published randomized controlled trials comparing outcomes after OPCAB and CCABG resulted in the following findings:

- There is no strong evidence that one treatment is superior with regard to preventing death from any cause, chest pain or reintervention for ischemia. There is evidence from one large, well performed study that the risk of cardiovascular death is higher at one year follow-up after OPCAB compared to CCABG. There is some evidence from large trials that patients undergoing OPCAB receive fewer grafts than patients undergoing CCABG, but this tendency is very small in studies performed in centres with a large experience in OPCAB. There is strong evidence that graft patency is lower after OPCAB, but not in very experienced centres.
- There is no evidence of a difference in peri-operative risk of mortality between the two treatments. There is strong evidence of a larger release of biochemical markers of

myocardial injury and of increased incidence of atrial fibrillation after CCABG but no difference in the incidence of clinically important myocardial infarctions.
There is conflicting evidence of increased need of inotropic or pressor drugs and of intra-aortic balloon pump after CCABG. There is strong evidence of increased release of biochemical markers of renal insufficiency after CCABG but not of postoperative need of dialysis.
There is conflicting evidence of differences in incidence of perioperative stroke. Limited evidence suggests that neuro-cognitive dysfunction is larger early after CCABG than after OPCAB. However, no difference is detected later than three months after the operation.
There is strong evidence of fewer chest infections and shorter ventilation times after OPCAB. Risk of peri-operative bleeding and need for transfusions is higher after CCABG than after OPCAB. There is conflicting evidence regarding increased risk of gastro-intestinal complications after CCABG.
There is strong evidence from a number of randomized, controlled trials that the inflammatory response and the oxidative stress is higher after CCABG than after OPCAB. However, the clinical significance of these findings remain unclear.
Finally, there is strong evidence that OPCAB is more cost-effective than CCABG at up to twelve months follow-up. Long term data on cost-effectiveness are not available.

5. References

[1] Roger VL, Go AS, Lloyd-Jones DM et al. Heart Disease and Stroke Statistics_2011 Update: A report from the American Heart Association. Circulation 2011;123:e18-e209

[2] Benetti FJ. Direct coronary surgery with sphenoid vein bypass without either cardiopulmonary bypass or circulatory arrest. J Cardiovasc Surg 1985;26:217-22

[3] Buffolo E, Andrade JC, Succi J et al. Direct myocardial revascularization without cardiopulmonary bypass. Thorac Cardiovasc Surg 1985:33;26-9

[4] Cleveland JC Jr, Shroyer AL, Chen AY, Peterson E, Grover FL. Off-pump coronary artery bypass grafting decreases risk-adjusted mortality and morbidity. Ann Thorac Surg. 2001;72(4):1282-8

[5] Magee MJ, Jablonski KA, Stamou SC, Pfister AJ, Dewey TM, Dullum MK, Edgerton JR, Prince SL, Acuff TE, Corso PJ, Mack MJ. Elimination of cardiopulmonary bypass improves early survival for multivessel coronary artery bypass patients. Ann Thorac Surg. 2002;73:1196-202

[6] van Dijk D, Spoor M, Hijman R, Nathoe HM, Borst C, Jansen EWL, Grobbee DE, de Jaegere PTP, Kalkman CJ for the Octopus Study Group. Cognitive and Cardiac Outcomes 5 Years After Off-Pump vs On-Pump Coronary Artery Bypass Graft Surgery. JAMA 2007;297(7):701-708

[7] Angelini GD, Taylor FC, Reeves BC, Ascione R.Early and midterm outcome after off-pump and on-pump surgery inBeating Heart Against Cardioplegic Arrest Studies (BHACAS 1 and 2): a pooled analysis of two randomised controlled trials. Lancet 2002; 359: 1194–99

[8] Czerny M, Baumer H, Kilo J, Zuckermann A, Grubhofer G, Chevtchik D, Wolner E, Grimm M. Complete Revascularization in Coronary Artery Bypass Grafting With and Without Cardiopulmonary Bypass. Ann Thorac Surg 2001;71:165–9

[9] Légaré J-F, Buth KJ, King S, Wood J, MD; Sullivan JA, Friesen HC, Lee J, Stewart K, Hirsch GM. Coronary Bypass Surgery Performed off Pump Does NotResult in Lower In-Hospital Morbidity Than Coronary Artery Bypass Grafting Performed on Pump. Circulation. 2004;109:887-892

[10] Lingaas PS, Hol PK, Lundblad R, Rein KA, Tønnesen TI, Svennevig JL, Hauge SN, Vatne K,Fosse E. Clinical and Angiographic Outcome of Coronary Surgery with and without Cardiopulmonary Bypass: A Prospective Randomized Trial. The Heart Surgery Forum 2003:302621

[11] Sajja LR, Mannam G, Chakravarthi RM, Sompalli S, Naidu SK, Somaraju B, Penumatsa RR. Coronary artery bypass grafting with or without cardiopulmonary bypass in patients with preoperative non–dialysis dependent renal insufficiency: A randomized study. J Thorac Cardiovasc Surg2007;133:378-88

[12] Puskas JD, Williams WH, Mahoney EM, Huber PR, Block PC, Duke PG, Stables JR, Glas KE, Marshall JJ, Leimbach ME, McCall SA, Petersen RJ; Bailey DE, Weintraub WS, Guyton RA. Off-pump vs conventional coronary artery bypass grafting: early and 1 year graft patency, cost, and quality-of-life outcomes. A randomized trial. JAMA 2004;291:1841-1849

[13] Straka Z, Widimsky P, Jirasek K, Stros P, Votava J, Vanek T, Brucek P, Kolesar M, Spacek R. Off-Pump Versus On-Pump Coronary Surgery: Final Results From a Prospective Randomized Study PRAGUE-4. Ann Thorac Surg 2004;77:789 –93

[14] Shroyer AL, Grover FL, Hattler B, Collins JF, McDonald GO, Kozora E, Lucke JC, Baltz JH, Novitzky D, for the Veterans Affairs Randomized On/Off Bypass (ROOBY) Study Group. On-Pump versus Off-Pump Coronary-Artery Bypass Surgery N Engl J Med 2009;361:1827-37.

[15] Karolak W, Hirsch G, Buth K, MSc, and J-F Legare. Medium-term outcomes of coronary artery bypass graft surgery on pump versus off pump: Results from a randomized controlled trial. Am Heart J 2007;153:689-95

[16] Ascione R, Williams S, Lloyd CT, Sundaramoorthi T, Pitsis AA, Angelini GD. Reduced postoperative blood loss and transfusion requirement after beating-heart coronary operations: A prospective randomized study. Ann Thorac Surg 1999;68:493– 8

[17] Paparella D, Galeone A, Venneri MT, Coviello M, Scrascia G, Marraudino N, Quaranta M, de Luca L, Schinosa T, Brister SJ, Activation of the coagulation system during coronary artery bypass grafting: Comparison between on-pump and off-pump techniques. J Thorac Cardiovasc Surg 2006;131:290-7

[18] Parolari A, Mussoni L, Frigerio M, Naliato M, Alamanni F, Galanti A, Fiore G, MD, Veglia F, Tremoli E, Biglioli P, Camera M. Increased prothrombotic state lasting as long as one month after on-pump and off-pump coronary surgery. J Thorac Cardiovasc Surg 2005;130:303-8

[19] Parolari A, Mussoni L, Frigerio M, Naliato M, Alamanni F, Polvani GL, Agrifoglio M, Veglia F, Tremoli E, Biglioli P, Camera M. The role of tissue factor and P-selectin in the procoagulant response that occurs in the first month after on-pump and off-pump coronary artery bypass grafting J Thorac Cardiovasc Surg 2005;130:1561-6

[20] Tanaka KA, Thourani VH, Williams WH, Duke PG, Levy JH, Guyton RA, Puskas JD Heparin anticoagulation in patients undergoing off-pump and on-pump coronary bypass surgery. J Anesth 2007;21:297–303

[21] Cheng DC, Bainbridge D, Martin JE, Novick RJ. The Evidence-based Perioperative Clinical Outcomes Research Group. Does Off-pump Coronary Artery Bypass Reduce Mortality, Morbidity, and Resource Utilization When Compared with Conventional Coronary Artery Bypass? A Meta-analysis of Randomized Trials. Anesthesiology. 2005;102(1):188-203

[22] Widimsky P, Straka Z, Stros P, Jirasek K, Dvorak J, Votava J, Lisa L, Budesinsky T, Kolesar M, Vanek T, Brucek P. One-Year Coronary Bypass Graft Patency A Randomized Comparison Between Off-Pump and On-Pump Surgery. Angiographic Results of the PRAGUE-4 Trial. Circulation. 2004;110:3418-3423

[23] Kochamba GS Yun KL, Pfeffer TA, Sintek CF, Khonsari S.Pulmonary Abnormalities After Coronary Arterial Bypass Grafting Operation: Cardiopulmonary Bypass Versus Mechanical Stabilization. Ann Thorac Surg 2000;69:1466 –70

[24] Nathoe HM, Dijk D, Jansen EWL, Suyker WJL, Diephuis JC, Boven WJ, Riviere AB, Borst C, Kalkman CJ, Grobbe DE, Buskens E, Jaegere PPT. A comparison of on-pump and off-pump coronary bypass surgery in low-risk patients. The New England Journal of Medicine 2003;348:394-402.

[25] Khan NE, De Souza A, Mister R, Flather M, Clague J, Davies S, Collins P, Wang D, Sigwart U, Pepper J. A Randomized Comparison of Off-Pump and On-Pump Multivessel Coronary-Artery Bypass Surgery. N Engl J Med 2004;350: 21-8.

[26] Møller CH, Perko MJ, Lund JT, Andersen LW, Kelbæk H, Madsen JK, Gluud, C, Steinbrüchel DA. Graft patency after off-pump versus on-pump coronary artery surgery in high-risk patients. Scandinavian Cardiovascular Journal, 2010; 44: 161–167

[27] Ascione R, Reeves BC, Taylor FC, Seehraa HK, Angelini GD.Beating heart against cardioplegic arrest studies (BHACAS 1 and 2): quality of life at mid-term follow-up in two randomised controlled trials. European Heart Journal 2004; 25: 765–770

[28] Bjorner JB, Kreiner S, Ware JE, Damsgaard MT, Bech P. Differential item functioning in the Danish translation of the SF-36. J Clin Epidemiol 1998;51:1189-202.

[29] Al-Ruzzeh S, George S, Bustami M, Wray J, Ilsley C, Athanasiou T, Amrani M. Effect of off-pump coronary artery bypass surgery on clinical, angiographic, neurocognitive, and quality of life outcomes: randomised controlled trial BMJ 2006;332:1365-72

[30] Jensen BO, Hughes P, Rasmussen LS, Pedersen PU, Steinbrüchel DA. Health-related quality of life following off-pump versus on-pump coronary artery bypass grafting in elderly moderate to high-risk patients: a randomized trial. European Journal of Cardio-thoracic Surgery 2006;30:294 – 299

[31] Tully PJ, Baker RA, Kneebone AS, Knight JL. Neuropsychologic and Quality-of-Life Outcomes After Coronary Artery Bypass Surgery With and Without Cardiopulmonary Bypass: A Prospective Randomized TrialJournal of Cardiothoracic and Vascular Anesthesia 2008;22:515-521

[32] Fattouch K, Guccione F, Dioguardi P, Sampognaro R, Corrado E, Caruso M, Ruvolo G. Off-pump versus on-pump myocardial revascularization in patients with ST-segment elevation myocardial infarction: A randomized trial. J Thorac Cardiovasc Surg 2009;137:650-7

[33] Gulielmos V, Menschikowski M, Dilla H-M, Ellera M, Thiele S, Tugtekina SM, Jarossb W, Schuelera S. Interleukin-1, interleukin-6 and myocardial enzyme response after coronary artery bypass grafting: a prospective randomized comparison of the

conventional and three minimally invasive surgical techniques. European Journal of Cardio-thoracic Surgery 2000;18:594-601
[34] Krejca M, Skiba J, Szmagala P, Gburek T, Bochenek A. Cardiac troponin T release during coronary surgery using intermittent cross-clamp with fibrillation, on-pump and off-pump beating heart. European Journal of Cardio-thoracic Surgery 1999;16: 337-341
[35] Chowdhury UK, Malik V, Rakesh Y Seth S, Ramakrishnan L, Kalaivani M, Reddy SM, Subramaniam GK, Govindappa R, Kakani M. Myocardial injury in coronary artery bypass grafting: On-pump versus off-pump comparison by measuring high-sensitivity C-reactive protein, cardiac troponin I, heart-type fatty acid–binding protein, creatine kinase-MB, and myoglobin release. J Thorac Cardiovasc Surg 2008;135:1110-9
[36] Malik V, Kale SC, Chowdhury UK, Ramakrishnan L, Chauhan S, Kiran U.Myocardial Injury in Coronary Artery Bypass Grafting On-Pump versus Off-Pump Comparison by Measuring Heart-Type Fatty-Acid–Binding Protein Release Tex Heart Inst J 2006;33:321-7
[37] Medved I, Anic D, Zrnic B, Ostric M Saftic I. Off-Pump versus On-Pump - Intermittent Aortic Cross Clamping - Myocardial Revascularisation:Single Center Expirience. Coll. Antropol. 2008;32:381–384
[38] Sahlman A, Ahonen J, Nemlander A, Salmenperä M, Eriksson H, Rämö J, Vento A. Myocardial metabolism on off-pump surgery; a randomized study of 50 cases. Scand Cardiovasc J 2003;37: 211–215,
[39] Selvanayagam JB, Petersen SE, Francis JM, Robson MD, Kardos A, Neubauer S, Taggart DP. Effects of Off-Pump Versus On-Pump Coronary Surgery on Reversible and Irreversible Myocardial Injury. A Randomized Trial Using Cardiovascular Magnetic Resonance Imaging and Biochemical Markers. Circulation. 2004;109:345-350.
[40] Serrano CV Jr, Souza JA, Lopes NH, Fernandes JL Nicolau JC, Blotta MHSL, Ramires JAF MD, Hueb WA. Reduced expression of systemic proinflammatory and myocardial biomarkers after off-pump versus on-pump coronary artery bypass surgery: A prospective randomized study. Journal of Critical Care 2010;25: 305–312
[41] van Dijk D, Nierich AP, Jansen EWL, Nathoe HM, Suyker WJL, Diephuis JC, van Boven W-J, Borst C, Buskens E, Grobbee DE, de Medina EOR, de Jaegere PTP, for the Octopus Study Group. Early Outcome After Off-Pump Versus On-Pump Coronary Bypass Surgery Results From a Randomized Study Circulation. 2001;104:1761-1766
[42] Vedin J, Jensen U, Ericsson A, Samuelsson S Vaage J. Pulmonary hemodynamics and gas exchange in off pump coronary artery bypass grafting Interact CardioVasc Thorac Surg 2005;4:493-497
[43] Hendrik M, Nathoe HM, Moons KGM, van Dijk D, Jansen EWL, Borst C, de Jaegere PTP, Grobbee DE, for the Octopus Study Group Risk and Determinants of Myocardial Injury During Off-Pump Coronary Artery Bypass Grafting. Am J Cardiol 2006;97:1482–1486
[44] Mantovani V Charles Kennergren C Bugge M, Sala A , Lönnroth P, Berglin E Myocardial metabolism assessed by microdialysis: A prospective randomized study in on- and off-pump coronary bypass surgery. International Journal of Cardiology 2010;143: 302–308

[45] Ascione R, Caputo M, Calori G, Lloyd CT, Underwood MJ,Angelini GD. Predictors of Atrial Fibrillation After Conventional and Beating Heart Coronary Surgery. A Prospective, Randomized Study. Circulation. 2000;102:1530-1535

[46] Møller CH, Perko MJ, Lund JT, Andersen LW, MD, Kelbæk H, Madsen JK, Winkel P, Gluud C, Steinbrüchel DA. No Major Differences in 30-Day Outcomes in High-Risk Patients Randomized to Off-Pump Versus On-Pump Coronary Bypass Surgery. The Best Bypass Surgery Trial. Circulation. 2010;121:498-504

[47] Wijeysundera DN, Beattie WS, Djaiani G, Rao V, Borger MA, Karkouti K, Cusimano RJ. Off-pump coronary artery surgery for reducing mortality and morbidity: meta-analysis of randomized and observational studies. J Am Coll Cardiol. 2005;46(5):872-82.

[48] Diegeler A, Hirsch R, Schneider F, Schilling L-O, MD, Falk V, Rauch T, Mohr FW. Neuromonitoring and Neurocognitive Outcome in Off-Pump Versus Conventional Coronary Bypass Operation. Ann Thorac Surg 2000;69:1162- 6

[49] van Dijk D, Jansen EWL, Hijman R, Nierich AP, Diephuis JC, Moons KGM, Lahpor JR, Borst C, Keizer AMA, Nathoe HM, Diederick E. Grobbee DE, De Jaegere PTP, Kalkman CJ, for the Octopus Study Group. Cognitive Outcome After Off-Pump and On-Pump Coronary Artery Bypass Graft Surgery. A Randomized Trial. JAMA. 2002;287(11):1405-1412

[50] Lee JD, Lee SJ, Tsushima WT, Yamauchi H, Lau WT, Popper J, Stein, A, Johnson D, Lee D, Petrovitch H, Dang CR. Benefits of Off-Pump Bypass on Neurologic and Clinical Morbidity: A Prospective Randomized Trial. Ann Thorac Surg 2003;76:18 -26

[51] Lloyd CT, Ascione R, Underwood MJ, Gardner F, Black A, Angelini GD. Serum S-100 protein release and neuropsycologic outcome during coronary revascularization on the beating heart: A prospective randomized study. J Thorac Cardiovasc Surg 2000;119:148-54

[52] Motallebzadeh R, Bland JM, Markus HS, Kaski JC, Jahangiri M. Neurocognitive Function and Cerebral Emboli: Randomized Study of On-Pump Versus Off-Pump Coronary Artery Bypass Surgery. Ann Thorac Surg 2007;83:475- 82

[53] Naseri MH, Pishgou B, Ameli J,Babaei E, Taghipour HR. Comparison of post-operative neurological complications between on-pump and off-pump coronary artery by-pass surgery Pak J Med Sci 2009;25:137-141

[54] Zamvar V, Williams D,Hall J, Payne N, Cann C, Young K, Karthikeyan S, Dunne J. Assessment of neurocognitive impairment after off-pump and on-pump techniques for coronary artery bypass graftsurgery: prospective randomised controlled trial. BMJ 2002;325:1268

[55] Selnes OA, Grega MA, Borowicz LM Jr, Barry S, Zeger S, Baumgartner WA, McKhann GM. Cognitive outcomes three years after coronary artery bypass surgery: a comparison of on-pump coronary artery bypass graft surgery and nonsurgical controls. Ann Thorac Surg. 2005 Apr;79(4):1201-9.

[56] Wandschneider W, Thalmann M, Trampitsch E, Ziervogel G, Kobinia G, Off-Pump Coronary Bypass Operations Significantly Reduce S100 Release: An Indicator for Less Cerebral Damage? Ann Thorac Surg 2000;70:1577–9

[57] Yin Y-q, Luo A-l, Guo X-y, Li L-h Huang Y-g. Postoperative neuropsychological change and its underlying mechanism in patients undergoing coronary artery bypass grafting. Chin Med J 2007;120:1951-1957

[58] Andersson LG, Ekroth R, Bratteby LE, Hallhagen S, Wesslen O. Acute renal failure in the patient undergoing cardiac operation. Prevalence, mortality rate, and main risk factors. J Thorac Cardiovasc Surg 1989;98:1107-12
[59] Abu-Omar Y, Ratatunga C. Cardiopulmonary by-pass and renal injury. Perfusion 2006; 21:209-213
[60] Ascione R, MD, Lloyd CT, Underwood MJ, Gomes WJ, Gianni D, Angelini GD. On-Pump Versus Off-Pump Coronary Revascularization: Evaluation of Renal Function. Ann Thorac Surg 1999;68:493- 8
[61] Tang ATM, Knotta J,. Nanson J, Hsua J, Hawa MP, Ohri SK. A prospective randomized study to evaluate the renoprotective action of beating heart coronary surgery in low risk patients. European Journal of Cardio-thoracic Surgery 2002;22:118–123
[62] Güler M, Kırali K, Toker ME, Bozbug N Ömeroglu SN , Akıncı E, Yakut C. Different CABG Methods in Patients With Chronic Obstructive Pulmonary Disease. Ann Thorac Surg 2001;71:152–7
[63] Covino E, Santise G, Di Lello F, De Amicis V, Bonifazi R, Bellino I, Spampinato N: Surgical myocardial revascularization (CABG) in patients with pulmonary disease: Beating heart versus cardiopulmonary bypass. J Cardiovasc Surg (Torino). 2001;42(1):23-6.
[64] Cox CM, Ascione R, Cohen AM, Davies IM, Ryder IG, Angelini GD. Effect of Cardiopulmonary Bypass on Pulmonary Gas Exchange: A Prospective Randomized Study. Ann Thorac Surg 2000;69:140 –5
[65] Syed A, Fawzy H, Farag A, Nemlander A, Comparison of Pulmonary Gas Exchange in OPCAB Versus Conventional CABG. HeartLung and Circulation 2004;13:168–172
[66] Raja SG, Haider Z, Ahmad M. Predictors of gastrointestinal complications after conventional and beatingheart coronary surgery. Surg J R Coll Surg 2003:221-228
[67] Formica F, Broccolo F, Martino A, Sciucchetti J, Giordano V, Avalli L, Radaelli G, Ferro O, Corti F, Cocuzza C, Paolini G. Myocardial revascularization with miniaturized extracorporeal circulation versus off pump: Evaluation of systemic and myocardial inflammatory response in a prospective randomized study. J Thorac Cardiovasc Surg 2009;137:1206-12
[68] Nesher N, Frolkis I, Vardi M, Sheinberg N, Bakir I, Caselman F, Pevni D, Ben-Gal Y, Sharony R, Bolotin G, Loberman D, Uretzky G, Weinbroum AA,. Higher Levels of Serum Cytokines and Myocardial Tissue Markers During On-Pump Versus Off-Pump Coronary Artery Bypass Surgery J Card Surg 2006;21:395-402
[69] Onorati F, Rubino AS, Nucera S, Foti D, Sica V, Santini F, Gulletta E, Renzulli A. Off-pump coronary artery bypass surgery versus standard linear or pulsatile cardiopulmonary bypass: endothelial activation and inflammatory response European Journal of Cardio-thoracic Surgery 2010;37: 897—904
[70] Wildhirt SM, Schulze C, Conrad NE, Schütz A, Reichart B. Expression von TNF-alpha und löslichen Adhäsionsmolekülen nach koronarchirurgischen Eingriffen mit und ohne extrakorporaler Zirkulation. Z Herz- Thorax- Gefäßchir 2001;15:7-13
[71] Johannson-Synnergren M, Nilsson F, Bengtsson A, Jeppson A, Wiklund L. Off-pump CABG reduces complement activation but does not significantly affect peripheral endothelial function: a prospective, randomized study. Scand Cardiovasc J 38; 53-58, 2004

[72] Gu YJ, Mariani MA, Oeveren W v , Grandjean JG, Boonstra PW. Reduction of the Inflammatory Response in Patients Undergoing Minimally Invasive Coronary Artery Bypass Grafting. Ann Thorac Surg 1998;65:420–4

[73] Kolackova M, Kudlova M, Kunes P, Lonsky V, Mandak J, Andrys C, Jankovicova K, Krejsek J. Early Expression of FcγRI (CD64) on Monocytes of Cardiac Surgical Patients and Higher Density of Monocyte Anti-Inflammatory Scavenger CD163 Receptor in "On-Pump" Patients. Mediators of Inflammation 2008; 235461

[74] Akila, D'souza AB, Prashant V, D'souza V. Oxidative injury and antioxidants in coronary artery bypass graft surgery:Off-pump CABG significantly reduces oxidative stress. Clinica Chimica Acta 2007;375:147–152

[75] Puskas JD, Williams WH, Duke PG, Staples JR, Glas KE, Marshall JJ, Leimbach M, Huber P, Garas S, Sammons BH, McCall SA, Petersen RJ, Bailey DE, Chu H, Mahoney EM, Weintraub WS, Guyton RA. Off-pump coronary artery bypass grafting providescomplete revascularization with reduced myocardial injury, transfusion requirements, and length of stay: A prospective randomized comparison of two hundred unselected patients undergoing off-pump versus conventional coronary artery bypass grafting. J Thorac Cardiovasc Surg 2003;125: 797-808

[76] Medved I, Anic D, Zrnic B, Ostric M Saftic I. Off-Pump versus On-Pump - Intermittent Aortic Cross Clamping - Myocardial Revascularisation: Single Center Expirience. Coll. Antropol. 2008;32:381–384

8

Re-Engineering in OPCAB Surgery

Murali P. Vettath, Et Ismail, Av Kannan and Athmaja Murali
Kozhikode Kerala
India

1. Introduction

Coronary artery bypass surgery is a procedure that started off with the first implantation of the internal mammary artery to the cardiac muscle in 1946 by Vineberg [Vineberg AM, 1954]. Later, the coronary anastomosis distal to the occlusion using the saphenous vein graft (SVG) or the internal mammary artery (IMA) was experimentally conceived by Murray [Murray et al, 1954]. Bailey et al [Bailey et al, 1957] were the first group to approach the problem of coronary occlusion in 1957. Though the pioneers of OPCAB were Goetz and colleagues [Goetz et al, 1961] and Kolessov [Kolessov VL, 1967] who performed the procedure in isolated cases. The first clinical series of consecutive patients was by Trapp and Bisarya [Trapp WG, Bisarya R,1975] and Ankeney [Ankeney JL,1975].
Then, with the development of direct coronary surgery, under the leadership of Favaloro [Favaloro RG,1968] and Green and coworkers [Green GE, Stertzer SH 1968], with procedures being performed in an arrested heart with the use of extracorporeal circulation, off-pump coronary surgery was abandoned. Thus the surgeons all over the world started performing CABG on the heart lung machine , and that became the standard of care for patients with coronary artery disease.
In 1981 Enio Buffolo [Buffolo E ,et.al,1985]from Brazil and Benneti [Benetti FJ,1985] from Argentina had started experimenting on this technique of Direct Myocardial revascularization. Both of them published their series around 1985 which rekindled the idea of OPCAB in the western world. It was probably the idea of minimally invasive direct coronary artery bypass graft (MIDCABG), introduced in the mid-1990s by Benneti [Benetti FJ ,1985,1995], that called attention to the possibility and advantages of not using CPB. Calafiore's [Calafiore AM,et al,1996,1998] publications re- enforced the advantages of the LAST(left anterior small thoracotomy) operation. The LIMA stitch was acclaimed as an extraordinary step in the development of off-pump coronary surgery, which allowed grafting of posterior branches of the coronary arteries. The introduction of stabilizers in the mid 1990s further facilitated the procedure[Borst C,1996]. Eric Jansen, was one of those surgeon in the mid nineties who was probably the man who had made the word -Octopus- so very popular in the rest of the world. The article published in 1991 by Benetti [Benetti F.J et al,1991] in Chest, gave confidence to the Cardiac surgeons around the world to perform OPCAB in all anterior vessels. But even then the circumflex territory became a danger zone for most surgeons to perform a safe coronary anastomoses. Though LIMA stitch was used quite often, it was the availability of the Positioners that that made the process of Verticalisation of the heart more comfortable.

By the end of the 90's, most of the surgeons in India and in the far east had been performing OPCAB in 90% of their Coronary artery patients, but by early 2000, there was a sharp decline in the numbers, as most of the surgeons did not find the comfort zone in OPCAB surgery, and that their patency rates were being questioned. In the 1990s the visibility of coronary anastomosis was again a doubtful proposition, and also converting, and going on to the pump became a recipe for disaster. Then came the comparative trials of OPCAB and ONCAB , which obviously brought in results which showed that both the techniques produce nearly the same results, and that the patency was a question of concern[Kim KB,et al,2001&.Puskas JD.et al,2001] The Rooby trial showed that, at 1 year of follow-up, patients in the off-pump group had worse composite outcomes and poorer graft patency than did patients in the on-pump group[A. Laurie Shroyer,et al,NEJM,2009]. The surgeons had then come to a conclusion that OPCAB is good in experienced hands and the results in that group of people have been outstanding.

The appeal of avoiding cardiopulmonary bypass with its direct and indirect physiological insult, the prospect of improved clinical outcomes, and the favorable economic impact gives OPCAB the potential of preference that may mark the dawn of a new era in our search for the optimal surgical strategy for the treatment of coronary artery disease.

OPCAB has been performed in many different ways. It's like different ways of skinning a cat. Ultimately, the gold standard of a perfect patent coronary anastomosis remains the corner stone of a good surgeon and a good operation. It is to be emphasized here that Coronary artery bypass surgery has a come a long way from performing them off pump, then on pump and now going back to off pump. But the most important point, one has to bear in mind is that , the surgeon has to do what he is most comfortable with and by which he would be able to give the best result.

The topic of Re-engineering in OPCAB came up , because, there was an engineering that was done during the early phase of OPCAB by the great pioneers of this procedure. But what happened along the way was that these procedures were not reproducible by lesser mortals like us and hence we had to re-engineer this procedure to suit us.

2. Theorotical reason of avoiding the pump

It is logical to suppose that avoiding CPB would abolish the SIRS (systemic inflammatory response syndrome)and its untoward physiological impact. [Gu Y.J, 1999]. Gu Y.J, investigated the inflammatory response with OPCAB, and found that complement activation and consequently systemic inflammatory response occurred (due to surgical trauma) but the extent and severity were curtailed.

Comparison with on-pump CABG confirms a limited and less severe form of inflammatory response. Strüber [Strüber M.,et al,1999&, Matata B.M.et al,2000] and Matata and their coworkers reported significant increases in the levels of specific biological markers of inflammation following on-pump CABG compared to OPCAB. The inflammatory indicators that were evaluated in both studies and their results are summarized:

- Activated complement factor 3a (C3a) demonstrated between 5- and 12-fold rise over the preoperative level after commencement of CPB, and minimal rise in the OPCAB patients.
- Proinflammatory interleukin 8 (IL-8) increased 5-folds with CPB whilst the level was only slightly altered with OPCAB.

- Tumor necrosis factor (TNF-) peaked 24–48 h after CPB at a significantly higher value compared to OPCAB patients who had no increase. Tumor necrosis factor receptors 1 and 2 were elevated to three times their preoperative level only with CPB.
- Different markers tested in each study (interleukin 6 and plasma elastase) were significantly elevated with CPB. OPCAB patients showed a blunted response.

The other variables of CPB such as haemodilution, non-pulsatile flow, and aortic cross-clamping, which may act in concert with SIRS to increase postoperative morbidity, are eliminated by the avoidance of CPB.

Thus avoiding the heart lung machine would be a logical solution in performing coronary artery bypass surgery

3. Myocardial preservation

Adequate myocardial preservation is crucial in CABG operations. Preoperative resuscitation of ischemic myocardium enables recruitment of hibernating myocardium and forms an important component of any myocardial protection strategy. The intraoperative strategy varies (within physiological boundaries) as much from patient to patient as it is from surgeon to surgeon, to the extent that a good clinical outcome becomes the ultimate determinant of the optimal strategy. Even with the same surgeon, the strategy is adapted to the patient and clinical scenario that a prescriptive regimen is not standard. The objective of intraoperative myocardial preservation is to enable efficient myocardial energy management by reducing cardiac metabolic demands on the one hand, while improving myocardial oxygen supply and utilization on the other [Buckberg G.D et.al,1996].

In on-pump CABG, cardioplegia or cross-clamp fibrillation are conventional methods of intraoperative myocardial protection. Cardioplegia favorably affects myocardial energy metabolism but results in the alteration of both the intra- and extracellular milieu and, together with CPB can precipitate changes in cardiac performance postoperatively [Mehlhorn U.,1995]. Cross-clamp fibrillation can increase the endocardial viability ratio and lead to similar changes in cardiac function. In both strategies of myocardial protection, a period of global myocardial ischemia is followed by reperfusion with oxygen-rich blood predisposing to reperfusion injury which manifests as myocardial stunning and arrhythmias in the early postoperative period.

Since deliberate induction of global ischemia is unnecessary in OPCAB, it is logical to suppose that iatrogenic biochemical injury to the myocardium would not occur. More so, the blunted inflammatory response with avoidance of CPB is characterised by low production of IL-8 which is involved in myocardial injury . In fact, Atkins et al. first suggested that OPCAB preserved cardiac function in 1984 [Atkins C.W .et al,1984]. In different prospective randomized studies, Ascione [Ascione R.et al,1999], Penttilä [Penttilä H.J.,et al,2001], Van Dijk [Van Dijk D..et al,2001], Czerny [Czerny M.,et al 2001], Bennetts [Bennetts J.S.et al,2002], and Masuda [Masuda M.et al,2002], and their collaborators reported minimal change in the biochemical markers of myocardial injury (troponin T and/or creatinine kinase-MB isoenzyme), and in some cases, better myocardial function after OPCAB compared to on-pump CABG. Changes in myocardial metabolism indicative of oxidative stress due to local ischemia when the target coronary artery is occluded to enable visualization for distal anastomoses have been reported in OPCAB [Matata B.M. et al 2002]. Compared to on-pump CABG, OPCAB is associated with better myocardial energy preservation, less oxidative stress and minimal myocardial damage [Penttilä H.J et al.2001].

However, emerging evidence suggests that intraoperative myocardial protection in OPCAB can provide an added advantage [.Guyton R.A. Et al,200 & Muraki S.et al.2001]. In their pioneering report, Trapp and Bisarya gave an exquisite description of coronary perfusion and the instantaneous improvement in the ECG and blood pressure during OPCAB. Vassiliades et al. [Vassiliades T.A .et al,2002] compared active coronary perfusion using a perfusion pump, with passive perfusion by a cannula connected from the aorta to the graft, and no coronary perfusion, after the distal anastomosis in a randomized clinical trial. They found lower troponin I levels with active and passive coronary perfusion, but cardiac performance was better with active coronary perfusion. The use of intracoronary shunt during OPCAB has also been shown to preclude left ventricular dysfunction [Yeatman M.et al 2002].

Reperfusion injury can occur from regional ischemia due to a combination of underlying coronary obstructive pathology, stabilization and anastomotic techniques, compounded by episodes of hypotension which precede revascularisation. The precarious normoxic and normothermic passive coronary perfusion may be insufficient to protect against myocardial damage in such clinical scenarios.

The concept of myocardial protection in OPCAB is less tedious. In most cases passive coronary perfusion with intracoronary shunts will suffice, but in the presence of heightened cardiac risk such as recent acute myocardial ischemia or infarction, and severely impaired left ventricular function active coronary perfusion is advantageous especially in multi-vessel revascularization.

The role of Intra-aortic balloon pump (IABP)in patients with Ischemic myocardium and in low ejection fraction would be discussed later in the chapter. As of today, apart from using intra coronary shunt, the use of aorto-coronnary shunts in some instances have been a disposable worth remembering.

Hemodynamic instability has been the major concern in performing OPCAB even today. Though we have been able to master the technique of positioning the heart by the use of various technique and devices, this still remains a major concern. Exposure of the coronary artery target sites requires the heart to be lifted, rotated, dislocated and displaced producing a distortion of cardiac geometry and consequently hemodynamic fluctuations frequently occur. As a result, the early reports of OPCAB described single or double grafts limited to anterior target sites. The corrective measures for these hemodynamic changes include volume loading, trendelenberg positioning, and displacement of the heart into the opened right pleura, use of inotropes, vasopressors, vasodilators, intra-aortic balloon pump, and right heart circulatory support [Mathison M.et al, 2000 &, Kim K.B. et al, 2001].

What we had **re-engineered** over the last five years is to avoid the Trendelenberg position. And we practice an **anti-Trendelenberg position** of the patient, where the patient lies on the table with the head end up. This is very useful in patients with ischemia, where the pulmonary artery (PA) pressure is high. This maneuver reduces the PA pressure, and there by reduces the left ventricular end diastolic pressure (LVEDP). This is exactly what the patient would do when he develops chest pain in his room. He sits up and tries to catch his breath. That is what we help him do in the operation theater as he is anaesthetised.

If the CVP is low and the right ventricle looks empty, then we give a fluid challenge to improve his preload. But we always try to avoid the Trendelenberg position.

In late nineties, the principle of OPCAB was to perform the coronary anastomosis at a heart rate of less than 60 per minute. Hence, the patients coming for surgery used to be well beta blocked, so that it would be easy to perform the anastomosis. But, most of these patients

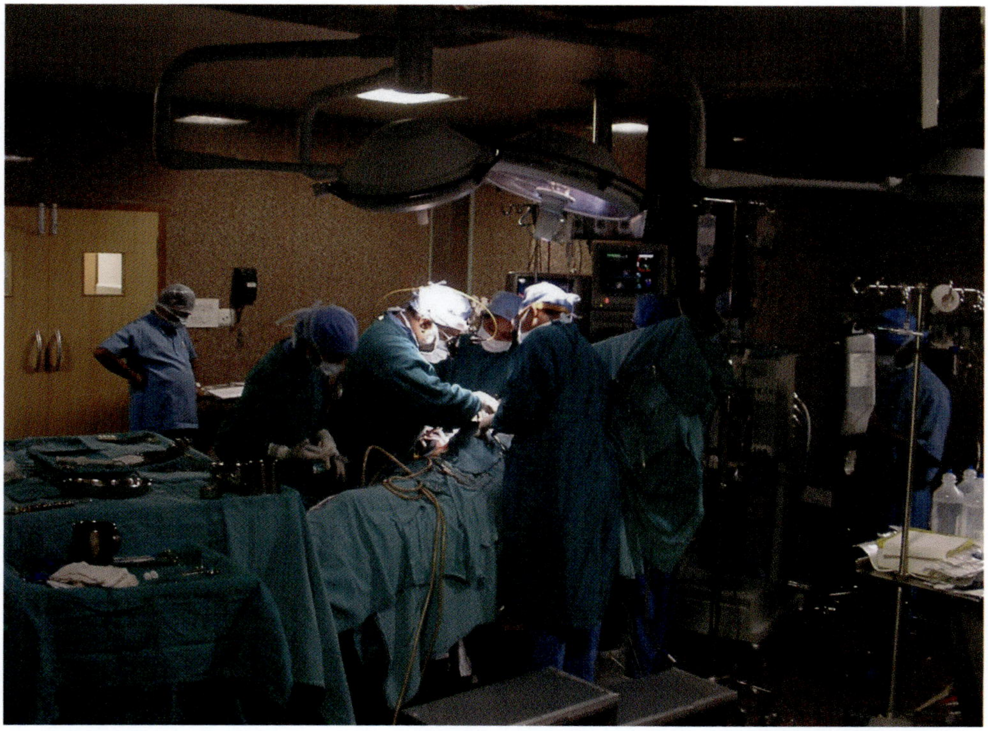

Fig. 1. Photo showing the operation table with the head end elevated and tilted to the side of the surgeon.

ended up having inotropes and vasoconstrictors to maintain hemodynamics. Ischemic patients when given either of them, they develop further ischemia and become bad.

What we had re-engineered here, was to increase the heart rate .To attain that, we use intermittent boluses of Injection Atropine (0.6mgs per milliliter), which is only a Chronotropic agent and not an Inotrope. Thus, avoiding unnecessary strain on the myocardium. We aim at a rate above 100 per minute and this keeps the heart briskly contracting and avoiding the usual hemodynamic collapse seen in the early days.

We do not use vasopressors or vasodilators in any of our patients undergoing OPCAB.The only drug the patient would be given intermittently is the Atropine injection. We use Glycerol trinitrate(GTN) in our patients after the distal anastomosis, and that too as an antihypertensive only.

Mueller et al. found no change in the hemodynamics during exposure of the posterior and anterior wall arteries, and only marginal change for the lateral wall artery with a 'no compression' technique [Mueller X.M et al,2002]. It has been suggested that the use of left ventricular apical suction device for cardiac positioning provokes less hemodynamic instability compared with pericardial retraction sutures [Sepic J.et al,2002].

The technique which we have developed is to cut down the pericardium on the right side, down to the inferior vena cava, and to leave the right pleura opened. We routinely open the left pleura to help in the mammary dissection. Hence, in all our patients we have all the three chambers- the mediastinum and both the pleural cavity, remaining in continuity with each other.

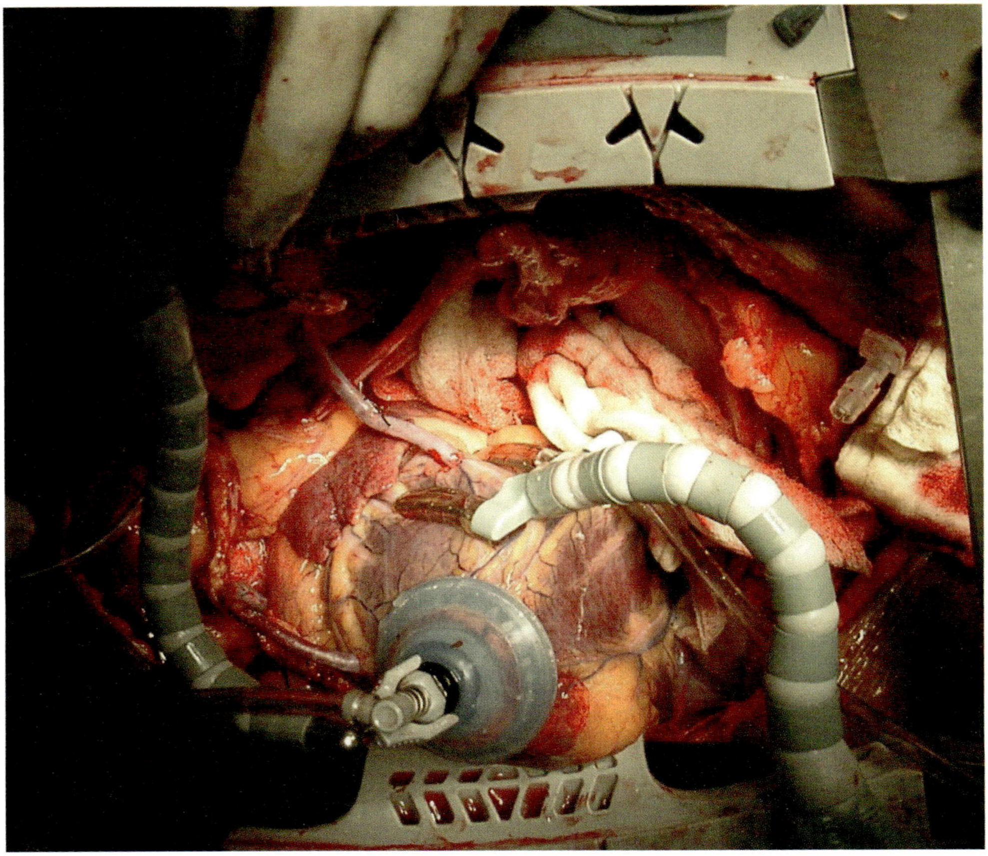

Fig. 2. Showing the Positioner verticalising the heart and the stabilizer used on the marginal circumflex.

We too routinely use the Positioner for lifting the apex of the heart. The suction pressure used is not more than 150-200 mm of Hg. The positioner is always used in an off apex position, so as to avoid sucking the Left anterior descending (LAD) coronary artery. We use this pressure to avoid excessive damage to the apex. We also watch the suction tube, to see if any blood is being sucked. In such cases , the positioner is removed and repositioned in a different place. In case of grafting of the circumflex and the Posterior descending artery (PDA) this heart is only Verticalized and not tilted to the right side. This lifting of the apex, increases the left and the right ventricular volume. And in case the PDA, is being grafted, then we tilt the head end down, so as to increase the visibility of the PDA. This probably would be the only time when the Trendelenberg position is used. By this time the LAD is already perfused, and this has relieved the ischemia. If the visibility of the circumflex is bad, then the table is dropped down to its maximum and the positioner moved to right a bit. With this maneuver, even the Atrioventricular groove could be visualized.

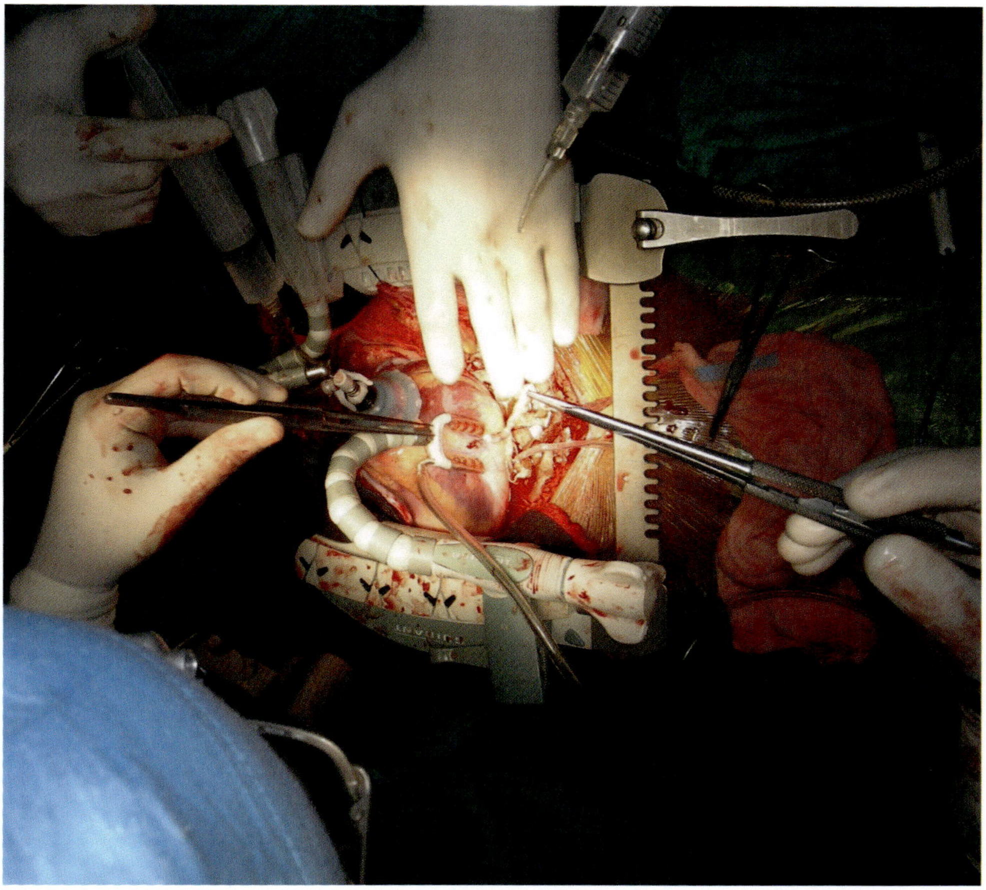

Fig. 3. Showing the heart totally verticalized by the use of the positioner, and the stabilizer in position around the PDA.

4. Quality of distal anastamosis

Performing vascular anastomoses on small arteries on a beating heart can be a daunting and frustrating adventure, and so far, no available method of target vessel stabilization can achieve a steady bloodless field comparable to an arrested heart. This was a major concern with OPCAB. The beating heart with a bloody operating field poses a major challenge to delicate tissue handling, and casts a shadow of uncertainty about the quality of the distal anastomosis. However, with the application of effective target vessel stabilization, and efficient visualization systems the early and mid-term patency of OPCAB has been encouraging

The stabilizers we use are the suction stabilizers. The position of the stabilizer is very. important to achieve a very stable anastomotic site to perform a good coronary anastomosis. We have tried all types of suction stabilizers, from the Medtronic -Octopus II, III and the Octopus IV. We are now using the Maquet, which was the previous Guidant - Acrobat

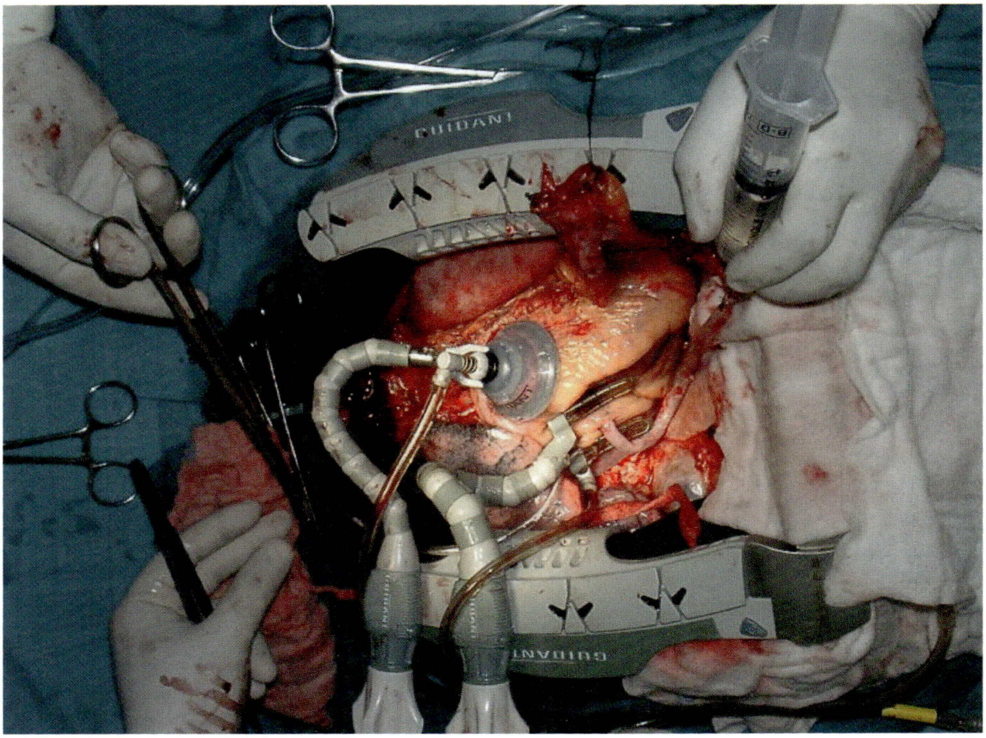

Fig. 4. Photograph showing the positioner on the RV free wall to graft the distal RCA or the acute marginal.

stabilizer. The Re- engineering in this is the pressure used for suction of these stabilizers. We use 100-150 mm of Hg on these stabilizers. The stabilizer is positioned according to the convenience of the surgeon. The position of our stabilizer is shown in the photographs. We do not use any suction while stabilizing the lateral wall, as the heart is allowed to fall on the stabilizer pods.

In order to achieve a stable bloodless field while accessing the coronary artery, we use the following technique. After stabilizing the coronary artery by using the acrobat stabilizer, we use a 5.0 polypropelene suture to run around the proximal part of the coronary artery, proximal to where the arteriotomy is planned to be made. The two ends of the 5.0 polypropylene are suspended using rubber shod . They are tightened just before the coronary arteriotomy is made. This is made using the bevel of a 18 gauge needle on a 2 ml syringe. After the nick is made on the coronary artery, the forward or the backward cutting scissors is used to open the coronary artery. A Castroveijo scissors is used to open the arteriotomy. The arteriotomy is usually one centimeter long. Then the intra-coronary shunt is inserted according to the size of the coronary artery. The shunt is to be deaired after inserting the proximal end first, then the snare is released and the then the distal end is inserted. Then the anastomosis of the coronary is performed using the conduits as preferred. We use shunts in nearly all the distal anastomosis.

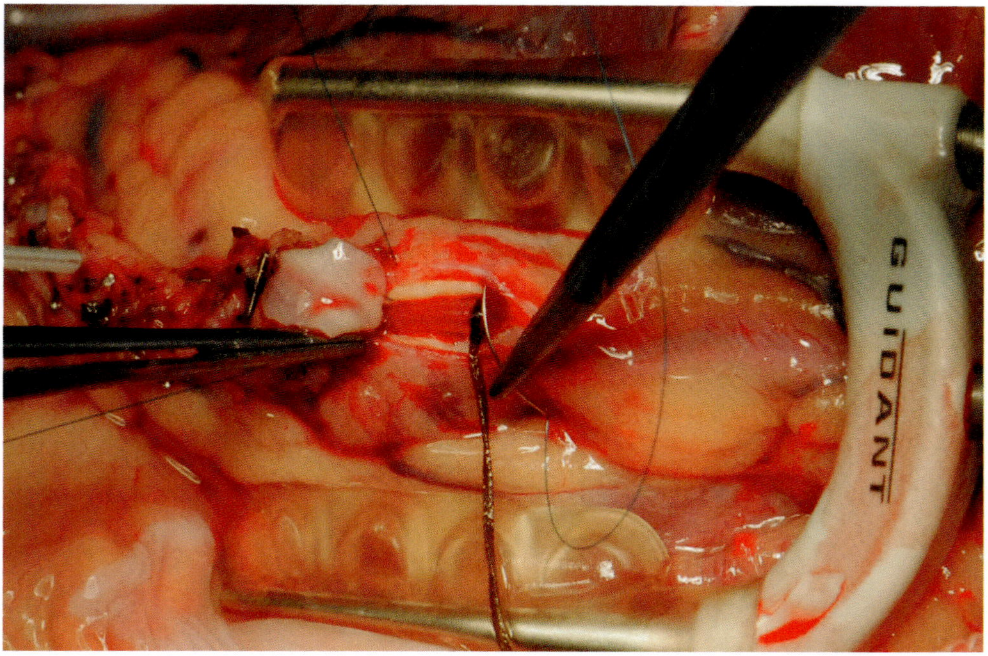

Fig. 5. Showing the clarity of the coronary anastamosis, while performing LIMA to LAD anastamosis.

5. Incomplete myocardial revascularisation

Early reports of OPCAB in the literature were uniformly consistent in the low number of grafts per patient [6,10]. The selection of patients with mainly single-vessel disease may, in part, explain this finding. But the persistence of lower average number of grafts in later comparative studies [Gundry S.R et al,1998 &Arom K.V.et al,2000] places OPCAB in a contentious position which detracts from its potential benefits. In their retrospective study, Gundry and colleagues reported a significantly lower mean number of grafts, and a two-fold increase in cardiac re-intervention rate during a 7-year period with off-pump performed without cardiac stabilization, compared to on-pump CABG. This finding has been corroborated by other reports , and exemplifies incomplete revascularization with OPCAB. Effective cardiac retraction, stabilization and visualization systems with patient positioning enables grafting of all graftable targets, making complete myocardial revascularization (CMR) attainable in OPCAB [Calafiore A.M et al 1995 & Cartier R et al, 2000], and this has been demonstrated in a recent prospective randomized study [Puskas J.D et al,2003]. However, incomplete myocardial revascularization with OPCAB is still reported in retrospective studies . Technical difficulties due to small caliber of target vessels or their intramyocardial course, poor exposure of target sites, precarious intraoperative hemodynamic state, electrophysiological instability and inexperience of the surgeon are some of the reasons for incomplete myocardial revascularization.

Today we have no contraindications for OPCAB , the intramyocardial coronary arteries, small coronary arteries and diffuse coronary arteries [Anil D Prabhu et al, 2007&2008], have

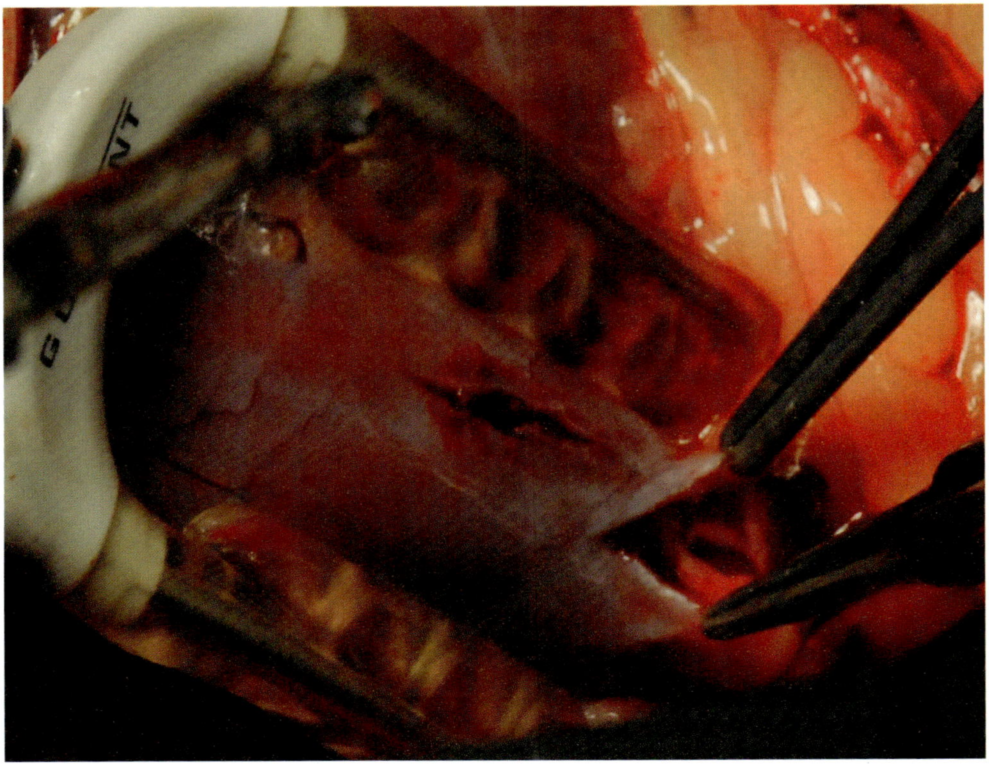

Fig. 6. Showing the dissection on the buried intramuscular coronary artery on the lateral wall of the heart.

been a thing of the past. Any patient who needs to undergo CABG would be able to have his coronary artery bypass surgery using the OPCAB technique.

6. High risk surgical patients

OPCAB has been demonstrated to offer prognostic advantage over on-pump CABG in patients with exaggerated surgical risk from complicated coronary artery disease and/or debilitating co-morbidities [Tashiro T et al,1996,Akiyama K.et al,1999,Yokoyama T. et al,2000 & Prifti E et al,2000]. More importantly, the preoperative optimization of high risk patients plays a crucial role in determining the clinical outcome for both methods of myocardial revascularization.
Acute myocardial infarction and depressed left ventricular function constitute a high surgical risk with on-pump CABG, because the myocardial damaging effects of CPB and the often cumbersome and, inefficient intraoperative myocardial protection do not prevent immediate postoperative cardiac dysfunction [Buckberg Get al,1996,Christenson J.T..et al,1997 &.D'Ancona G,2001]. OPCAB achieves comparatively better outcomes in patients who have myocardial revascularization soon after recent AMI [Locker C,2001]. Mohr et al. [Mohr R et al 1999] reported a mortality of 1.7% with 1- and 5-year actuarial survival rates of 94.7 and 82.3%, respectively, in a series of 57 patients in which 56% had emergency surgery

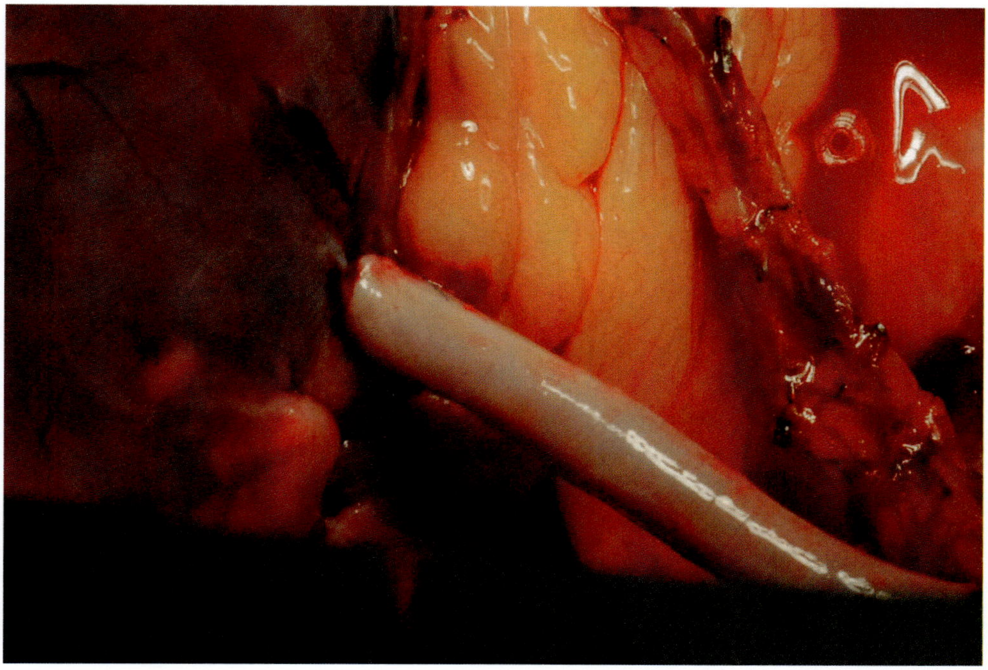

Fig. 7. Showing the vein graft after anastomosis on the coronary artery.

within 48 hr of acute myocardial infarction and some were in cardiogenic shock. OPCAB decreases the operative risk in the presence of impaired left ventricular function [Nakayama Y.et al,2003]

Preoperative renal impairment is an independent predictor of poor prognosis after on-pump CABG [Ascione R et al 1999]]. OPCAB preserves renal function better than on-pump CABG [Ascione R.et al,2001], and available evidence favors the preferential use of OPCAB for patients with chronic renal for a better early clinical outcome.

Patients with coexisting chronic obstructive airway disease derive better early clinical benefit from CABG performed without CPB compared with on-pump surgery [Güler M et al,2001], although in low-risk patients, OPCAB induces impairment of the mechanics of the respiratory system, lung and chest wall similar to on-pump CABG [Roosens C et al,2002].

Elderly patients are considered high risk surgical patients because of their reduced functional capacity and the presence of co-morbidities. Correspondingly, the outcome of on-pump CABG in this group is characterized by increased morbidity and mortality [Montague N.T et al,,1985,,Mullany C.J et al,1980 & Hirose H,2000]. Interestingly, OPCAB has been shown to improve the clinical outcome in this growing population of surgical patients [Boyd W.D et al, 1999, Stamou S.C et al, 2000, Al-Ruzzeh S et al, 2001 & Hoff S.J.et al, 2002]. Specifically, the incidence of stroke, perioperative myocardial infarction, duration of mechanical ventilation, blood transfusion, length of intensive care and hospital stay, and mortality are decreased.

7. Vettath's anastamotic obturator

In patients with diffusely diseased coronary arteries and in patients with diseased aortas, OPCAB has remained a life saver. We had developed the Vettaths anastomotic obturator (VAO) (Murali.P.Vettath,2003,2004) - which , is is an aortic anastomosis enabling device. This allows the surgeon to avoid the side clamp on the aorta, when a no touch technique is required in cases of diseased aorta. In patients with plaquey aortas, where a saphenous vein top end is to be connected, this could be used to make an anastomosis on a no plaquey zone in the aorta. The technique is to identify a soft spot and make two purse string sutures with 3.0 polypropylene around the intended zone of anastomosis. The purse strings are about a centimeter in diameter. A stab wound is made using a no.11 blade and an aortic punch is used to make a punch hole on the aorta. The VAO is then inserted into the hole and one of the 3.0 purse strings are used to snare the bleeding around the VAO if it persists. The aortic systolic pressure may be maintained at around 100 mm of Hg. The advantage is that this allows the surgeon to perform a hand sewn anastomosis on the vein graft. This is like the devices that are available in the market, like the Heartstring and the Enclose device. This is like an instrument and is made of steel and can be reused and could help in avoiding a stroke in elderly patients. We have performed more than 500 top ends using this device and is a good one to have in the armamentarium of a cardiac surgeon. This is also a good tool to use in redo CABG, when a proximal anastomosis could be made on the hood of the old vein graft.

The VAO is also a useful tool in cases where a combined aortic valve replacement is done with a CABG. Here it is useful when the side clamp needs to be avoided.

8. Diffusely diseased coronary arteries

The diffusely diseased coronary arteries have been a curse in the south East-Asian population, and more so in patients with Indian origin. This is seen in these patients in the younger age group and they are usually termed inoperable. The disease is so diffuse that grafting area in the coronary arteries are studded with plaques. We had developed our own technique of Vettath's technique of long mammary patch on LAD without endarterectomy on beating heart. We had performed this on more than 200 patients since the last 9 years. We have also published the same (Murali Vettath,2008) in couple of journals. In fact we have been reviewing these patients with coronary angiograms and the results have been quite gratifying.

9. Vettath's technique of long mammary patch

A single stabilizer is used if the arteriotomy is <4 cm. If it exceeds >4 cm, two stabilizers (one facing each other) are used for coronary stabilization. The arteriotomy extends distally to reach the normal lumen of LAD. Proximal extent of arteriotomy is kept just short of the most severe proximal lesion to avoid competitive flow from native LAD.

Distal coronary perfusion during anastomosis is maintained using conventional intracoronary shunts (Clearview, Medtronic Inc, Minneapolis, MN, USA). If the arteriotomy exceeds 3-4 cm, cut ends of aorto- coronary shunts (Quickflow, Medtronic Inc, Minneapolis, MN, USA) are used. These may be tailored to use in arteriotomies upto 6-7 cms. In this technique, hither to undescribed (Vettath's modification of aorto-coronary shunts), the distal perfusion tips of aorto- coronary shunts are cut and inserted into the coronary artery. The

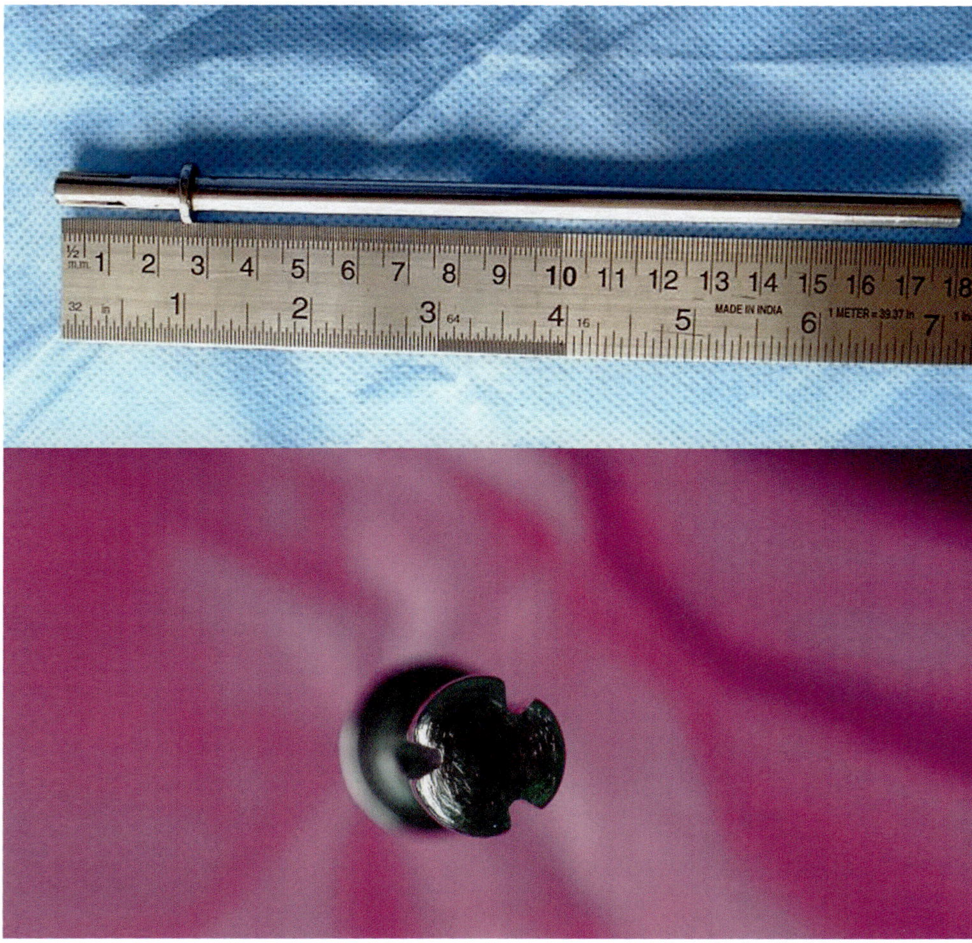

Fig. 8. Shows the Vettath's anastomotic obturator , the whole length of the device and the working end of the piece that goes into the aorta.

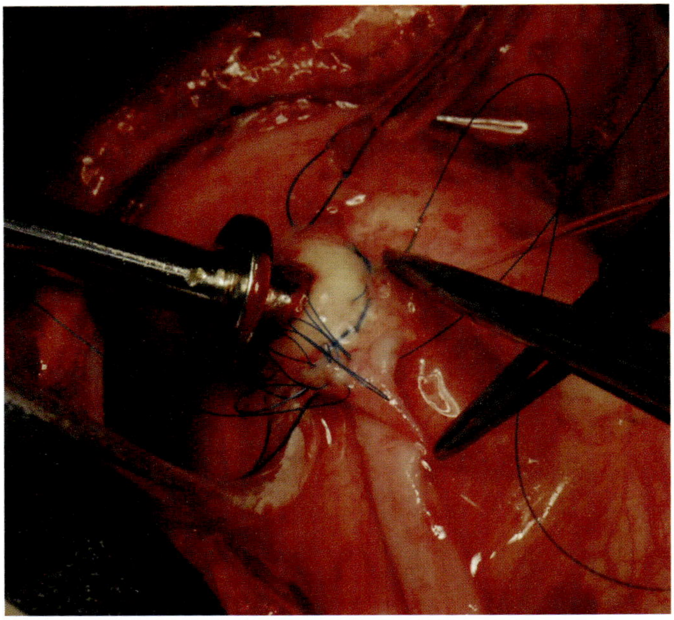

Fig. 9. Shows the close up of the top end anastomosis in progress using the VAO

bulb is inserted into the end from where the blood flows (i.e., into distal coronary lumen if the flow is retrograde and vice-verse). If the shunt does not sit inside the coronary (or it bowstrings), it is tacked down with a tacking suture taken in the midpoint of arteriotomy. This tacking suture is taken out at the end of anastomosis, along with the shunt. We use 7-0 polypropylene for this tacking suture. Occasionally, when native coronary flow is negligible and/or coronary lumen is <1 mm, the LAD is snared proximally with circumferential suture and LIMA to LAD anastomose was done. LIMA is slit to match the coronary arteriotomy and LIMA to LAD anastomosis is performed using 7-0 polypropylene. The plaques are excluded from the lumen of the reconstructed LAD. Diagonals and perforators are included in the new lumen. Posterior 25% of reconstructed coronary artery is formed by native coronary artery and anterior 75% by LIMA . Approximately 10 minutes were taken to construct a 2cm patch and an additional 5 minute per each added centimeter of patch was taken for anastomosis.

The advantage of this technique is that the intima is left intact and no injury is made on it. The avoidance of endarterectomy is a definite reason for the patency in our study. We also do not add any anticoagulants or anything other medications, than those used for the normal CABG patients. Also that in spite of our long anastomosis, patients remain quite stable all along the anastomotic time.This technique of long patch has also been described by Takanashi [S.Takanashi,2003.]

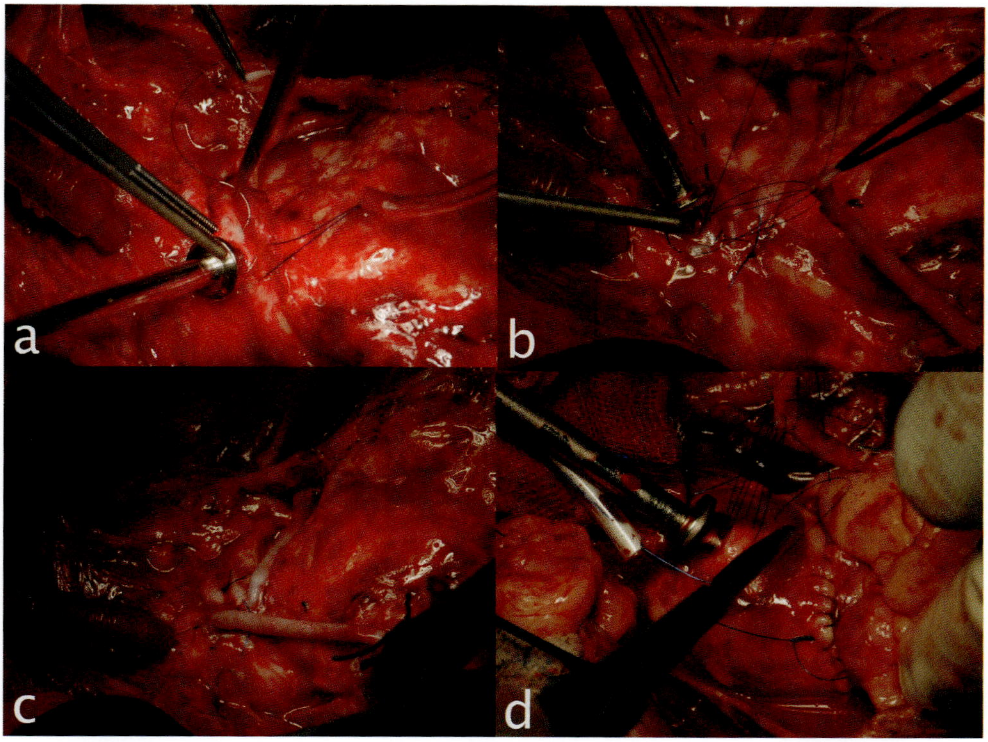

Fig. 10. Shows:
(a) The VAO is inserted into the vein hood of the blocked vein graft. In a re do CABG- On pump.
(b) The suturing being done on the top end of the vein graft.
(c) The anastomosed vein graft s in position.
(d) The top end of the vein graft in a CABG plus AVR done without using side clamp

10. Role of IABP in OPCAB

The use of intra-aortic balloon pump (IABP) either preoperatively or intraoperatively, to reduce operative risk and to facilitate posterior vessel OPCAB has been well documented. IABP has been useful in high-risk patients with left main coronary artery disease (> 75% stenosis), intractable resting angina, post infarction angina, left ventricular dysfunction (ejection fraction < 35%), or unstable angina.
Preoperative IABP counterpulsation has been shown to have better outcomes compared with perioperative or postoperative insertion in critical patients, and off-pump surgical procedures have been advocated to reduce mortality in high-risk patients.
In patients with high risk factors, higher mortality and morbidity rates have been demonstrated in spite of massive pharmacologic support combined with postoperative IABP support. IABP therapy results in a more favorable myocardial blood supply, increased stroke volume and cardiac output through augmentation of the diastolic pressure, and afterload reduction (Christenson, 1997, 1999).Intraoperative or postoperative IABP insertion has been reported to be associated with higher operative mortality rate and device-related complication rate, as compared with preoperative use of IABP.

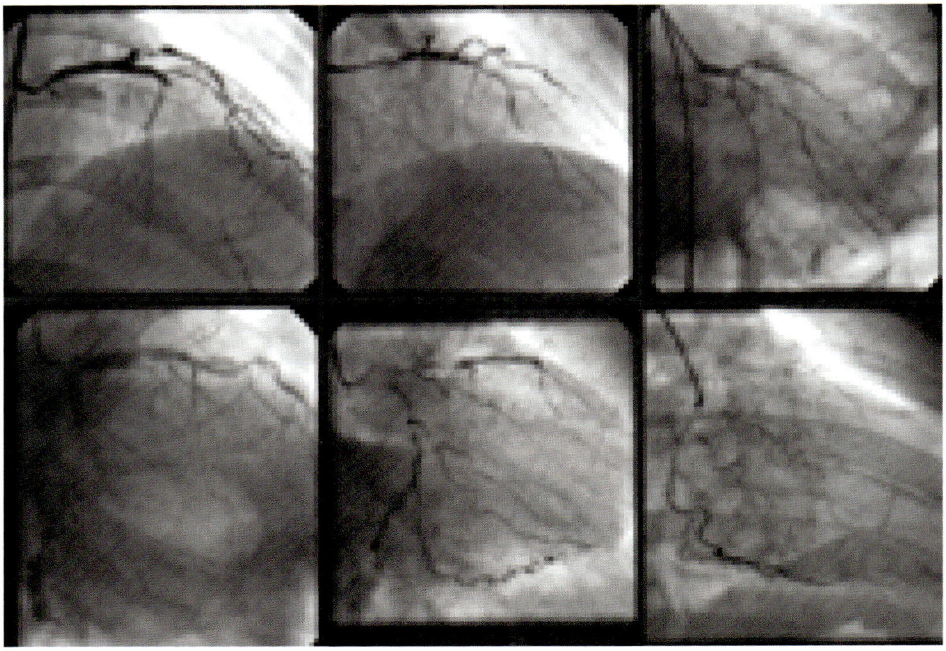

Fig. 11. Shows the Coronary angiograms of patients, showing diffusely diseased coronary arteries.

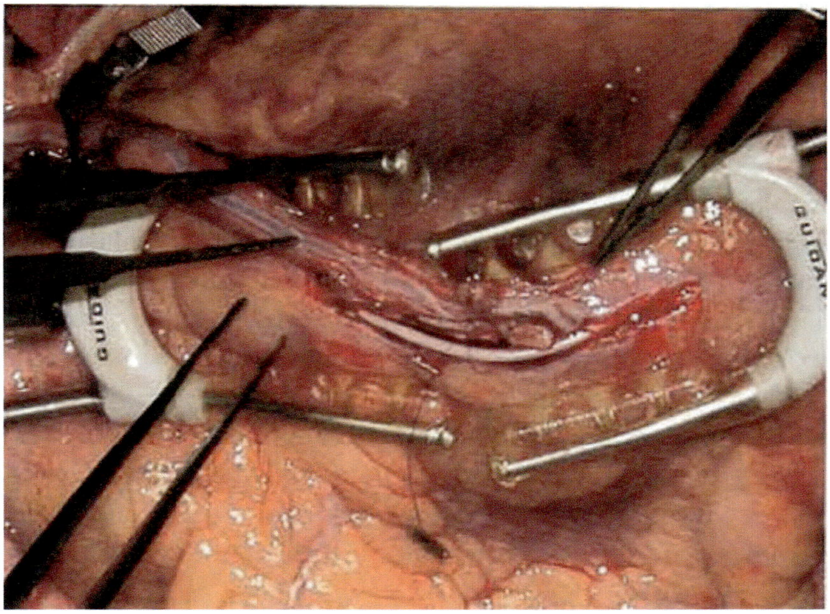

Fig. 12. Showing the Double stabilizer technique while performing the long mammary patch anastomosis of LIMA on the LAD without enadarterectomy.

Any patient who has a hemodynamic compromise or has an inclination to crash, gets an IABP inserted sheath less.(8 or &7 Fr). We had the IABP inserted in the early days when we had the patient included in one of the high risk group like- left main coronary artery disease (> 75% stenosis), intractable resting angina, ST depression more than 2.5mm,Post-infarction angina, Left ventricular dysfunction (ejection fraction < 35%), or unstable angina.

We had noticed that the use of IABP was not high in the left main disease group and low ejection fraction group, but was high in patients with ongoing ischemia. Hence we re-engineered our use of IABP such that every patient undergoing OPCAB gets a femoral arterial line and this is used for monitoring along with the radial arterial line. When a patient becomes ischemic during lifting the heart and while positioning for lateral wall grafting, then the heart is repositioned, and a sheathless IABP inserted. This is then used till the distal anastomosis is over. Once the anastomosis is complete and the heart repositioned for top end anastomosis, then the IABP is kept on standby mode. Then after the top end anastomosis is over, the heparin is reversed. Once the reversal is over and when the patient remains hemodynamically stable, we remove the IABP on the table, after inserting another femoral arterial line in the other groin. This technique has been very useful and we have been following this for the past four years, with excellent results. In fact this technique is being sent for publication. We have not had to reintroduce any IABP in any of these patients over the last four years.

TOTAL NO. OF OFF PUMP (OPCAB)

FROM	TO	OFF PUMP CASES	CONVERSION	IABP	MORTALITY
07-2002	12-2002	47	NIL	NIL	NIL
01-2003	12-2003	177	12	1	NIL
01-2004	12-2004	238	6	NIL	1
01-2005	12-2005	300	NIL	6	3
01-2006	12-2006	248	NIL	10	4
01-2007	12-2007	261	1	13	NIL
01-2008	12-2008	228	NIL	24	2
01-2009	12-2009	282	NIL	15	1
01-2010	12-2010	338	NIL	22	1
TOTAL		2155	19	97	12

TOTAL IABP USAGE - 2.5%
FIRST 1000 PATIENTS HAD CONVERSION OF 1.8% & MORTALIT Y OF 0.8%
SECOND 1000 PATIENTS HAD CONVERSION OF 0.1% &MORTALITY OF 0.4%

11. Results

We had analyzed the results of our last 2000 OPCAB patients. It was noticed that we had a higher rate of conversion onto the heart lung machine in our first thousand, when compared the second thousand. Probably, that was our initial learning curve which was seen in our technique, which we have developed and standardized. The use of IABP had been low in the early years, and probably the reason for the increased conversion on to the Heart lung machine. But as we understood the use of IABP, we found it more user friendly. Also the need

for the balloon pump only for distal anastomosis did come as a surprise to us. In the last 1600 odd patients, we had to convert only one patient on to the heart lung patient (That too when the patient developed intractable Ventricular arrhythmia). The mortality of the second thousand patients had come down by half and we have been able to maintain that result.
Our results of the different parameters like the use of ionotropes, number of grafts, Renal failure, perioperative Myocardial infarction etc, in comparison with our two groups of patients have been elucidated in the Table below.

ROLE OF IABP IN OPCAB

	FIRST 1000	2ND 1000
CONVERSION	1.8%	0.1%
NO OF GRAFTS	3.5%	3.9%
INOTROPIC USE	75%	2%
RENAL FAILURE	3%	0.2%
PERI OP MI	<1%	0.4%
STROKE	0.4%	0.2%
MORTALITY	0.8%	0.4%
IABP	16	40

12. Conclusion

The advance that has been made in the surgical management of coronary artery disease has placed us in a vantage position of judging the outcome of our management techniques not only by morbidity and mortality incurred, but also by the potential of our treatment modality to cause harm. This is why OPCAB has generated renewed, widespread and sustained interest. The resurgence of OPCAB has also ignited a keen enthusiasm in the refinement of CPB techniques and the management of on-pump CABG patients. In most practices, OPCAB is paradoxically dependent on, and guaranteed by the presence of the CPB machine. We would like to stress here that OPCAB is not for everyone. It is definitely not for the faint hearted surgeon, It needs a Team with a MINDSET. And the team has to gear itself from being able to perform CABG on full Cardiopulmonary bypass, with cross clamp and cardoplegia, to performing CABG on pump with a beating heart, and then going on to just cannulating the aorta, and then stabilizing the heart and performing OPCAB, to doing a full OPCAB. This should be a slow transition, than a sudden change. Then the results would be good. There has been numerous article comparing OPCAB with ONCAB, but in our opinion, a surgeon performing OPCAB would not have to perform ONCAB, what ever the coronary anatomy is, if he sets his mind to it.

In our last 12 years of OPCAB experience and over 2500 OPCABs, we have been able to perform the last 1600 OPCABs with only one conversion to the heart lung machine. That was when patient developed intractable arrhythmia. Hence in our opinion, intractable arrhythmia is the only reason for conversion. The mortality in the first one thousand patients have been 0.8% and in the second thousand is 0.4%.This proves to say that OPCAB has definitely reduced the mortality in coronary surgery. And if trained well we would be able to perform the same in patients with any ejection fraction.

13. References

Akiyama K., Ogasawara K., Inoue T., Shindou S., Okumura H., Negishi N., Sezai Y. Myocardial revascularization without cardiopulmonary bypass in patients with operative risk factors. Ann Thorac Cardiovasc Surg 1999;5:31-35

Al-Ruzzeh S., George S., Yacoub M., Amrani M. The clinical outcome of off-pump coronary artery bypass surgery in the elderly patients. Eur J Cardiothorac Surg 2001;20:1152-1156.

A. Laurie Shroyer, Ph.D., Frederick L. Grover, M.D., Brack Hattler, M.D., Joseph F. Collins, Sc.D., Gerald O. McDonald, M.D., Elizabeth Kozora, Ph.D., John C. Lucke, M.D., Janet H. Baltz, R.N., and Dimitri Novitzky, M.D., Ph.D. for the Veterans Affairs Randomized On-Pump versus Off-Pump Coronary-Artery Bypass Surgery.On/Off Bypass (ROOBY) Study Group.N Engl J Med 2009; 361:1827-1837.

Anil D Prabhu, MCh, Ismail E Thazhkuni, PhD, Sunil Rajendran, MRCS, Ranjish A Thamaran, MS, Kannan A Vellachamy, MD, Murali P Vettath, MD. Mammary patch reconstruction of left anterior descending coronary artery.*Asian Cardiovasc Thorac Ann 2008;16:313-317*

Anil D. Prabhu, MCh, Rafeek A. Karim, MCh, Sunil Rajendran, FRCS, Ismail E. Thazhkuni, PhD, Ranjish A. Thamaran, MS, Kannan A. Vellachami, MD,Murali P.Vettath, MCh. Vettath's technique of long mammary patch reconstruction of a diffusely diseased left anterior descending coronaryartery without endarterectomy on the beating heart.The Heart Surgery Forum #2007-1155 11 (2) P 64-67, 2008 doi: 10.1532/HSF98.20071155 http://cardenjennings.metapress.com

Ankeney JL. To use or not use the pump oxygenator in coronary bypass operations Ann Thorac Surg 1975;19:108-109.

Arom K.V., Flavin T.F., Emery R.W., Kshettry V.R., Janey P.A., Petersen R.J. Safety and efficacy of off-pump coronary artery bypass grafting. Ann Thorac Surg 2000;69:704-710.

Ascione R., Lloyd C.T., Gomes W.J., Caputo M., Bryan A.J., Angelini G.D. Beating versus arrested heart revascularization: evaluation of myocardial function in a prospective randomized study. Eur J Cardiothorac Surg 1999;15:685-690.

Ascione R., Lloyd C.T., Underwood M.J., Gomes W.J., Angelini G.D. On-pump versus off-pump coronary revascularization: evaluation of renal function. Ann Thorac Surg 1999;68:493-498.

Ascione R., Nason G., Al-Ruzzeh S., Ko C., Ciulli F., Angelini G.D. Coronary revascularization with or without cardiopulmonary bypass in patients with preoperative nondialysis-dependent renal insufficiency. Ann Thorac Surg 2001;72:2020-2025

Atkins C.W., Boucher C.A., Pohot G.M. Preservation of interventricular septal function in patient having coronary artery bypass grafts without cardiopulmonary bypass. Am Heart J 1984;107:304-309.

Bailey CP, May A, Lemon WM. Survival after coronary endarterectomy I men . JAMA 1957;167:641.

Benetti FJ. Direct coronary surgery with saphenous vein bypass without either cardiopulmonary bypass or cardiac arrest J Cardiovasc Surg 1985;26:217-222.

Benetti FJ. Video assisted coronary bypass surgery J Cardiovasc Surg 1995;10:620-625.

Benetti F.J., Naselli C., Wood M., Geffner L. Direct myocardial revascularization without extracorporeal circulation. Experience in 700 patients. Chest 1991;100:312-316

Bennetts J.S., Baker R., Ross I.K., Knight J.L. Assessment of myocardial injury by troponin T in off-pump coronary artery grafting and conventional coronary artery graft surgery. ANZ J Surg 2002;72:105-109.

Borst C, Jansen EW, Tulleken CA, et al. Coronary artery bypass grafting without cardiopulmonary bypass and without interruption of native coronary flow using a novel anastomosis site restraining device ("Octopus") J Am Coll Cardiol 1996;27:1356-1364.

Boyd W.D., Desai N.D., Del Rizzo D.F., Novick R.J., McKenzie F.N., Menkis A.H. Off-pump surgery decreases postoperative complications and resource utilization in the elderly. Ann Thorac Surg 1999;68:1490-1493

Buckberg G.D., Allen B.S. Myocardilal protection management during adult cardiac operations. In: Baue A.E., Geha A.S., Hammond G.L., Laks H., Naunheim K.S., eds. Glenn's thoracic and cardiovascular surgery. Stamford: Apple & Lange, 1996:1653-1687.

Buckberg G.D., Allen B.S. Myocardilal protection management during adult cardiac operations. In: Baue A.E., Geha A.S., Hammond G.L., Laks H., Naunheim K.S., eds. Glenn's thoracic and cardiovascular surgery. Stamford: Apple & Lange, 1996:1653-1687.

Buffolo E, Andrade JCS, Succi JE, et al. Direct myocardial revascularization without cardiopulmonary bypass Thorac Cardiovasc Surg 1985;33:26-29

Calafiore AM, Gianmarco GD, Teodori G, et al. Left anterior descending coronary artery grafting via left anterior small thoracotomy without cardiopulmonary bypass Ann Thorac Surg 1996;61:1658-1665.

Calafiore AM, Vitolla G, Mazzei V, et al. The Last operation technique and results before and after stabilization era. Ann Thorac Surg 1998;66:998-1001.

Calafiore A.M., Di Giammarco G., Teodori G., Mazzei V., Vitolla G. Recent advances in multivessel coronary grafting without cardiopulmonary bypass. Heart Surg Forum 1998;1:20-25.

Cartier R., Brann S., Dagenais F., Martineau R., Couturier A. Systematic off-pump coronary artery revascularization in multivessel disease: experience of three hundred cases. J Thorac Cardiovasc Surg 2000;119:221-229.

Christenson J.T., Simonet F., Badel P., Schmuziger M. Evaluation of preoperative intra-aortic balloon pump support in high risk coronary patients. Eur J Cardiothorac Surg 1997;11:1097-1103.

Christenson J., Simonet F., Badel P., Schmuziger M. The effect of preoperative intra-aortic balloon pump support in patients with coronary artery disease, poor left-ventricular function (LVEF < 40%) and hypertensive LV hypertrophy. Thorac Cardiovasc Surg 1997;45:60-64.

Christenson J., Simonet F., Badel P., Schmuziger M. Optimal timing of preoperative intraaortic balloon pump support in high-risk coronary patients. Ann Thorac Surg 1999;68:934-939

Czerny M., Baumer H., Kilo J., Zuckermann A., Grubhofer G., Chevtchik O., Wolner E., Grimm M. Complete revascularization in coronary artery bypass grafting with and without cardiopulmonary bypass. Ann Thorac Surg 2001;71:165-169.

D'Ancona G., Karamanoukian H., Ricci M., Kawaguchi A., Bergsland J., Salerno T. Myocardial revascularization on the beating heart after recent onset of acute myocardial infarction. Heart Surg Forum 2001;4:74-79.

Favaloro RG. Saphenous vein graft in the surgical treatment of coronary artery disease J Thorac Cardiovasc Surg 1968;58:178-185.

Goetz RH, Rohman M, Haller JD, et al. Internal mammary-coronary anastomosis. A nonsuture method employing tantalum rings J Thorac Cardiovasc Surg 1961;41:378-386.

Green GE, Stertzer SH, Reppert EH. Coronary artery bypass graft Ann Thoracic Surg 1968;5:443-450

Güler M., Kirali K., Toker M.E., Bozbuga N., Ömeroglu S.N., Akinci E., Yakut C. Different CABG methods in patients with chronic obstructive pulmonary disease. Ann Thorac Surg 2001;71:152-157.

Gundry S.R., Romano M.A., Shattuck O.H., Razzouk A.J., Bailey L.L. Seven-year follow-up of coronary artery bypasses performed with and without cardiopulmonary bypass. J Thorac Cardiovasc Surg 1998;115:1273-1278.

Gu Y.J., Mariani M.A., Boonstra P.W., Grandjean J.G., Oeveren W.V. Complement activation in coronary artery bypass grafting patients without cardiopulmonary bypass: the role of tissue injury by surgical incision. Chest 1999;116:892-898.

Guyton R.A., Thourani V.H., Puskas J.D., Shanewise J.S., Steele M.A., Palmer-Steele C.L., Vinten-Johansen J. Perfusion-assisted direct coronary artery bypass: selective graft perfusion in off-pump cases. Ann Thorac Surg 2000;69:171-175.

Hoff S.J., Ball S.K., Coltharp W.H., Glassford D.M., Jr., Lea J.W., IV, Petracek M.R. Coronary artery bypass in patients 80 years and over: is off-pump the operation of choice?. Ann Thorac Surg 2002;74:S1340-S1343.

Kim KB, Lim C, Lee C, et al. Off-pump coronary artery bypass may decrease the patency of saphenous vein grafts Ann Thorac Surg 2001;72:1033-1037.

Kim K.B., Lim C., Ahn H., Yang J.K. Intraaortic ballon pump therapy facilitates posterior vessel off-pump coronary artery bypass grafting in high-risk patients. Ann Thorac Surg 2001;71:1964-1968.

Kolessov VL. Mammary artery coronary anastomosis as method of treatment for angina pectoris J Thorac Cardiovasc Surg 1967;54:535-544.

Locker C., Shapira I., Paz Y., Kramer A., Gurevitch J., Matsa M., Pevni D., Mohr R. Emergency myocardial revascularization for acute myocardial infarction: survival benefits of avoiding cardiopulmonary bypass. Eur J Cardiothorac Surg 2000;17:234-2385.

Masuda M., Morita S., Tomita H., Kurisu K., Nishida T., Tominaga R., Yasui H. Off-pump attenuates myocardial enzyme leakage but not postoperative brain natriuretic peptide secretion. Ann Thorac Cardiovasc Surg 2002;8:139-144.

Matata B.M., Sosnowski A.W., Galiñanes M. Off-pump bypass graft operation significantly reduces oxidative stress and inflammation. Ann Thorac Surg 2000;69:785-791.

Mathison M., Buffolo E., Jatene A.D., Jatene F., Reichenspurner H., Matheny R.G., Shennib H., Akin J.J., Mack M.J. Right heart circulatory support facilitates coronary artery bypass without cardiopulmonary bypass. Ann Thorac Surg 2000;70:1083-1085.

Mehlhorn U., Allen S.J., Adams D.L., Davies K.L., Gogola G.R., de Vivie R., Laine G.A. Normothermic continuous antegrade blood cardioplegia does not prevent myocardial edema and cardiac dysfunction. Circulation 1995;92:1940-1946.

Mohr R., Moshkovitch Y., Shapira I., Amir G., Hod H., Gurevitch J. Coronary artery bypass without cardiopulmonary bypass for patients with acute myocardial infarction. J Thorac Cardiovasc Surg 1999;118:50-56.

Montague N.T., Kouchoukos N.T., Wilson T.A., Bennett A.L., Knott H.W., Lochridge S.K., Erath H.G., Clayton O.W. Morbidity and mortality of coronary bypass grafting in patients 70 years of age and older. Ann Thorac Surg 1985;39:552-557.

Mueller X.M., Chassot G., Zhou J., Eisa K.M., Chappuis C., Tevaearai H.T., von Seggesser L.K. Hemodynamics optimization during off-pump coronary artery bypass: the 'no compression' technique. Eur J Cardiothorac Surg 2002;22:249-254.

Mullany C.J., Darling G.E., Pluth J.R., Orszulak T.A., Schaff H.V., Ilstrup D.M., Gersh B.J. Early and late results after isolated coronary artery bypass surgery in 159 patients aged 80 years and older. Circulation 1990;82(5 Suppl):IV229-IV236.

Hirose H. Coronoary artery bypass grafting in the elderly. Chest 2000;117:1262-1270

Muraki S., Morris C.D., Budde J.M., Velez D.A., Zhao Z., Guyton R., Vinten-Johanson J. Experimental off-pump coronary artery revascularization with adenosine-enhanced reperfusion. J Thorac Cardiovasc Surg 2001;121:570-579.

Murray G,Porcheron R, Hilario J, Rosemblau W. Anastamosis of a systemic artery to the coronary artery. Can Med Assoc J 1954;594:71.

Nakayama Y., Sakata R., Ura M., Itoh T. Long-term results of coronary artery bypass grafting in patients with renal insufficiency. Ann Thorac Surg 2003;75:496-500.

Penttilä H.J., Lepojärvi M.V.K., Kiviluoma K.T., Kaukoranta P.K., Hassinen I.E., Peuhkurinen K.J. Myocardial preservation during coronary surgery with and without cardiopulmonary bypass. Ann Thorac Surg 2001;71:565-571.

Prifti E., Bonacchi M., Giunti G., Frati G., Proietti P., Leacche M., Salica A., Sani G., Brancaccio G. Does on-pump/beating-heart coronary artery bypass grafting offer better outcome in end-stage coronary artery disease patients?. J Card Surg 2000;15:403-410.

Puskas JD, Thourani VH, Marshall JJ, et al. Clinical outcomes, angiographic patency and resource utilization in 200 consecutive off-pump coronary bypass patients Ann Thorac Surg 2001;71:1477-1484.

Puskas J.D., Williams W.H., Duke P.G., Staples J.R., Glas K.E., Marshall J.J., Leimbach M., Huber P., Garas S., Sammons B.H., McCall S.A., Petersen R.J., Bailey D.E., Chu H., Mahoney E.M., Weintraub W.S., Guyton R.A. Off-pump coronary artery bypass grafting provides complete revascularization with reduced myocardial injury, transfusion requirements, and length of stay: a prospective randomized comparison of two hundred unselected patients undergoing off-pump versus conventional coronary artery bypass grafting. J Thorac Cardiovasc Surg 2003;125:797-808

Roosens C., Heerman J., De Somer F., Caes F., Van Belleghem Y., Poelaert J.I. Effects of off-pump coronary surgery on the mechanics of the respiratory system, lung, and chest wall: comparison with extracorporeal circulation. Crit Care Med 2002;30:2430-2437.

Sepic J., Wee J.O., Soltesz E.G., Hsin M.K., Cohn L.H., Laurence R.G., Aklog L. Cardiac positioning using an apical suction device maintains beating heart hemodynamics. Heart Surg Forum 2002;5/volume-nr>:279-284

Stamou S.C., Dangas G., Dullum M.K., Pfister A.J., Boyce S.W., Bafi A.S., Garcia J.M., Corso P.J. Beating heart surgery in octogenarians: perioperative outcome and comparison with younger age groups. Ann Thorac Surg 2000;69:1140-1145.

Strüber M., Cremer J.T., Gohrbandt B., Hagl C., Jankowski M., Völker B., Rückoldt H., Martin M., Haverich A. Human cytokine responses to coronary artery bypass grafting with and without cardiopulmonary bypass. Ann Thorac Surg 1999;68:1330-1335.

Shuichiro Takanashi, Toshihiro Fukui, Yasuyuki Hosoda, and Yoshihiro Shimizu. Off-pump long onlay bypass grafting using left internal mammary artery for diffusely diseased coronary artery.Ann. Thorac. Surg., Aug 2003; 76: 635 - 637.

Svedjeholm R., Huljebrant I., Hkanson E., Vanhanen I. Glutamate and high dose glucose–insulin–potassium (GIK) in the treatment of severe cardiac failure after cardiac operations. Ann Thorac Surg 1995;59:S23-S30.

Tashiro T., Todo K., Haruta Y., Yasunaga H., Tachikawa Y. Coronary artery bypass grafting without cardiopulmonary bypass for high-risk patients. Cardiovasc Surg 1996;4:207-211.

Trapp WG, Bisarya R. Placement of coronary artery bypass graft without pump-oxygenator Ann Thorac Surg 1975;19:1-9.

Van Dijk D., Nierich A.P., Jansen E.W.L., Nathoe H.M., Suyker W.J.L., Diephuis J.C., van Boven W., Borst C., Buskens E., Grobbee D.E., de Medina E.O.R., de Jaegere P.P.T. Early outcome after off-pump versus on pump coronary bypass surgery. Circulation 2001;104:1761-1766.

Vassiliades T.A., Nielsen J.L., Lonquist J.L. Coronary perfusion methods during off-pump coronary bypass: results of a randomized clinical trial. Ann Thorac Surg 2002;74:S1383-S1389.

Vettath, Murali P; Kannan, A.V.; Sheen Peecheeyen, C.S.; Baburajan, A.K.; Vahab, Abdul and Sujith, M.P.

Vettath's anastamotic obturator: A simple proximal anastamotic device. Murali P Vettath. The heart surgery forum #2003-73305 6 (5), 2003 Online address: www.hsforum.com/vol6/issue5/2003-73305.html

Vettath P Murali. Vettath's anastamotic obturator – our experience of 269 proximal anastamosis.(2004). Heart Lung and Circulation, 13. pp. 288-290. Heart Lung and Circulation 2004; 13:288–290

Vineberg AM . Development of anastomosis between coronary vessels and transplanted mammary artery: Med Assoc J 1954;594:71

Yeatman M., Caputo M., Narayan P., Ghosh A.K., Ascione R., Ryder I., Angelini G.D. Intracoronary shunts reduce transient intraoperative myocardial dysfunction during off-pump coronary operations. Ann Thorac Surg 2002;73:1411-1417.

Yokoyama T., Baumgartner F.J., Gheissari A., Capouya E.R., Panagiotides G.P., Declusin R.J. Off-pump versus on-pump coronary bypass in high-risk subgroups. Ann Thorac Surg 2000;70:1546-1550.

9

Strategies for the Prevention of Postoperative Atrial Fibrillation in Cardiac Surgery

Estella M. Davis[1], Kathleen A. Packard[1], Jon T. Knezevich[1], Thomas M. Baker[2] and Thomas J. Langdon[2]
[1]*Creighton University School of Pharmacy and Health Professions*
[2]*Alegent Health, Cardiovascular and Thoracic Surgery*
USA

1. Introduction

Atrial fibrillation (AF) occurs in 15% to 50% of patients after cardiac surgery (Bradley et al., 2005; Dunning et al., 2006). Postoperative atrial fibrillation (POAF) most often develops between the second and fifth postoperative day, with a peak incidence in the first two to three days. While POAF can be self-limiting, it may also be associated with hemodynamic compromise, postoperative stroke, perioperative myocardial infarction (MI), ventricular arrhythmias, and heart failure (Echahidi et al., 2008; Kaireviciute et al., 2009). The development of POAF is associated with, on average, an additional hospital length of stay (LOS) of 1 to 1.5 days (Kim et al., 2001; Zimmer et al., 2003). Some studies, however, report that POAF increases hospital LOS by almost 5 days (Aranski et al., 1996; Gillespie et al., 2006). POAF is also associated with higher hospital costs with an average increase of $10,000-$12,600 per hospitalization (Gillespie et al., 2006; Aranski et al., 1996).

Practice guidelines for the prevention of POAF in patients undergoing cardiac surgery exist which include the American College of Chest Physicians (ACCP) 2005 POAF Guidelines, the ACCP 2005 Recommendations for the Role of Cardiac Pacing for POAF, the American College of Cardiology (ACC)/American Heart Association (AHA)/European Society of Cardiology (ESC) 2006 Atrial Fibrillation Guidelines, the ACC/AHA 2004 Coronary Artery Bypass Graft Surgery (CABG) Guidelines, the Canadian Cardiovascular Society (CCS) Consensus Conference Statements on AF, and the European Association for Cardio-Thoracic Surgery (EACTS) 2006 POAF Guidelines and updated ESC/EACTS 2010 AF Guidelines (Bradley et al., 2005; Maisel & Epstein 2005; Dunning et al., 2006; Fuster et al., 2006; Eagle et al., 2004; Mitchell et al., 2005; Kerr & Roy, 2004; European Society of Cardiology ([ESC], 2010) (Table 1).

The guidelines are consistent in that they all strongly recommend using beta-blockers to reduce POAF incidence (ACCP 2005 POAF Guidelines Strength A, ACC/AHA/ESC 2006 AF Guidelines and ACC/AHA 2004 CABG Guidelines Class I, Canadian Cardiovascular Society AF/POAF Consensus Class I, and ESC 2010 AF Guidelines Class I). The Surgical Care Improvement Project (SCIP) National Quality Measures also state that all patients undergoing cardiac surgery should receive a beta-blocker during the perioperative period if they were on a beta-blocker prior to arrival (Surgical Care Improvement Project [SCIP] Version 3.0a, 2009). Most institutions have incorporated this requirement into their prospective preoperative order sets for all patients without contraindications to beta-blockers.

Medication or Class	Canadian CV Society Consensus Conference:AF Following Cardiac Surgery (Mitchell et al., 2005a); Canadian CV Society Consensus Conference:AF Executive Summary (Kerr & Roy, 2004)		ACCP 2005 POAF Guidelines (Bradley et al., 2005) ACCP CHEST 2005 Cardiac Pacing (Maisel & Epstein, 2005)			ACC/AHA/ESC 2006 AF Guidelines (Fuster et al., 2006); ACC/AHA 2004 CABG Guidelines (Eagle et al., 2004)		ESC 2010 AF Guidelines (ESC 2010)	
	Class	**Level of Evidence**	**Strength**	**Quality of Evidence**	**Net Benefit**	**Class**	**Level of Evidence**	**Class**	**Level of Evidence**
Pacing	I	C - Temporary ventricular epicardial pacing electrode wires placed at time of cardiac surgery to allow for backup pacing as necessary	B	Good	Biatrial pacing Small/weak	-	-	IIb	A - Biatrial pacing
	IIa	A - Atrial pacing (with or without a ventricular lead) should be considered in pts with symptomatic bradycardia							
	IIa	B - Atrial pacing if not on BB before surgery							
	IIa	B - The proportion of time the ventricles are paced should be minimize in pts with intrinsic AV conduction							

	IIa III	B - Temporary atrial pacing should be considered following heart surgery B - Atrial pacing for the prevention of AF in the absence of symptomatic bradycardia is not recommended							
Off pump CABG	-	-	-	-	-	-	-	A *(last noted in Dunning et al., 2006)	1a/b *(last noted in Dunning et al., 2006)
Posterior Pericardiotomy	-	-	-	-	-	-	-	B *(last noted in Dunning et al., 2006)	1b *(last noted in Dunning et al., 2006)
Beta-Blockers	I IIa	A - BB before surgery, should be continued through operative period A - If not on BB before surgery	A	Fair	Substantial	I (Fuster) I (Eagle)	A (Fuster) B (Eagle)	Class I	A B - If used, BB are recommended to be continued until day of surgery
Sotalol	-	-	B	Good	Intermediate	IIb - consider if BB contraindicated (Eagle)	B (Fuster,Eagle)	Class IIb	A - May be considered, but associated with risk of proarrhythmia
Amiodarone	IIa	A - If not on BB before surgery	B	Good	Intermediate	IIa - consider in patients at high risk for POAF IIa - consider in patients at high risk for POAF if BB contraindicated	A (Fuster) B (Eagle)	Class IIa	A - Preoperative amiodarone should be considered for pts at high risk for POAF
Magnesium	IIa	B - If not on BB before surgery	D	Low	None	-	-	-	-
Dexamethasone	-	-	I	Low	Conflicting	-	-	IIb	B - Corticosteroids may be considered, but are associated with risk

ACCP= American College of Chest Physicians, ACC= American College of Cardiology, AHA= American Heart Association, ESC= European Society of Cardiology AF = atrial fibrillation, BB = beta-blocker, CABG = coronary artery bypass graft, CV = cardiovascular, EACTS = European Association for Cardiothoracic Surgery, POAF= postoperative atrial fibrillation, pts = patients

Table 1. International Guideline Recommendations for Therapies for the Prevention of POAF in Patients Undergoing Cardiac Surgery

Though there are no studies examining POAF prophylaxis for patients intolerant of beta-blockers, effective alternatives include sotalol and amiodarone, depending upon the contraindication. The guidelines further specify that amiodarone may be given as an alternative or considered in patients at high risk for POAF (Fuster et al., 2006; Eagle et al., 2004; ESC, 2010; Mitchell et al., 2005a; Kerr & Roy, 2004). Only the previous 2006 EACTS and Canadian guidelines support the use of magnesium and state that it may be given in addition to other strategies to reduce POAF(Dunning et al., 2006; Mitchell et al., 2005a; Kerr & Roy, 2004). Additionally, the most recent ESC guidelines include consideration of corticosteroids for the prevention of POAF (ESC, 2010).

The practice guidelines also recommend utilization of non-pharmacologic strategies for the prevention of POAF in cardiac surgery patients (Table 1). The most common strategy referred to in the guidelines is cardiac pacing. The most recent 2010 ESC AF guidelines and ACCP statement from 2005 recommend that biatrial pacing should be considered for prophylaxis (ESC, 2010, Maisel & Epstein, 2005). The CCS statement also recommends that atrial pacing with or without a ventricular lead should be considered in patients with symptomatic bradycardia (Class 2A recommendation based on Level A evidence) and that atrial pacing should be considered if a patient is not on a beta-blocker before surgery (Class 2A recommendation based on Level B evidence) (Mitchell et al., 2005a; Kerr & Roy, 2004). Lastly, the CVS guidelines strongly recommend placing temporary ventricular epicardial pacing electrode wires at the time of surgery to allow for backup pacing as necessary (Class 1 recommendation based on Level C evidence) (Mitchell et al., 2005a; Kerr & Roy, 2004). Other non-pharmacologic strategies mentioned in the guidelines include the use of off-pump CABG, posterior pericardiotomy, and introperative maze ablation (Mitchell et al., 2005a; Kerr & Roy, 2004; ESC, 2010).

2. Pathogenesis of POAF

The underlying mechanisms for the development of POAF after cardiac surgery are not precisely known, but are thought to be multifactorial (Figure 1) (Banach et al., 2010). It has been proposed that certain causative mechanisms alter atrial refractoriness and slow atrial conduction which results in multiple reentry wavelets circulating within the atria (Baker & White, 2007a). Some of these mechanisms include pericardial inflammation, excessive production of catecholamines, and volume and pressure changes. Numerous predisposing factors such as advanced age, hypertension, diabetes, left atrial enlargement, left ventricular hypertrophy, intraoperative and postoperative factors such as atrial injury or ischemia, are all thought to impact the development of POAF. Once these conditions exist, a triggering event such as premature atrial contraction, electrolyte imbalance, and/or enhanced adrenergic or vagal stimulation initiates POAF. Neurohormonal activation is more widely recognized as a cause of POAF based on studies linking elevated norepinephrine and epinephrine concentrations to the development of POAF (Baker & White, 2007a; Kalman et al., 1995). Hence, the majority of interventions that reduce the incidence of POAF modulate sympathetic and parasympathetic systems or alter cardiac conduction (Table 1).

While the mechanisms involved in the development of POAF are multifactorial, there is increasing evidence that inflammation also plays a role. Such inflammation may be induced by extracorporeal circulation or cardiopulmonary bypass (CPB) with subsequent elevations of C-reactive protein (CRP), interleukin-6 (IL-6), and the complement system (Echahidi et al., 2008; Gaudino et al., 2003; Bruins et al., 1997; Canbaz et al., 2008). Angiotensin II has been

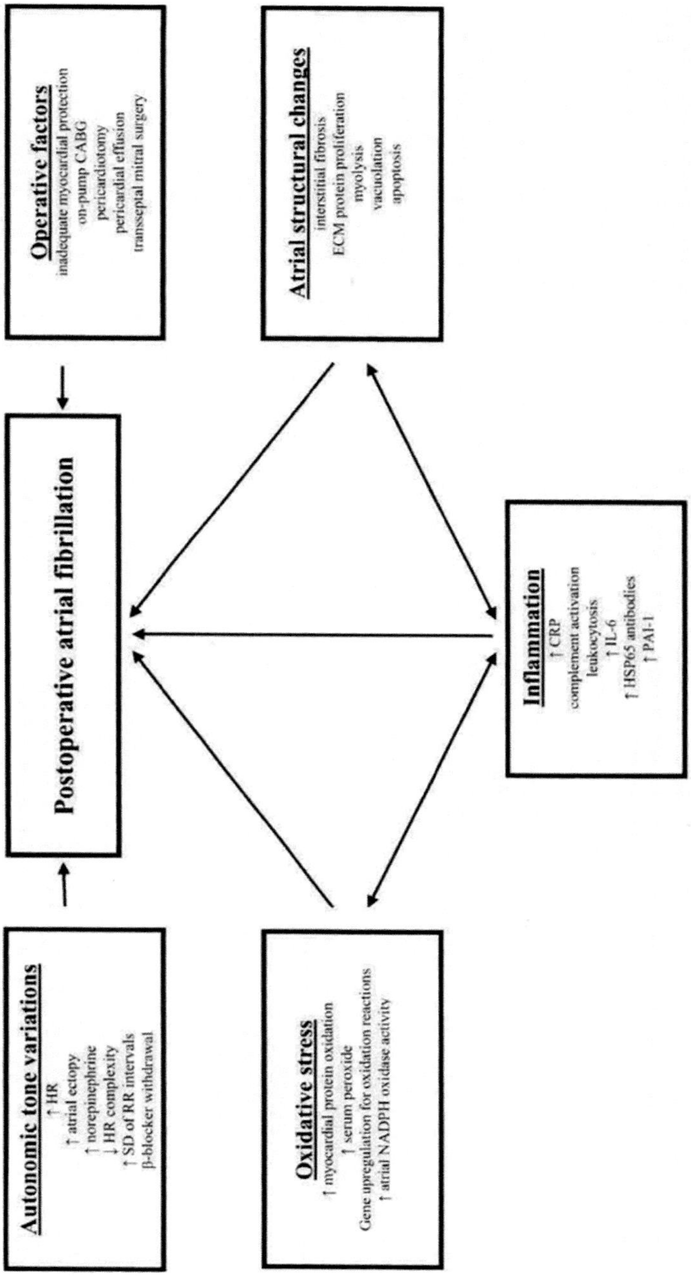

HR= heart rate, SD= standard deviation, NADPH= nicotinomide adenine dinucleotide phosphate, CABG= coronary artery bypass grafting, ECM= extracellular matrix, CRP= C-reactive protein, IL-6= interleukin-6, HSP= heat shock protein, PAI= plasminogen activator inhibitor

Fig. 1. Pathogenesis of postoperative atrial fibrillation (Banach et al., 2010)

shown to increase the production of proinflammatory cytokines, adhesion molecules, and selectins (Erlich et al., 2006; Boos et al., 2006). White blood cell count may also be a predictor of POAF (Lamm et al., 2006). The degree of inflammation postoperatively can negatively affect atrial conduction and duration of atrial fibrillation (Ishii et al., 2005; Tselentakis et al., 2006).
Oxidative stress has also been implicated in the pathogenesis of atrial fibrillation as the atrial tissue undergoes oxidative challenge during CPB (Rodrigo et al., 2008). Patients with POAF have been shown to have increased acute myocardial oxidation when compared to patients that did not experience POAF (Ramlawi et al., 2007). Specifically, nicotinamide adenine dinucleotide phosphate (NADPH) oxidase, an enzyme associated with the formation of the reactive oxygen species, superoxide, was found to be independently associated with increased risk of POAF (Kim et al., 2008). This may be due to damage of cardiac myocytes through lipid peroxidation, breakdown of cell membrane, decreased mitochondrial function, calcium overload, and apoptosis (Elahi et al., 2008). Because NADPH is activated by numerous mediators including tumor necrosis factor- α (TNF-α) (Griendling et al., 2000), it has been proposed as a link between inflammation and oxidative stress in POAF.
Based on these newly identified pathways, emerging pharmacologic therapies for the prevention of POAF have been under investigation including HMG Co-A reductase inhibitors (statins), renin-angiotensin-aldosterone-system modulators (including angiotensin converting enzyme inhibitors (ACEIs) and angiotensin receptor blockers (ARBs)), corticosteroids, omega-3 fatty acids, ascorbic acid, N-acetylcysteine, and sodium nitroprusside.
The guidelines suggest additive therapies can be considered for patients at high risk of developing POAF. Risk factors that have been identified to increase the risk of POAF include advanced age, history of atrial fibrillation, COPD, valvular surgery, hypertension, poor left ventricular function, chronic renal insufficiency, diabetes mellitus, rheumatic heart disease, withdrawal of preoperative beta-blockers or ACEIs, and increased aortic cross-clamp and CPB time (Mathew et al., 2004; Baker et al., 2007b; Nisanoglu et al., 2007). No simple criteria exist that allow patients to be classified as high risk for the development of POAF. A risk index model (Multicenter Study of Perioperative Ischemia Atrial Fibrillation Risk Index) (Table 2) was developed to identify subjects at high risk for POAF (Mathew et al., 2004). Patients receiving a risk score less than 14 were considered low risk, 14-31 were considered medium risk, and greater than 31 were considered high risk for developing POAF. Comparison of the predictive ability of the model revealed that the incidence of atrial fibrillation was similar in the derivation and validation cohorts across the three risk groups, and the area under the receiver operating characteristic curve applied to the final model was 0.77 (where >0.75 represents a model with good discriminate power). This risk scoring tool has been used to stratify patients into risk groups that may benefit from add-on prophylactic therapy (Barnes et al., 2006).

3. Pharmacologic therapies for the prevention of POAF in cardiac surgery

3.1 Established pharmacologic therapies

3.1.1 Beta-blockers

Beta-blockers work at the myocardium antagonizing the effects of catecholamines and have been studied extensively for the prevention of POAF. Meta-analyses have shown significant reduction in POAF incidence with the use of beta-blocker therapy, resulting in recommendation for their use as first-line therapy (Bradley et al., 2005; Dunning et al.; 2006, Fuster et al., 2006; Eagle et al., 2004, Kerr & Roy, 2004; [ESC], 2010). The largest meta-

Predictor of POAF after CABG	Risk Score Point Assignment
Age (Y)	
<30	6
30-39	12
40-49	18
50-59	24
60-69	30
70-79	36
≥80	42
History of AF	7
History of COPD	4
Concurrent valve surgery	6
Withdrawal of postoperative treatment	
BB	6
ACEI	5
BB treatment	
Preoperative and postoperative	-7
Postoperative	-11
Preoperative and postoperative ACEI treatment	-5
Postoperative treatment	
Potassium supplementation	-5
NSAIDs	-7
	= [a]Total Points

[a]Risk Groups based on summative total point assignment using predictors from table:
Low risk = Score < 14, Medium risk = Score 14-31, High risk = Score >31

ACEI = angiotensin converting enzyme inhibitor, AF = atrial fibrillation, BB = beta-blocker, CABG = coronary artery bypass graft, COPD = chronic obstructive pulmonary disease, NSAIDs = non-steroidal anti-inflammatory drugs, POAF = postoperative atrial fibrillation

Table 2. Multicenter Study of Perioperative Ischemia Atrial Fibrillation Risk Index (Mathew et al., 2004)

analysis was published in 2002 by Crystal et al. that included 27 randomized controlled trials with 3,840 patients (Crystal et al., 2002). Use of beta-blocker therapy decreased the incidence of POAF from 33% in the control group compared to 19% in the group receiving beta-blockade. This corresponded to a number needed to treat (NNT) of seven patients. A large retrospective analysis of the Society of Thoracic Surgeons (STS) database containing 629,877 patients, demonstrated a reduction in mortality rate with use of peri-operative beta-blockers (Ferguson et al., 2002). It has been shown that patients receiving perioperative beta-blockers have reduced mortality compared to control (3.4% versus 2.8%, OR 0.8, 95% CI 0.78 - 0.82; p<0.001). Efficacy of beta-blockade in the prevention of POAF has been theorized to decrease hospital LOS. However, two beta-blocker trials reporting effect on LOS demonstrated a non-significant reduction in LOS (-0.66 days; 95% CI, -2.04-0.72) (Cybulsky et al., 2000; Wenke et al., 1999).

The importance of beta-blockers is also affirmed by the two to five-fold increase in the incidence of POAF when beta-blockers are discontinued postoperatively (Kalman et al., 1995; Jideus et al., 2000; Ali et al., 1997). The increase in POAF is thought to be caused by beta-blocker withdrawal and mediated by an upregulation of beta adrenergic receptors and sympathetic stimulation (Kalman et al., 1995). Beta-blocker withdrawal is significantly associated with a greater than two-fold risk of developing POAF in cardiac surgery patients (Adjusted OR 2.17, 95% CI 1.11-4.25, p=0.04) (Lertsburapa et al., 2008). Thus, timing of beta-blocker administration appears play an important role and evidence supports the continuation of beta-blocker therapy from the preoperative stage through postoperative management. The guidelines emphasize the importance of reinitiating beta-blockers postoperatively without delay (Bradley et al., 2005).

In addition, the mode of administration of beta-blocker therapy has been evaluated in the prevention of POAF. Intravenous administration of metoprolol has demonstrated superiority to oral administration when accessing for the prevention of POAF. This is theorized to be a result of diminished gastrointestinal absorption with oral administration early after surgery. This phenomenon has been demonstrated by Halonen et al., when a significant reduction (p=0.036) of POAF occurrence by 11.3% was noted to occur in patients assigned to receive intravenous metoprolol therapy compared to patients assigned oral therapy (Halonen et al., 2006).

Controversy exists around selection of the most effective beta-blocker in reducing POAF. Two studies have demonstrated improved efficacy of carvedilol when compared to metoprolol (Acikel et al., 2008; Haghjoo et al., 2007). This was confirmed by approximately 18%-20.4% less episodes of POAF in those patients assigned to receive carvedilol.

Despite the overwhelming evidence to support beta-blocker therapy in the prevention of POAF, contraindications to this therapy exist. Alternative pharmacologic and non-pharmacologic modalities are warranted for patients who cannot tolerate or have the following contraindications to beta-blockers: bradycardia (<45 bpm), heart block, cardiac failure, severe peripheral edema, sick-sinus syndrome, bronchospastic disease (non-selective beta-blockers), and hypotension (SBP < 100 mmHg) with myocardial infarction.

3.1.2 Amiodarone

Amiodarone, a class III antiarrhythmic agent, has shown efficacy in the prevention of POAF. Its activity is demonstrated through blockade of alpha and beta-adrenergic receptors as well as sodium, calcium and potassium channels. Only beta-blockers have more safety and efficacy data to support their effectiveness in the prevention of POAF. Most randomized, controlled trials have supported the efficacy of amiodarone over placebo in the prevention of POAF by showing reduction of occurrence between 12% to 51% (Auer et al., 2004a; Barnes et al., 2006; Daoud et al., 1997; Guarnieri et al., 1999; Giri et al., 2001; White et al., 2002; Yazigi et al., 2002; Tokmakoglu et al., 2002; White et al., 2003; Mitchell et al., 2005a; Budeus et al., 2006; Zebis et al., 2007). Therefore, amiodarone has been granted a class IIa recommendation for POAF prophylaxis, behind beta-blockers, according to the ACC/AHA/ESC 2006 AF Guidelines, ACC/AHA 2004 CABG Guidelines, 2004 CCS AF/POAF Consensus statement, and ESC 2010 (Fuster et al., 2006; Eagle et al., 2004; Kerr & Roy, 2004; ESC, 2010). Additionally, the guidelines support amiodarone as prophylactic therapy in patients unable to tolerate beta-blockers or in high-risk patients with or without beta-blocker therapy (Bradley et al., 2005).

Two trials evaluating amiodarone versus placebo have demonstrated clear reduction of POAF occurrence (Mitchell et al., 2005b; Daoud et al., 1997). Compared to placebo, amiodarone reduced POAF incidence by 13.4%-19%. Effectiveness between amiodarone versus other pharmacological agents has been established. Two meta-analysis have been conducted evaluating the efficacy of amiodarone in POAF in which a statistically significant decrease in incidence was established (Bagshaw et al., 2006; Haan et al., 2002). Comparisons of amiodarone effectiveness have been made with agents such as beta-blockers (propranolol, metoprolol, and bisoprolol), sotalol, digoxin, and diltiazem. No clear superiority has been established amongst comparative trials. Amiodarone has been given in direct combination with metoprolol, magnesium, and atrial septal pacing in Bachmanns's Bundle (Auer et al., 2004a; Cagli et al.; 2006, White et al., 2003). All of these studies showed amiodarone in direct combination with the previous pharmacologic and non-pharmacologic options to be superior than that of placebo, with absolute reductions in the incidence of POAF by 20% to 24% (Auer et al., 2004a; Cagli et al., 2006; White et al., 2003). Combination therapy with amiodarone and beta-blockers has been well validated. A meta-analysis also found that amiodarone also significantly reduces the LOS by 0.91 days (95% CI, -1.59- -0.24) (Crystal et al., 2002).

Various dosing regimens using IV and/or oral amiodarone with varying administration times have been used in the POAF prevention trials. A meta-analysis evaluating 14 randomized, controlled trials in 2,864 patients, stratified into low (<3 g), medium (3-5 g), or high (>5 g) and timing was divided into preoperative or postoperative administration, found that cumulative doses of >3 g may be more effective than lower doses and preoperative initiation of amiodarone may be unnecessary (Buckley et al., 2007).

Amiodarone is effective for the prevention of POAF, however it has a complex side effect profile that includes QTc interval prolongation, pulmonary and liver toxicity, thyroid abnormalities, and visual disturbances. Patients with any of these pre-existing conditions may be placed at more risk with the addition of amiodarone for the prevention of POAF and the risk versus benefit must be evaluated for each patient. Side effects of amiodarone are typically associated with large cumulative doses and prolonged use. However, dosing regimens for prophylaxis tend to be short in duration, use lower cumulative dosing, and may use more convenient oral doses with or without a short course of IV amiodarone to avoid side effects associated with IV administration. The safety of amiodarone in patients undergoing cardiac surgery has been evaluated in a meta-analysis reviewing 18 randomized controlled trials (Patel et al., 2006). Results showed that amiodarone use was significantly associated with increased risk of hypotension (OR 1.79; 95% CI 1.04-3.09) and bradycardia (OR 2.33; 95% CI 1.41-3.61), especially when the intravenous formulation was utilized in high doses (greater than 1 gram). Therefore, clinicians should be cautious using amiodarone, especially in combination therapy with beta-blockers or other therapies that may cause bradycardia or hypotension. Finally, if amiodarone therapy is added to a patient's medication profile, physical and laboratory exams should be conducted and evaluated for the presence of drug-drug interactions or medication side effects.

3.1.3 Sotalol

Sotalol, a class III antiarrhythmic that possess beta-blocking activity, has been shown to be an effective pharmacological agent for the prevention of POAF. Within the primary literature, sotalol has demonstrated absolute reductions in the incidence of POAF between 13% - 16% (Auer et al., 2004a; Janssen et al., 1986; Suttorp et al., 1991; Weber et al., 1998; Evrard et al., 2000). Despite its demonstrated effectiveness, sotalol is contraindicated in patients with severe renal insufficiency and should be avoided in patients with heart failure. Furthermore, because of its propensity to cause torsades de pointes, it should be avoided in patients with congenital long QT syndrome or a baseline corrected QT interval greater than 440 msec. Due to its beta-blocking properties, sotalol is contraindicated in patients intolerant of beta-blockers. Because of the aforementioned limitations of this agent, sotalol has been granted a class IIb recommendation for POAF prophylaxis behind beta-blockers according to the ACC/AHA/ESC 2006 AF Guidelines and the ACC/AHA 2004 CABG Guidelines (Fuster et al., 2006; Eagle et al., 2004). The most recent 2010 ESC guidelines have assigned a Class IIb recommendation for sotalol due to its proarrhythmic risk (ESC, 2010). However, the earlier 2006 EACTS guidelines gave sotalol a stronger grade A recommendation based upon its comparative efficacy trials versus beta-blockers (Dunning et al., 2006) similar to ACC recommendations.

Patel and Dunning evaluated seven different randomized trials comparing sotalol to conventional beta blockers (Patel et al., 2005). Out of the seven trials evaluated, five studies demonstrated a statistically significant reduction in POAF for those patients assigned to sotalol compared to conventional beta-blockade. The number of patients needed to be treated with sotalol to prevent POAF over that of conventional beta-blocker therapy was found to be 10. Conversely, because of the pro-arrythmic properties of sotalol, conventional beta-blocker therapy may be a safer option.

3.1.4 Magnesium

POAF has been associated with decreased postoperative magnesium levels (Kalman et al., 1995). In fact, plasma magnesium concentration levels less that 0.9 mmol have been found to be an independent predictor of POAF (OR 6.7) when using multivariate logistic regression models (Treggiari-Venzi et al., 2000). Multiple large, randomized, controlled trials with magnesium have failed to demonstrate superiority to usual care with no magnesium in the prevention of POAF. These trials included various delivery forms of magnesium including: IV infusion (Treggiari-Venzi et al., 2000; Serafimovski et al., 2008; Caspie et al., 1995; Bert et al., 2001; Zangrillo et al., 2005), IV infusion based on serum levels (Wilkes et al., 2002), magnesium supplementation in maintenance fluids (Colquhoun et al., 1993) and in supplementation through cardioplegia solution (Shakerinia et al., 1996). Surprising lower cumulative doses of magnesium supplementation (mean cumulative dose 8.2 g) have shown to be more effective in reducing the incidence of POAF (OR 0.36, 95% CI 0.23-0.56), compared to higher doses (mean cumulative dose 15 g) (OR 0.99, 95% CI 0.70-1.41) (Henyan et al., 2005). Results from the same meta-analysis found that preoperative administration of magnesium was more effective at decreasing the incidence of POAF (OR 0.46, 95% CI 0.31-0.67) compared to intraoperative or postoperative administration. Results from several meta-analysis (Woodend et al., 1998; Burgess et al., 2006; Shiga et al., 2004; Miller et al., 2005; Alghamdi et al., 2005; Henyan et al., 2005; Shepard et al., 2008) have shown inconsistent efficacy with magnesium use. A few studies have demonstrated a significant benefit of magnesium when compared to usual care with absolute reductions in the incidence of POAF by 16% to 34% (Nurozler et al., 1996; Maslow et al., 2000; Kohno et al., 2005). However, at this time there is a lack of statistically significant data to support magnesium supplementation as monotherapy compared to that of beta-blocker, amiodarone, or sotalol therapy in the treatment of POAF (Bert et al., 2001; Solomon et al., 2000; Cagli et al., 2006). Only the CCS consensus statement includes magnesium as a Class IIa recommendation, however no other guidelines strongly recommend its use for the prevention POAF (Kerr & Roy, 2004). Magnesium therapy may be considered in combination with amiodarone and/or B-blocker therapy for those patients deemed at high risk or intolerant to the latter medications. If magnesium is utilized in the prevention of POAF, doses of 2.5-5 g have been most commonly utilized (Nurozler et al., 1996; Maslow et al., 2000; Kohno et al., 2005). When utilized in combination with B-blockers, clinicians should monitor for hypotension as combination therapy has been shown to significantly increase the risk of hypotension compared to B-blocker therapy alone (24.4% versus 43.5%, p=0.01) (Solomon et al., 2000). Finally, it should be noted that magnesium levels need to be monitored carefully throughout cardiac surgery and postoperatively regardless if magnesium is being utilized as a pharmacological agent for the prophylaxis of POAF.

4. Emerging pharmacologic therapies for the prevention of POAF in cardiac surgery

4.1 HMG Co-A reductase inhibitors

HMG Co-A reductase inhibitors (statins) may possess pleiotropic activity beyond lipid lowering effects and may be protective against POAF. They have been shown to reduce oxidative stress by inhibiting oxidant enzymes, up-regulate antioxidant enzymes, and enhance nitric oxide bioavailability (Paraskevas, 2008). It is also proposed that they possess direct antiarrhythmic effects mediated through cell membrane stabilization, down-regulation of the renin-angiotensin-aldosterone-system (RAAS), and protection of ischemic myocardium (Howard & Barnes, 2008). They also have been shown to reduce the expression of inflammatory mediators (i.e. interleukin-6 (IL-6), interleukin-8 (IL-8), tumor necrosis factor- α (TNF-α), C-reactive protein (CRP), cyclooxygenase 2) and decrease the expression of CD11b with consequential decreased adherence to endothelial cells of vein grafts (Chello et al., 2006; Patel et al., 2007). Therefore, statins may favorably impact the acute inflammatory response and alter atrial refractoriness or sympathetic activation that could lead to POAF after cardiac surgical procedures.

Many trials have evaluated the effect of statins on the incidence of POAF in cardiac surgery patients. Prospective, randomized trials found an absolute reduction in the incidence of POAF of 14% to 22% with statins compared to placebo or usual care (Chello et al., 2006; Patti et al, 2006; Song et al., 2008; Ji et al., 2009). The largest and most robust of these three trials was the Atorvastatin for Reduction of MYocardial Dysrhythmia After cardiac surgery study (ARMYDA-3) in which a significant reduction in POAF of 22% and a reduction in LOS of 0.6 days was observed with a statin compared to placebo (Patti et al., 2006). This study enrolled only patients who had no previous history of statin use and these patients could have less risk of pre-existing atherosclerotic disease and subsequently been at lower risk for developing POAF.

Other statin trials in CABG patients are observational, cohort studies with conflicting results of no benefit (Thielmann et al., 2007; Mithani et al., 2009) or a significant reduction in the incidence of POAF (Lertsburapa et al., 2008; Subramaniam et al., Mariscalco et al., Ozaydin et al., 2007; Miceli et al., 2009a; Kinoshita et al., 2010).

One study evaluated the combination of a statin and beta-blocker on the incidence of POAF. Monotherapy with atorvastatin or a beta-blocker reduced the risk of POAF by 61% (OR 0.39; 95% CI 0.18-0.85) and 82% (OR 0.19; 95% CI 0.08-0.44), respectively. However, the combination of atorvastatin plus a beta-blocker performed better by reducing the risk of POAF by 90% (OR 0.10; 95% CI 0.02-0.25) (Patti et al., 2006). The combination of preoperative and postoperative beta-blocker and amiodarone prophylaxis in 40% of patients may have also influenced the positive results in the statin group (Lertsburapa et al., 2008).

A few studies have been conducted to determine the optimal prophylactic dose of statins. Kourlioros et al found that simvastatin 40 mg and atorvastatin 40 mg had the greatest effect on POAF (Kourlioros et al., 2008). Simvastatin 20 mg and atorvastatin 20 mg maintained efficacy compared to control, but no difference was found at 10 mg or 80 mg of either drug. Lertsburapa et al analyzed patients by converting their statin dose to atorvastatin equivalents. Relative statin doses ≥40 mg of atorvastatin resulted in the greatest reduction in POAF by 55% (OR 0.45; 95% CI 0.21-0.99) (Lertsburapa et al., 2008). The 20 mg atorvastatin dose still showed a significant benefit (OR 0.6; 95% CI 0.23-0.99), while the < 20 mg dose showed no significant benefit (OR 0.75; 95% CI 0.47-1.20). Mithani et al found in their multivariate analysis that POAF was less common among patients taking higher doses of statins compared to those taking simvastatin < 20 mg/day (28% versus 34%, p=0.03). (Mithani et al., 2009) Comparing statins, only one prospective, observational study found that POAF was less frequent in patients receiving pravastatin compared to atorvastatin (9.5% versus 34.9%, p=0.0257) or no statins (9.5% versus 34.2%, p=0.0025). (Tamura et al., 2010)

A long-term study found that statins' benefit may extend beyond the immediate postoperative period and in outcomes other than POAF. Statins reduced the composite endpoint of death, MI, and unstable angina at both 60 days (OR 0.09; 95% CI 0.01-0.70, p=0.02) and one year post-CABG (OR 0.26; 95% CI 0.015-0.4, p<0.0001) (Dotani et al., 2000). Kaplan-Meier 30 day atrial fibrillation-free survival curves also indicated benefit with statins (Patti et al., 2006; Mariscalco et al., 2007; Ozaydin et al., 2007; Song et al., 2008). One meta-analysis confirmed the protective benefit of preoperative statins for POAF and early all cause mortality. This study also found a significant reduction in the risk of stroke by 26% with statins when compared to controls (OR 0.74; 95% CI 0.60-0.91) (Laikopoulos et al., 2008, Chen et al., 2010). While statins appear to reduce POAF in the short term setting in cardiac surgery patients, a recent meta-analysis found that longer term (≥ 6 months of follow-up) use of statins in cardiac patients was not associated with a significant reduction in AF (OR 0.95; 95% CI 0.88-1.03, p=0.24), however only one of the 22 studies was in CABG patients (Rahimi et al., 2011).

Statins have shown benefit in reducing the risk of POAF, LOS, mortality, and 30 day atrial fibrillation-free survival. It is less clear which statin, what dose, and for what duration will achieve the greatest benefit. While the combination of statins and standard beta-blocker therapy is safe, certain statins, such as simvastatin, should only be used in reduced doses with the combination of amiodarone due to risk of myalgias or rhabdomyolysis (FDA Alert 2008). Larger, prospective, randomized control trials are necessary to confirm that statins are effective in reducing the occurrence of POAF in addition to beta-blockers.

4.2 Renin-angiotensin-aldosterone-system (RAAS) modulators

An increasing number of investigations are being conducted to evaluate the association between the RAAS, the inflammatory process, and atrial fibrillation. Interruption of the RAAS by angiotensin-converting enzyme inhibitors or angiotensin II receptor blockers prevents the production of the regulatory hormone angiotensin II, which plays a key role in controlling blood pressure, vascular smooth muscle tone, aldosterone release, and sodium resorption from the renal tubules (Boos et al., 2006). Beyond these actions, angiotensin II has been implicated in increasing the production of pro-inflammatory cytokines (i.e. IL-6, IL-8, TNF-α), adhesion molecules, selectins, and the recruitment of neutrophils (Boos et al., 2006). Histologic evidence exists that persistent and paroxysmal atrial fibrillation leads to altered angiotensin II receptor expression (Erlich et al., 2006; Boos et al., 2006). Genetic polymorphisms in the angiotensinogen gene are also two to three times more likely to have non-familial atrial fibrillation (Tsai et al., 2004), further supporting the role RAAS plays in the development of atrial fibrillation. ACEIs and ARBs have been shown to reduce the incidence of atrial fibrillation in patients with congestive heart failure, hypertension, or post MI (Makkar et al., 2009).

Three potential mechanisms have been suggested to explain the antiarrhythmic benefits of ACEIs and ARBs against atrial fibrillation. It is proposed that they improve left ventricular hemodynamics, reduce atrial stretch, suppress angiotensin-induced fibrosis, and direct modulation of potassium and calcium ion channel function. These ACEI/ARB-induced changes decrease atrial vulnerability and may diminish the initiation of atrial fibrillation (Erlich et al., 2006).

Few prospective, controlled studies have been conducted to assess the efficacy of ACEIs or ARBs in reducing the incidence of POAF in cardiac surgery patients (White et al., 2007a; Ozaydin et al., 2008a). One study randomized patients to an active intervention of ACEI or combination of ACEI/ARB and then compared these two treatment groups to a historical control. Greater than 85% of patients randomized to ACEI or combination were also on beta-blockers preoperatively and 97% of patients in the historical control group were on beta-blockers (Ozaydin et al., 2008a). Despite the high percentage of preoperative beta-blocker use in the control group, the combination of an ACEI/ARB or an ACEI alone proved superior to usual care with absolute reductions in the incidence of POAF compared to controls by 23% and 21%, respectively. There was no difference in the magnitude of the reduction of the incidence of POAF using the combination of an ACEI/ARB compared to an ACEI alone. The authors also found that both the combination ACEI/ARB or ACEI alone significantly reduced the risk of POAF by 72% and 66%, respectively (RR 0.28; 95% CI 0.09-0.83 and RR 0.34; 95% CI 0.12-0.93, respectively). The other study examined the effect of ACEI or ARBs on development of POAF from a nested cohort of patients from the AFIST II and III trials (White et al., 2007a). This study also found that preoperative use of ACEIs or ARBs were protective in reducing the risk of POAF by 29%, however the magnitude of the reduction was not statistically significant (adjusted OR 0.71; 95% CI 0.42-1.20). The clinical reduction in risk of POAF in patients on ACEIs or ARBs could have been influenced by 84% of the total population of patients receiving postoperative beta-blockade and 38% receiving amiodarone for POAF prophylaxis, therefore it remains unclear from that study the independent effect ACEIs or ARBs on POAF. Multivariate logistic regression analysis found that postoperative beta-blocker (adjusted OR 0.47, 95%CI 0.24-0.89) and prophylactic amiodarone (adjusted OR 0.32, 95%CI 0.18-0.57) were both negative predictors of POAF, thus decreasing the risk for POAF by 53% and 68%, respectively (White et al., 2007a).

Cohort studies conducted to evaluate the risk factors associated with the development of POAF in cardiac surgery patients found that preoperative and postoperative use of ACEIs or ARBs decreased the risk of POAF by 38% (OR 0.62; 95% CI 0.48-0.79; $p<0.001$) and that withdrawal of ACEI or ARB increases the risk of POAF by 1.7 times (OR 1.69; 95% CI 1.38-2.08; $p<0.001$) (Mathew et al., 2004) while another study in cardiac surgery patients with EF ≤ 50% confirmed this association that both ACEIs decreased the risk of POAF by 73% (OR 0.27, 95% CI 0.12-0.62, $p=0.002$) and ARBs by 79% (OR 0.21; 95% CI 0.07-0.62, $p=0.005$) (Ozaydin et al., 2010). Unfortunately, three other cohort studies did not confirm a protective effect of ACEIs or ARBs with no significant reduction in the risk of POAF compared to controls (Coleman et al., 2007; Miceli et al., 2009b; Rader et al., 2010). The largest of these cohort studies, evaluating over 10,000 patients, found that preoperative ACEI doubled the risk of death (OR 2.00, 95% CI 1.17-3.42; $p= 0.013$) and that preoperative ACEIs were an independent predictor of mortality ($p = 0.04$), postoperative renal dysfunction ($p= 0.0002$), use of inotropic drugs ($p < 0.0001$), and new onset POAF ($p < 0.0001$). (Miceli et al., 2009b) A

significant reduction may not have been observed in these studies as patients were propensity score matched for common predictors of atrial fibrillation. Thus groups could have been at high risk for the development of POAF (Coleman et al., 2007; Rader et al., 2010).
Further prospective, controlled trials are needed evaluate the impact of ACEIs or ARBs on the development of POAF. These studies will provide more definitive evidence concerning the effectiveness of ACEIs and ARBs in the prevention of POAF following cardiac surgical procedures. If ACIEs or ARBs are used in combination with standard therapies for the prevention of POAF, they must be used with caution or avoided in patients with renal dysfunction or electrolyte abnormalties, specifically hyperkalemia.

4.3 Corticosteroids

Corticosteroids have been traditionally utilized in cardiac surgeries to reduce inflammation in an effort to achieve early extubation, enhance pulmonary function recovery, or decrease postoperative nausea and vomiting. Inflammatory biomarkers increase in patients undergoing cardiothoracic surgery and inflammation appears to play a role in the development of POAF.
Studies evaluating corticosteroids have used various types of intravenous (IV) steroids, doses, and regimens. Two studies used beta-blockers postoperatively in all of their patients found that corticosteroids were superior to placebo with absolute reductions in the incidence of POAF of 18% to 30% (Prasongsukarn et al., 2005; Halonen et al., 2007). However other trials failed to show a significant benefit (Chaney et al., 1998; Halvorsen et al., 2003) in reducing incidence of POAF compared to placebo or usual care. Halonen et al further reported that after adjusting for potential unbalanced confounders, that hydrocortisone continued to be effective in reducing the risk of POAF by 46% (HR 0.54; 95% CI 0.35-0.83) with treatment of only 5.6 patients needed to prevent one occurrence of POAF (Halonen et al., 2007). The authors further performed a meta-analysis combining results from their trial with two other similar trials for a total of 621 patients (Prasongsukarn et al., 2005; Halvorsen et al., 2003). They found that corticosteroid therapy significantly reduced the risk of POAF by 33% (OR 0.67; 95% CI 0.54-0.84) (Halonen et al., 2007). Two other meta-analyses confirmed this finding where corticosteroids significantly reduced the risk of POAF by 29% (OR 0.71; 95% CI 0.59-0.87) and 45% (OR 0.55; 95% CI 0.39-0.78) and show a significant decrease in LOS with steroids of 0.6 days and 1.6 days (Whitlock et al., 2008; Baker et al., 2007b).
At this time, specific dosing of corticosteroids that may confer optimal protection against POAF is unkown. Baker et al converted the steroid dosing to dexamethasone equivalence based on total cumulative dose and relative potencies and found that reduction in POAF appeared greatest in patients receiving intermediate doses of corticosteroids (50-120 mg dexamethasone equivalent), while lower (≤ 8 mg dexamethasone equivalent) and higher (236-2850 mg dexamethasone equivalent) dosing resulted in blunted effects (Baker et al., 2007b). The most recent meta-analysis by Ho et al converted steroid dosing to hydrocortisone equivalence and found a significant reduction of POAF in patients receiving low (< 1,000 mg hydrocortisone equivalent) and intermediate (1,000-10,000 mg hydrocortisone equivalent) doses of steroids (Ho & Tan, 2009).
While corticosteroids can attenuate biomarkers shown to regulate the inflammatory response leading to the development of POAF, they are also associated with side effects that may inhibit their widespread use. Cardiac surgery patients who have received

corticosteroids have been shown to have peak white blood cell counts were higher up to 14 days postoperatively, higher blood glucose and larger insulin requirements (Sano et al., 2006), greater risk of wound and infectious complications (Whitlock et al., 2008). Therefore it may be necessary to avoid corticosteroids in patients with uncontrolled hyperglycemia, infection, or edema.

Corticosteroids can target the inflammatory process for the prevention of POAF in patients undergoing cardiac surgery. While some studies found a reduction in the incidence of POAF using corticosteroids as prophylaxis in cardiac surgery patients receiving standard beta-blocker therapy, there is no consensus on which steroid, dose, and duration has the greatest benefit. Only the 2010 European guidelines recommend corticosteroids for prophylaxis of POAF in cardiac surgery patients and include suggested dosing in dexamethasone equivalent for the prevention of POAF with a Class 2B recommendation, stating however that there is risk associated with using them (ESC, 2010). The most relevant risk in hospitalized patients after cardiac surgery includes steroid-induced hyperglycemia or leukocytosis. Corticosteroids may play a future role in targeting the inflammatory process in patients undergoing cardiothoracic surgery, however larger clinical trials are necessary to confirm if corticosteroids are effective in reducing the occurrence of POAF in addition to beta-blockers.

4.4 Omega-3 fatty acids

The ability of omega-3 fatty acids to reduce the occurrence of POAF is thought to result from a stabilizing effect on the myocardium, anti-inflammatory properties, and possibly antioxidant activity (Kris-Etherton et al., 2002; Korantzopoulos et al., 2006). Calo et al performed a prospective, randomized, open label study in 160 patients assessing the impact of N-3 polyunsaturated fatty acids (PUFA) 2 g/day on the incidence of POAF in cardiac surgery patients (Calo et al., 2005). Approximately 60% of patients in both groups were on preoperative beta-blockers. They found a significant reduction in incidence of POAF (15.2% versus 33.3%, respectively, p=0.013) and mean LOS (7.3 $\pm$ 2.1 days versus 8.2 $\pm$ 2.6 days, respectively, p=0.017) in patients receiving PUFA compared to control patients. Another small prospective, randomized study found that administration of IV PUFA at 100 mg fish oil/kg/day significantly reduced the incidence of POAF compared to control (17.3% vs. 30.6%, p<0.05) however this study did not mention the percentage of patients on beta-blocker therapy (Heidt, et al., 2009). Similar to other new agents showing studies with conflicting results for the prevention of POAF in cardiac surgery patients, two small, prospective, randomized, double blind, placebo controlled studies found no benefit using PUFA ~ 2 g/day therapy (Heidarsdottir et al., 2010; Saravanan et al., 2010). Further studies are warranted to determine if omega-3 fatty acids are viable add-on prophylactic therapy or alternative for patients unable to take beta-blockers.

4.5 Ascorbic acid

The ability of ascorbic acid (vitamin C) to prevent POAF is thought to occur due its antioxidant properties and potential to attenuate inflammation and electrical remodeling (Korantzopoulos et al., 2005). Vitamin C has been studied in prospective trials for the prevention of POAF in cardiac surgery patients (Carnes et al., 2001; Eslami et al., 2007). Both studies demonstrated significant benefit using vitamin C compared to usual care with an absolute reduction in POAF between 19-22%, but no reduction in mean LOS. Both studies also had substantial rates of both pre- and postoperative beta-blocker utilization. Due to the low cost and relative safety of this drug, larger placebo-controlled trials appear to be warranted.

4.6 N-Acetylcysteine

N-acetylcysteine (NAC) has been theorized to prevent POAF based on its antioxidant activity as a free radical scavenger and ability to reduce cellular damage in the atrium (Carnes et al., 2007). Two recent studies, which were randomized and placebo-controlled, found conflicting results with NAC in the prophylaxis of POAF (El-Hamamsy et al, 2007; Ozaydin et al., 2008b). The first study failed to demonstrate a significant reduction in the incidence of POAF (7% with NAC versus 12% with placebo, p=0.7). A more recent study, which included valve surgeries, did show a significant benefit with NAC compared to placebo (5% versus 21%, p=0.01). After controlling for perioperative beta-blocker use, NAC was still associated with a significant reduction in POAF (OR 0.17, 95% CI 0.04-0.69, p=0.01). Neither study found a significant reduction in LOS. Both studies reported substantial preoperative beta-blocker use while Ozaydin et al also reported substantial postoperative beta-blocker utilization. Two conflicting meta-analyses have been recently published, one that found a statistically significant reduction in POAF with NAC use (36%, 95% CI 2-58%, total n=1,338) and one larger one that did not (OR 0.67, 95% CI 0.37-1.22, p=0.19, total n=1,407) (Baker et al., 2009; Wang et al., 2011). Large, prospective, randomized clinical trials are necessary to determine if NAC is effective in reducing the occurrence of POAF in addition to beta-blockers.

4.7 Sodium nitroprusside

One pilot study evaluated sodium nitroprusside as an agent for POAF prophylaxis compared to placebo (Cavolli et al., 2008). This study demonstrated a significant reduction in the incidence of POAF when compared to placebo (12% versus 36%, p=0.005) and a significant reduction in mean LOS (7.3 $\pm$ 0.7 days versus 9.1 $\pm$ 1.2 days, p<0.001). The authors suggest that nitric oxide (NO) function may be disrupted due to ischemia-reperfusion injury and that administration of NO donors such as nSNP could recover this function. SNP may also reduce POAF by reducing left atrial stretching due to preload and afterload reduction. This study also showed a significant reduction in serum CRP levels in patients given SNP when compared to placebo (p<0.05), suggesting some possible effects on inflammation. Though not significant, more patients randomized to SNP received preoperative beta-blockers when compared to the placebo group (68% versus 58% p=0.303). Postoperative beta-blocker use was not addressed. Likewise, patients in this study had relative preserved ejection fractions (60-61%). Currently, SNP is routinely used in institutions for the management of postoperative hypertension. Patients receiving this medication may also experience an additional benefit of arrhythmia prevention.

4.8 Dofetilide

Dofetilide has been compared to placebo for postoperative atrial tachycardia (POAT) prophylaxis in one study (Serafimovski et al., 2008). The investigators found that patients receiving dofetilide prophylaxis experienced a significant reduction in the incidence of POAT, including atrial fibrillation and atrial flutter, when compared to placebo (18% versus 36%, p<0.017). There was no significant decrease in mean LOS. Although the use of postoperative beta-blockers was not reported, the authors conclude that the dofetilide group experienced a significant decrease in POAT independent of concomitant beta-blocker use based on multivariate logistic regression accounting for preoperative beta-blocker use. Due to cost, stringent prescribing and monitoring guidelines, and lack of robust head to head trials, dofetilide is not currently recommended as first line POAF prophylaxis. Like sotalol, it also carries a greater risk of Torsades and should be avoided in patients with prolonged QT intervals. It could be considered for add on therapy in high risk patients or in patients intolerant of beta-blockers but should first be compared to other traditional class III antiarrhythmics such as amiodarone or sotalol in head to head trials.

4.9 Levosimendan

Levosimendan is an intravenous calcium sensitizer agent that is used for the treatment of acute decompensated heart failure. It increases myocardial contraction without increasing myocardial oxygen consumption and produces coronary and peripheral vasodilation (Lilleberg et al., 1998). While the drug is not approved and will not be pursued for FDA approval in the US, it has been shown in one study to significantly reduce the incidence of POAF and increase stroke volume in patients with ejection fraction $\leq$30% when compared to milrinone (50% for milrinone, 5% for levosimendan started post anesthesia, and 35% for levosimendan started after cross clamp release, $p<0.01$) (De Hert et al., 2008). Very few patients in this study, however, were taking preoperative beta-blockers (~13-14%) and all patients received dobutamine after the release of the cross clamp.

5. Unestablished pharmacologic therapies for the prevention of POAF in cardiac surgery

5.1 Propafenone, procainamide, digoxin and calcium channel blockers

Given the availability of just a few trials with inconsistent results, propafenone is not currently recommended as first-line for POAF prophylaxis (Bradley et al., 2005; Dunning et al., 2006; Fuster et al., 2006; Eagle et al., 2004). Its use may be limited by its proarrhythmic effects in patients with structural heart disease. Current available evidence also does not support the use of procainamide for POAF prophylaxis. Although based on limited evidence, preoperative "digitalization" was historically used to prevent POAF. Currently, digoxin does not have an indication for POAF prophylaxis but can be used for rate control once atrial fibrillation occurs (Bradley et al., 2005). Only the non-dihydropyridine calcium channel blockers (non-DHP-CCB) diltiazem and verapamil, have evidence supporting their effectiveness for POAF prophylaxis from a meta-analysis evaluating twelve small studies encompassing 719 patients (Wijeysundera et al., 2003). However, two other meta-analyses found a non-significant reduction (Andrews et al., 1991) and even an increase in the risk of POAF (Woodend et al., 1998) with the CCBs. Because of this and the risk of atrioventricular block and low-output syndrome, especially in combination with beta-blockers, the guidelines recommend against routine use of CCBs for POAF prophylaxis and that the non-DHP-CCBs, diltiazem or verapamil, be reserved for rate control only once POAF has occurred (Bradley et al., 2005; Eagle et al., 2004).

5.2 Thiazolidinediones

Thiazolidinediones (TZDs) may affect POAF through pleiotropic anti-inflammatory activity against macrophage activation and pro-inflammatory cytokines (Consoli & Devangelio, 2005; Ricote et al., 1998). One study evaluated a nested cohort study of diabetic patients from the AFIST I, II, and III trials (Giri et al., 2001; White et al., 2003; White et al., 2007a) assessed whether the use of TZDs affected the incidence of POAF in diabetic patients who were also receiving beta- blockers and amiodarone (Anglade et al., 2007). In addition to substantial pre- and postoperative beta-blocker use, 43.8% of control patients and 35% of

TZD patients received amiodarone. Despite this, the study was unable to show a significant reduction in POAF. This may have been due to a lack of power due to small sample size, dilution of effect from concomitant beta-blocker and/or amiodarone use, or increased fluid retention associated with TZD use. In this same analysis, statins did demonstrate a significant reduction in POAF (28% versus 37%, $p<0.05$). This suggests that the most likely reason TZDs were of no benefit is due to their risk of fluid accumulation thereby attenuating any anti-inflammatory effect (Lertsburapa K, 2008). At this time, TZDs can not be recommended as an option for POAF prophylaxis, either alone or in combination with beta-blockers.

5.3 Triiodothyronine

The rationale behind the use of triiodothyronine (T3) for POAF prophylaxis lies in the observation that CPB results in a euthyroid sick or low T3 state (Klemperer et al., 1996). The mechanism by which T3 may prevent POAF is unknown (Reichert & Verzino, 2001). Interestingly, it has been shown that POAF is more common in patients with subclinical hypothyroidism when compared to those with normal thyroid function, after adjustments for other variables (Park et al., 2009). One demonstrated that intravenous administration of T3 starting at the time of cross clamp removal significantly decreases the incidence of POAF when compared to placebo (24% versus 46%, $p=0.009$) (Klemperer et al., 1996). All patients had a left ventricular ejection fraction of less than 40%. While T3 administration was associated with significantly higher postoperative cardiac indices and lower systemic vascular resistance, there was no significant difference in LOS (Klemperer et al., 1995). The authors previously reported data from this same study but included those patients with a history of preoperative atrial fibrillation (Klemperer et al., 1995). In this earlier study, there were no significant differences in the incidence of SVT between the two treatment groups. The authors do not report postoperative beta-blocker use but suggest that because the study population was more ill (ejection fraction <40%), beta-blockade may not be as effective and add-on therapy would be warranted. None of the guidelines currently recommend the use of T3 due to low quality of evidence (Bradley et al., 2005). Until more data becomes available supporting its for POAF prophylaxis, it should not be routinely utilized.

6. Non-pharmacologic strategies for the prevention of POAF in cardiac surgery

6.1 Pacing

The use of right atrial, left atrial, bi-atrial and pacing of the Bachman's bundle all have been evaluated in their merit in reducing post-operative supraventricular arrhythmias. The mechanism of atrial fibrillation is in part believed to be related to changes in the substrate on a temporary basis which causes lengthening of the P-R interval thereby allowing re-entrant POAF (Fan et al., 2003). There is evidence that bi-atrial pacing is beneficial especially in the age group over 70 (Gerstenfeld et al., 2001). While bi-atrial pacing has demonstrated some success it is noted the right atrial pacing alone is less favorable (Chung et al., 1996). Pacing thresholds and stability of the pacing wire has become problematic and alternate sources of pacing locations have been sought out (Goette et al., 2002). Bachman's bundle, a thick fibrous strip of muscle at the roof of both atria that crosses the intra-atrial septum has been demonstrated to have low pacing thresholds for at least five days post-operatively. This site may reduce intra-atrial conduction times thus reducing POAF (Goette et al., 2002).

In a meta-analysis of 10 clinical trials it was demonstrated that atrial pacing at the right atrium, left atrium or Bachman's bundle produced a decrease in atrial fibrillation (Fan et al., 2003). These 10 studies are limited by multiple pacing protocols, including using complex algorithms, fixed pacing and flexible algorithms. Eight of these studies demonstrated that bi-atrial pacing reduced the odds of POAF by 54% (OR=0.46; 95% CI 0.3-0.71). There was a significant lack of use of beta-adrenergic blocking drugs used in the post-operative phase in the meta-analysis at 56%. In a small group of patients (n=80) who underwent valvular surgery it was found that bi-atrial synchronous pacing for 72 hours decreased atrial fibrillation from 45% in the control group to 20% in the paced group (p=0.02) (Debrunner et al., 2004). It is noted that only 30% of this small group were exposed to pre-operative beta-adrenergic blockade, and post-operative use was not collected.
Pacing of the atria is not without risk. In a randomized trial of 100 patients it was found that atrial fibrillation occurred in 27.5% of the paced patients and 28.6% of the control group (Chung, 2003). There was an increase in atrial ectopy (10 fold increase) in the group of patients whom developed atrial fibrillation (Chung, 2003). It was hypothesized that inconsistent pacing in the atria, under sensing and intermittent loss of capture were factors in the increase in ectopy (Chung, 2003). A sub-analysis of patients paced at a lower rate (80 bpm) and use of an algorithm that maintained the atrial rate 50 ms above the intrinsic rate, demonstrated no difference in atrial fibrillation rates (Chung, 2003).
The most recent 2010 European AF guidelines recommend that biatrial pacing should be considered for prophylaxis (Class 2B recommendation based on Level A evidence) (ESC, 2010). Earlier publication in 2006 by EACTS for the guidelines for POAF after cardiothoracic surgery in 2006 (Grade A recommendation based on Level 1B studies) and in 2005 by the American College of Chest Physicians (ACCP) (Strength: B, Evidence: good, Net Benefit: small/weak) both similarly recommend biatrial pacing for prophylaxis (Dunning et al., 2006; Maisel & Epstein, 2005). (Table 1) Specifically, the 2005 ACCP guideline specifically recommends not using unilateral pacing of the right or left atrium. (Strength: I, Evidence: fair, Net Benefit: small/weak) (Maisel & Epstein, 2005). Furthermore, the 2006 EACTS guidelines recommend that temporary pacing should be used in high risk patients receiving beta-blockers and amiodarone for prophylaxis as protection from complications of bradycardia (Grade A recommendation based of Level 1B studies). The CCS guideline also recommends considering atrial pacing with or without a ventricular lead in patients with symptomatic bradycardia (Class 2A recommendation based on Level A evidence) and those patients who are not on a beta-blocker before surgery (Class 2A recommendation based on Level B evidence) (Mitchell et al., 2005a; Kerr & Roy, 2004). Last, the CCS guidelines strongly recommend placing temporary ventricular epicardial pacing electrode wires at the time of surgery to allow for backup pacing as necessary (Class 1 recommendation based on Level C evidence) (Mitchell et al., 2005a; Kerr & Roy, 2004).

6.2 Posterior pericardiotomy

The pathophysiology of posterior pericardiotomy is based upon adequate drainage of the pericardial space thereby reducing pericardial effusion (Biancari, 2010). Only the earlier European guidelines do include posterior pericardiotomy as a non-pharmacologic option for the prevention of POAF (Grade B recommendation based on Level 1B studies) (Dunning et al., 2006). A recent meta-analysis evaluating 763 patients found that patients who had a posterior pericardiotomy significantly reduced POAF (10.8% versus 28.1%, p=0.003; OR. 0.33, 95% CI 0.16–0.69) and early (6.9% versus 46.2% p<.0001) or late (0% versus 11.3%, p=0.0001) pleural effusion (Biancari & Mahar, 2010). The authors noted several limitations to the studies favoring pericardiotomy, including no data regarding hemodynamic instability, re-operation for bleeding and use of drugs for prevention of POAF (Biancari & Mahar, 2010). Posterior pericardiotomy however is not risk free. Potential risks include cardiac herniation as well as compromise of grafts protruding thought the pericardiotomy (Biancari & Mahar, 2010).

6.3 Coronary bypass surgery without the use of cardiopulmonary bypass ("Off-pump" CABG)

The introduction of cardiac surgery without the use of cardiopulmonary bypass, also referred to as "off-pump", has been hypothesized to lower the incidence of POAF. The multiple mechanisms hypothesized to cause POAF may all be avoided when coronary bypass surgery is completed without the use of the cardiopulmonary bypass circuit. Salamon et al evaluated a series of over 2500 patients with 252 undergoing "off-pump" coronary bypass surgery (Salamon et al., 2003). Patient on cardiopulmonary bypass had higher rates of atrial fibrillation and concluded that avoiding cardiopulmonary bypass did not aid in the reduction of AF. Another retrospective analysis by Enc and colleagues in 670 patients undergoing conventional compared to "off-pump" coronary bypass surgery, found a lower, but non-significant reduction in POAF respectively (16.1% versus 14.6%) (Enc et al., 2004).
Elimination of the use of cardiopulmonary bypass in cardiac surgery has shown inconsistent results from meta-analyses and studies. Only the European EACTS 2006 guidelines supports its use as a non-pharmacologic option are the 2006 EACTS guidelines and include earlier meta-analysis that show conflicting results (Dunning et al., 2006). Focus for the prevention of POAF in cardiac surgery patients should focus on the use more standard prophylactic regimens including beta-blockers, rather than explicit avoidance of cardiopulmonary bypass.

6.4 Pericardial fat pad

Two other novel non-pharmacologic options that have been studied include preservation of pericardial fat pad and regulation of body temperature during cardiac surgery which targets disruption of AV node and inflammation, respectively. The anterior fat pad is commonly disrupted to provide clear field of view while applying the cross clamp during cardiac surgery. The anterior fat pad is known to possess parasympathetic ganglia as well as vagal pathways (Singh et al., 1996). The fat pads located at the superior vena cava-atrial junction contain post ganglionic fibers that lead to the sino-atrial node (Carlson et al., 1992). The fat pads located at the pulmonary vein-left atrium contain post ganglionic fibers that innervate the atrio-ventricular node (Quan et al., 2001). These fat pads are analogous to dog physiology and has been determined that ablation of these fibers in dogs reduces susceptibility of POAF. In a study of 55 patients where the fat pad was preserved, a significant reduction of POAF was observed (Cummings et al., 2004). A significant limitation of this research includes a small sample size and not accounting for the use of beta-adrenergic blocking drugs. Secondarily the rate of atrial fibrillation in "off-pump" cardiac surgery remains a significant problem despite no manipulation of the epicardial fat pads (Salamon et al., 2003).

6.5 Regulation of body temperature during surgery

The other novel non-pharmacologic strategy is to regulate body temperature to limit systemic effects of the inflammatory cascade during cardiac surgery. Adams and colleagues identified that hypothermia decreases sympathetic activation which lowers plasma norepinephrine levels and neuropeptide Y levels (Adams et al., 2000). A study randomized patients into two groups including mild hypothermia (34° C) and moderate hypothermia (28° C) and found no difference in the incidence of POAF between the groups, thus did not validate this pathophysiologic basis of POAF (Adams et al., 2000). The study was completed without benefit of knowledge regarding use of beta blockers or other adjunct measures to prevent POAF which could influence the outcome of that study.. It should be noted that POAF is still common in beating heart surgery with normothermia, therefore negating the use of hypothermia as a valid tool in prevention of POAF.

6.6 Maze procedure during open-heart surgery

The surgical maze procedure, or Cox-maze procedure, uses surgical incisions in the atria to form scar tissue to interrupt possible macroreentrant circuits (Cox et al., 1991). Alternative energy sources including radiofrequency or cryothermia have been incorporated to create lesions blocking atrial conduction without surgical incision into the atria. These procedures can be effective in restoring sinus rhythm, however when it is combined with other open heart operations to treat chronic AF, operative morbidity is consistently increased (Banach, et al., 2010). It is usually only performed on patients needing open-heart surgery for other issues, such as valve replacement or repair or CABG. The Canadian and most recent European guidelines both mention surgical ablation, however it should only be considered in patients with symptomatic AF already undergoing cardiac surgery (Kerr & Roy, 2004; ESC, 2010). The Canadian guidelines additionally mention that it should be considered in patients with previous AF who are undergoing mitral valve surgery, who may be at higher risk of POAF (Kerr & Roy, 2004)

7. Conclusion

For the prevention of postoperative atrial fibrillation in patients undergoing cardiac surgery, pharmacologic prophylaxis with beta-blockers and amiodarone are widely utilized. Evidence based guidelines also support the use of sotalol, magnesium, and atrial pacing. While these agents reduce the incidence of POAF, they do not eliminate it. Thus, there is a need for additional effective therapies. Other strategies that may be beneficial for prophylaxis include dofetilide, renin-angiotensin-aldosterone-system modulators, statins, corticosteroids, omega-3 fatty acids, ascorbic acid, N-acetylcysteine, sodium nitroprusside, levosimendan or intraoperative maze procedure in symptomatic AF patients undergoing cardiac surgery. For most of these strategies, there is a need for additional large scale, adequately powered, clinical studies to determine the benefit before they can be considered for routine use. Identification of high risk patients undergoing cardiac surgery and use of appropriate pharmacologic and non-pharmacologic therapies may further reduce the incidence of POAF and lead to improvements in the overall morbidity and burden to the health care system.

8. References

Acikel, S.; Bozbas, H.; Gultekin, B.; Aydinalp, A.; Saritas, B.; Bal, U.; Yildirir, A.; Muderrisoglu, H.; Sezgin, A. & Ozin, B. (2008). Comparison of efficacy of metoprolol and carvedilol for preventing atrial fibrillation after coronary bypass surgery. *International Journal of Cardiology*, Vol.126, pp. 108-113, ISSN 0167-5273

Adams, D.; Heyer, E.; Simon, A.; Delphin, E.; Rose, E.; Oz, M.; McMahon, D. & Sun, L. (2000). Incidence of atrial fibrillation after mild or moderate hypothermic cardiopulmonary bypass. *Critical Care Medicine*, Vol.28, No.2, pp. 309-311, ISSN 0090-3493

Alghamdi, A.; Al-Radi, O. & Latter, D. (2005). Intravenous magnesium for prevention of atrial fibrillation after coronary artery bypass surgery a systemic review and meta-analysis. *Journal of Cardiac Surgery*, Vol.20, pp. 293-299, ISSN 1540-8191

Ali, I.; Sanalla, A. & Clark, V. (1997). Beta-blocker effects on post-operative atrial fibrillation. European Journal of Cardiothoracic Surgery, Vol.11, pp. 1154-115-7, ISSN 1010-7940

Andrews, T.; Reimold, S.; Berlin, J. & Antman, E. (1991). Prevention of supraventricular arrhythmias after coronary artery bypass surgery. *Circulation*, Vol.84, Suppl. III, pp. 236-244, ISSN 0009-7322

Anglade, M.; Kluger, J.; White, M.; Aberle, J. & Coleman, C. (2007). Thiazolidinedione use and post-operative atrial fibrillation a US nested case-control study. *Current Medical Research and Opinion*, Vol.23, No.11, pp. 2849-2855, ISSN 0300-7995

Aranski, S.; Shaw, D.; Adams, D.; Rizzo, R.; Couper, G.; VanderVliet, M.; Collins, J.; Cohn, L. & Burstin, H. (1996) Predictors of atrial fibrillation after coronary artery surgery. Current trends and impact on hospital resources. *Circulation*, Vol.94, pp. 390-397, ISSN 0009-7322

Auer, J.; Weber, T.; Berent, R. Puschmann, R.; Hartl, P.; Ng, C.; Schwarz, C.; Lehner, E.; Strasser, U.; Lassnig, E.; Lamm, G. & Eber, B. (2004a). A comparison between oral antiarrhythmic drugs in the prevention of atrial fibrillation after cardiac surgery: the pilot study of prevention of postoperative atrial fibrillation (SPPAF), a randomized, placebo-controlled trial. *The American Heart Journal*, Vol.147, pp. 636-643, ISSN 0002-8703

Auer, J.; Weber, T.; Berent, R.; Lamm, G.; Ng, C.; Hartl, P; Strasser, U. & Eber, B. (2004b). Use of Hmg-coenzyme a-reductase inhibitors (statins) and risk reduction of atrial fibrillation after cardiac surgery: results of the SPPAF study: a randomized placebo-controlled trial. *European Heart Journal*, Vol.25, Suppl.353, Abstract 2045, ISSN 1522-9645

Bagshaw, S.; Galbraith, P.; Mitchell, L.; Sauve, R.; Exner, D. & Ghali, W. (2006). Prophylactic amiodarone for prevention of atrial fibrillation after cardiac surgery: a meta-analysis. *The Annals of Thoracic Surgery*, Vol.82, pp. 1927-1937, ISSN 0003-4975

Banach, M.; Kourliouros, A.; Reinhart, K.; Benussi, S.; Mikhailidis, D.; Jahangiri, M.; Baker, W.; Galanti, A.; Rysz, J.;Camm, J.; White, C. & Alfieri, O. (2010). Postoperative atrial fibrillation - what do we really know? *Current Vascular Pharmacology*, Vol.8, No. 4, pp. 553-572, ISSN 1875-6212

Barnes, B.; Kirkland, E.; Howard, P.; Grauer, D.; Gorton, M.; Kramer, J.; Muehlebach, G. & Reed, W. (2006). Risk-stratified evaluation of amiodarone to prevent atrial fibrillation after cardiac surgery. *The Annals of Thoracic Surgery*, Vol.82, pp. 1332-1337, ISSN 0003-4975

Baker, W. & White, C. (2007a). Post-cardiothoracic surgery atrial fibrillation: a review of preventive strategies. *The Annals of Pharmacotherapy*, Vol.41, pp.587-598, ISSN 1060-0280

Baker, W.; White, C.; Kluger, J.; Denowitz, A.; Konecny, C. & Coleman, C. (2007b). Effect of perioperative corticosteroid use on the incidence of postcardiothoracic surgery atrial fibrillation and length of stay. *Heart Rhythm*, Vol.4, pp.461-468, ISSN 1547-5271

Baker, W.; Anglade, M.; Baker, E.; White, C.; Kluger, J. & Coleman, C. (2009). Use of N-acetylcysteine to reduce post-cardiothoracic surgery complications: a meta-analysis. *European Journal of Cardiothoracic Surgery*, Vol.35, pp. 521-527, ISSN 1873-734X

Barnes, B.; Kirkland, E.; Howard, P.; Grauer, D.; Gorton, M.; Kramer, J.; Muehlebach, G. & Reed W. (2006). Risk-stratified evaluation of amiodarone to prevent atrial fibrillation after cardiac surgery. *Annals of Thoracic Surgery*, Vol.82, pp. 1332-1337, ISSN 0003-4975

Bert, A.; Reinert, S. & Singh, A. (2001). A beta-blocker, not magnesium, is effective prophylaxis for atrial tachyarrhythmias after coronary artery bypass graft surgery. *Journal of Cardiothoracic and Vascular Anesthesia*, Vol.15, No.2, pp. 204-209, ISSN 1532-8422

Biancari, F. & *Mahar, M.* (2010). Meta-analysis of randomized trials on the efficacay of posterior pericardiotomy in preventing atrial fiibrillation after coronary bypass surgery. *The Journal of Thoracic and Cardiovascular Surgery*, Vol.139, pp. 1158-1161, ISSN 0022-5223

Boos, C.; Anderson, R. & Lip, G. (2006). Is atrial fibrillation an inflammatory disorder? *European Heart Journal*, Vol.27, pp. 136-149, ISSN 1522-9645

Bradley, D.; Creswell, L.; Hogue, C.; Epstein, A.; Prystowsky, E. & Daoud, E. (2005). American college of chest physicians guidelines for the prevention and management of Postoperative atrial fibrillation after cardiac surgery. *Chest*, Vol.128, No.2, pp. 39S-47S, ISSN 1931-3543

Bruins, P.; Velthuis, H.; Yazdanbakhsh, A.; Jansen, P.; van Hardevelt, F.; de Beaumont, E.; Wildevuur, C.; Eijsman, L,.; Trouwborst, A. & Hack, C. (1997). Activation of the complement system during and after cardiopulmonary bypass surgery: postsurgery activation involves C-reactive protein and is associated with postoperative arrhythmia. *Circulation*, Vol.96, No.10, pp. 3542-3548, ISSN 0009-7322

Buckley, M.; Nolan, P.; Slack, M.; Tisdale, J.; Hilleman, D. & Copeland, J. (2007). Amiodarone prophylaxis for atrial fibrillation after cardiac surgery: meta-analysis of dose response and timing of initiation. *Pharmacotherapy*, Vol.27, pp. 360-368, ISSN 1060-0280

Budeus, M.; Hennersdorf, M.; Perings, S.; Rohlen, S.; Schnitzler, S.; Felix, O.; Reimert, K.; Feindt, P.; Gams, E.; Lehmann, N.; Weineke, H.; Sak, S.; Erbel, R. & Perings, C. (2006). Amiodarone prophylaxis for atrial fibrillation of high-risk patients after coronary bypass grafting: a prospective, double-blinded, placebo-controlled, randomized study. *European Heart Journal* Vol.27, pp.1584-1591, ISSN 1522-9645

Burgess, D.; Kilborn, M. & Keech, A. (2006). Interventions for prevention of post-operative atrial fibrillation and its complications after cardiac surgery: a meta-analysis. *European Heart Journal*, Vol.27, pp. 2846-2857, ISSN 1522-9645

Cagli, K.; Ozeke, O.; Ergun, K.; Ergun, K.; Budak, B.; Demirtas, E.; Birincioglu, C. & Pac, M. (2006). Effect of low-dose amiodarone and magnesium combination on atrial fibrillation after coronary surgery. *Journal of Cardiac Surgery*, Vol.21, pp. 458-464, ISSN 1540-8191

Calo, L.; Bianconi, L.; Colivicchi, F.; Lamberti, F.; Loricchio, M.; de Ruvo, E.; Meo, A.; Pandozi, C.; Staibano, M. & Santini, M. (2005). N-3 fatty acids for the prevention of atrial fibrillation after coronary artery bypass surgery: a randomized, controlled trial. *Journal of the American College of Cardiology*, Vol.45, pp. 1723-1728, ISSN 1936-8798

Canbaz, S.; Erbas, H.; Huseyin, S. & Duran, E. (2008). The role of inflammation in atrial fibrillation following open heart surgery. *The Journal of International Medical Research*, Vol.36, pp. 1070-1077, ISSN 1473-2300

Carlson, M.; Geha, A.; Hsu, J.; Martin, P.; Levy, M.; Jacobs, G. & Waldo, A. (1992). Selective stimulation in of parasympathetic nerve fibers in the human sinoatrial node. *Circulation*, Vol.85, pp. 1311-1317, ISSN 0009-7322

Carnes, C.; Ching, M.; Nakayama, T.; Nakayama, H.; Baliga, R.; Piao, S.; Kanderian, A.; Pavia, S.; Hamlin, R.; McCarthy, P.; Bauer, J. & Van Wagoner, D. (2001). Ascorbate attenuates atrial pacing-induced peroxynitrite formation and electrical remodeling and decreases the incidence of postoperative atrial fibrillation. *Circulation Research*, Vol.89, pp. e32-38, ISSN 0009-7330

Carnes, C.; Janssen, P.; Ruehr, M.; Nakayama, H.; Nakayama, T.; Haase, H.; Bauer, J.; Chung, M.; Fearon, I.; Gillinov, A.; Hamlin, R. & Van Wagoner, D. (2007). Atrial glutathione content, calcium current, and contractility. *The Journal of Biological Chemistry*, Vol.282, pp. 28063-28073, ISSN 0021-9258

Caspie, J.; Rudis, E.; Bar, I.; Safadi, T. & Saute, M. (1995). Effects of magnesium on myocardial function after coronary artery bypass grafting. *The Annals of Thoracic Surgery*. Vol.59, pp. 942-947, ISSN 0003-4975

Cavolli, R.; Kaya, K.; Aslan, A.; Emiroglu, O.; Erturk, S.; Korkmaz, O.; Oguz, M.; Tasoz, R. & Ozyurda, U. (2008). Does sodium nitroprusside decrease the incidence of atrial fibrillation after myocardial revascularization? A pilot study. *Circulation*, Col.118, pp.476-481, ISSN 0009-7322

Chaney, M.; Nikolov, M.; Blakeman, B.; Bakhos, M. & Slogoff, S. (1998). Pulmonary effects of methylprednisolone in patients undergoing coronary artery bypass grafting and early tracheal extubation. *Anesthesia and Analgesia*, Vol.87, pp. 27-33, ISSN 0003-2999

Chen, W.; Krishnan G.; Sood, N.; Kluger, J. & Coleman, C. (2010). Effect of statins on atrial fibrillation after cardiac surgery: a duration- and dose-response meta-analysis. *The Journal of Thoracic and Cardiovascular Surgery*, Vol.140, pp. 364-72, ISSN 0022-5223

Chung, M.; Augostini, R.; Asher, C.; Pool, D.; Grady, T.; Zikri, M.; Buehner, S.; Weinstock, M. & McCarthy, P. (1996). A randomized, controlled study of atrial overdrive pacing for the prevention of atrial fibrillation after coronary bypass surgery [Abstract]. *Circulation*, Vol.94, Supplement I, pp. I-90, ISSN 0009-7322

Chung, M. (2003). Proarrhythmic effects of post-operative pacing intended to prevent atrial fibrillation: evidence from a clinical trial. *Cardiac Electrophysiology Review*, Vol.7, No. 2, pp. 143-146, ISSN 1385-2264

Coleman, C.; Makanji, S.; Kluger, J. & White, C. (2007). Effect of angiotensin-converting enzyme inhibitors or angiotensin receptor blockers on the frequency of post-cardiothoracic surgery atrial fibrillation. *The Annals of Pharmacotherapy*, Vol.41, pp. 433-437, ISSN 1060-0280

Colquhoun, I.; Berg, G.; El-Fiky, M.; Hurle, A.; Fell, G. & Wheatley, D. (1993). Arrhythmia prophylaxis after coronary artery surgery. *European Journal of Cardiothoracic Surgery,* Vol.7, pp. 520-523, ISSN 1010-7940

Consoli, A. & Devangelio, E. (2005). Thiazolidinediones and inflammation. *Lupus*, Vol.14, No.9, pp. 794-797, ISSN 0961-2033

Cox, J.; Schuessler, R.; D'Agostino, H.; Stone, C.; Chang, B.; Cain, M.; Corr, P. & Boineau, J. (1991). The surgical treatment of atrial fibrillation. III. Development of a definitive surgical procedure. *Journal of Thoracic and Cardiovascular Surgery, Vol.*101, No.4, pp. 569–83, ISSN 0022-5223

Crystal, E.; Connolly, S.; Sleik, K.; Ginger, T.; & Yusuf, S. (2002). Interventions on prevention of postoperative atrial fibrillation in patients undergoing heart surgery: a meta-analysis. *Circulation*, Vol.106, pp. 75-80, ISSN 0009-7322

Cummings, J.; Akhrass, R.; Dery, M.; Biblo, L. & Quan, K. (2004). Preservation of the anterior fat pad paradoxically decreases the incidence of post-operative atrial fibrillation in humans. *Journal of American College of Cardiology*, Vol.43, No.6, pp. 994-1000, ISSN 1936-8798

Cybulsky, I.; Connolly, S.; Lamy, A.; Roberts, R.; O'brien, B.; Carroll, S.; Crystal, E.; Thorpe, K. & Gent M. (2000). Beta-blocker length of stay study (BLOSS): a randomized trial of metoprolol for reduction of post-operative length of stay. *The Canadian Journal of Cardiology*, Vol.16, Abstract, pp. 238F, ISSN 0828-282X

Daoud, E.; Strickberger, S.; Man, K.; Goyal, R.; Deeb, G.; Bolling, S.; Pagani, F.; Bitar, C.; Meissner, M.; & Morady, F. (1997). Preoperative amiodarone as prophylaxis against atrial fibrillation after heart surgery. *The New England Journal of Medicine*, Vol.337, pp. 1785-1791, ISSN 0028-4793

Debrunner, M.; Naegeli, B.; Genoni, M.; Turina, M. & Bertel, O. (2004). Prevention of atrial fibrillation after cardiac valvular surgery by epicardial, biatrial synchronous pacing. *European Journal of Cardio-Thoracic Surgery, Vol.*25, pp. 16-20, ISSN 1010-7940

DeHert, S.; Lorsomradee, S.; Eede, H.; Cromheecke, S. & Van der Linden, P. A randomized trial evaluating different modalities of levosimendan administration in cardiac surgery patients with myocardial dysfunction. (2008). *Journal of Cardiothoracic and Vascular Anesthesia* Vol.22, No.5, pp. 699-705, ISSN 1532-8422

Dotani, M.; Elnicki, D.; Jain, A. & Gibson, C. (2000). Effect of preoperative statin therapy and cardiac outcomes after coronary artery bypass grafting. *The American Journal of Cardiology*, Vol.86, pp. 1128-1130, ISSN 1879-1913

Dunning, J.; Treasure, T.; Versteegh, M.; Samer, A. & the EACTS Audit and Guidelines Committee. (2006.) Guidelines on the prevention and management of de novo atrial fibrillation after cardiac and thoracic surgery. *European Journal of Cardiothoracic Surgery*, Vol.30, pp. 852-872, ISSN 1010-7940

Eagle, K.; Guyton, R.; Davidoff, R.; Edwards, F.; Ewy, G.; Gardner, T.; Hart, J.; Herrmann, H.; Hillis, L.; Hutter, A.; Lytle, B.; Marlow, R.; Nugent, W.; Orszulak, T.; Antman, E.; Smith, S.; Alpert, J.; Anderson, J.; Faxon, D.; Fuster, V.; Gibbons, R.; Gregoratos, G.; Halperin, J.; Hiratzka, L.; Hunt, S.; Jacobs, A. & Ornato, J. (2004). ACC/AHA 2004 Guideline update for coronary artery bypass graft surgery: summary article. A report of the American college of cardiology/American heart association task force on practice guidelines (Committee to update the 1999 guidelines for coronary artery bypass graft surgery). *Journal of the American College of Cardiology*, Vol.44, pp. e213-310, ISSN 1936-8798

Echahidi, N.; Pibarot, P.; O'Hara, G. & Mathieu, P. (2008). Mechanisms, prevention, and treatment of atrial fibrillation after cardiac surgery. *Journal of American College of Cardiology*, Vol.51, No.8, pp. 793-801, ISSN 1936-8798

Elahi, M.; Flatman, S. & Matata, B. (2008). Tracing the origins of postoperative atrial fibrillation: the concept ofoxidative stress-mediated myocardial injury phenomenon. *European Journal of Cardiovascular Prevention and Rehabilitation*, Vol.15, pp.735-741, ISSN 1741-8275

El-Hamamsy, I.; Stevens, L.; Carrier, M.; Pellerin, M.; Bouchard, D.; Demers, P.; Cartier, R.; Page, P. & Perrault, L. (2007). Effect of intravenous N-acetylcysteine on outcomes after coronary artery bypass surgery: a randomized, double-blind, placebo-controlled clinical trial. *Journal of Thoracic and Cardiovascular Surgery*, Vol.133, No.1, pp. 7-12, ISSN 0022-5223

Enc, Y.; Ketenci, B.; Ozsoy, D.; Camur, G.; Kayacioglu, I.; Terzi, S. & Cicek, S. (2004). Atrial fibrillation after surgical revascularization: is there any difference between on-pump and off-pump? *European Journal of Cardiothoracic Surgery*, Vol.26, pp. 1129-1133, ISSN 1010-7940

Erlich, J.; Hohnloser, S. & Nattel, S. (2006). Role of angiotensin system and effects of its inhibition in atrial fibrillation: clinical and experimental evidence. *European Heart Journal*, Vol.27, pp. 512-518, ISSN 1522-9645

Eslami, M.; Badkoubeh, R.; Mousavi, M.; Radmehr, H.; Salehi, M.; Tavakoli, N. & Avadi, M. (2007). Oral ascorbic acid in combination with beta-blockers. *Texas Heart Institute Journal*, Vol.34, pp. 268-274, ISSN 0730-2347

European Society of Cardiology. (2010). Guidelines for the management of atrial fibrillation: The Task Force for the Management of Atrial Fibrillation of the European Society of Cardiology (ESC). *European Heart Journal*, Vol.31, No.19, pp. 2369-2429, ISSN 1522-9645

Evrard, P.; Gonzalez, M.; Jamar, J.; et al. (2000). Prophylaxis of supraventricular arrhythmias after coronary artery bypass grafting with low-dose sotalol. *The Annals of Thoracic Surgery*, Vol.70, pp. 151-156, ISSN 0003-4975

Fan, K.; Lee, K. & Lau, CP. (2003). Mechanisms of biatrial pacing for prevention of postoperative atrial fibrillation-insights from a clinical trail. *Cardiac Electrophysiology Review*, Vol.7, No.2, pp. 147-153, ISSN 1573-725X

FDA Alert 8/8/2008. Information for Healthcare Professionals - Simvastatin (marketed as Zocor and generics), Ezetimibe/Simvastatin (marketed as Vytorin), Niacin extended-release /Simvastatin (marketed as Simcor), used with Amiodarone (Cordarone, Pacerone) Available from http://www.fda.gov/Drugs/DrugSafety/PostmarketDrugSafetyInformationforPatientsandProviders/ucm118869.htm.

Ferguson, J.; Coombs, L. & Peterson, E. (2002). Society of thoracic surgeons national adult cardiac surgery database: pre-operative beta-blocker use and mortality and morbidity following CABG surgery in north america. *Journal of the American Medical Association*, Vol.287, pp. 2221-2227, ISSN 0098-7484

Fuster, V.; Ryden, L.; Cannom, D.; Crijns, H.; Curtis, A.; Crijns, H.; Curtis, A.; Ellenbogen, K.; Halperin, J.; Le Heuzey, J.; Kay, G.; Lowe, J.; Olsson, S.; Prystowsky, E.; Tamargo, J.; Wann, S.; Smith, S.; Jacobs, A.; Adams, C.; Anderson, J.; Antman, E.; Halperin, J.; Hunt, S.; Nishimura, R.; Ornato, J.; Page, R.; Riegel, B.; Priori, S.; Blanc, J.; Budaj, A.; Camm, A.; Dean, V.; Deckers, J.; Despres, C.; Dickstein, K.; Lekakis, J.; McGregor, K.; Metra, M.; Morais, J,.; Osterspey, A.; Tamargo, J. & Zamorano, J. (2006). ACC/AHA/ESC 2006 Guidelines for the management of patients with atrial fibrillation - executive summary: a report of the American college of cardiology/American heart association task force on practice guidelines and the European society of cardiology committee for practice guidelines (writing committee to revise the 2001 guidelines for the management of patients with atrial fibrillation): developed in collaboration with the European heart rhythm society. *Circulation,* Vol.114, pp.700-752, ISSN 0009-7322

Gerstenfeld, E.; Khoo, M.; Cook, J.; Lancey, R.; Rofino, K.; Vander Salm, T. & Mittleman, R. (2001). Effectiveness of bi-atrial pacing for reducing atrial fibrillation after coronary artery bypass graft surgery. *Journal of Interventional Cardiac Electrophysiology*, Vol.5, No.3, pp. 275-283, ISSN 1572-8595

Gillespie, E.; White, C.; Kluger, J.; Rancourt, J.; Gallagher, R. & Coleman, C.(2006). Cost-effectiveness of amiodarone for prophylaxis of atrial fibrillation after cardiothoracic surgery. *Pharmacotherapy*, Vol.26, pp. 499-504, ISSN 0277-0008

Giri, S.; White, C.; Dunn, A.; Felton, K.; Freeman-Bosco, L.; Reddy, P.; Tsikouris, J.; Wilcox, H. & Kluger, J. (2001). Oral amiodarone for the prevention of atrial fibrillation after open heart surgery, the Atrial Fibrillation Suppression Trial (AFIST): a randomized placebo-controlled trial. *The Lancet*, Vol.357, pp. 830-836, ISSN 0099-5355

Goette, A.; Mittag, J.; Friedl, A.; Busk, H.; Jepsen, M.; Hartung, W.; Huth, C. & Klein H. (2002). Pacing of Bachmann's bundle after coronary artery bypass grafting. *Pacing and Clinical Electrophysiology: PACE*, Vol.25, No.7, pp. 1072-1078, ISSN 1540-8159

Griendling, K.; Sorescu, D. & Ushio Fukai, M. (2000). NAD(P)H oxidase: role in cardiovascular biology and disease. *Circulation Research*, Vol.86, pp. 494-501, ISSN 0009-7330

Gaudino, M.; Andreotti, F.; Zamparelli, R.; Di Castelnuovo, A.; Nasso, G.; Burzotta, F.; Iacoviello, L.; Donati, M.; Schiavello, R.; Maseri, A. & Possati, G. (2003). The -174G/C interleukin-6 polymorphism influences postoperative interleukin-6 levels and postoperative atrial fibrillation. Is atrial fibrillation an inflammatory complication? *Circulation* 2003;Vol.108, Suppl 1:II, pp. 195-199, ISSN 0009-7322

Guarnieri, T.; Nolan, S.; Gottlieb, S.; Dudeck, A. & Lowry, D. (1999). Intravenous amiodarone for the prevention of atrial fibrillation after open heart surgery: the amiodarone reduction in coronary heart (ARCH) trial. *Journal of the American College of Cardiology*, Vol.34, pp. 343-347, ISSN 1936-8798

Haan, C. & Geraci, S. (2002). Role of amiodarone in reducing atrial fibrillation after cardiac surgery in adults. *The Annals of Thoracic Surgery*, Vol.73, pp. 1665-1669, ISSN 0003-4975

Haghjoo, M.; Saravi, M.; Hashemi, M.; Hosseini, S.; Givtaj, N.; Ghafarinejad, M.; Khamoushi, J.; Emkanjoo, Z.; Fazelifar, A.; Alizadeh, A. & Sadr-Ameli, M. (2007). Optimal beta-blocker for prevention of atrial fibrillation after on-pump coronary artery bypass graft surgery. *Heart Rhythm*, Vol.4, pp. 1170-1174, ISSN 1547-5271

Halonen, J.; Hakala, T.; Auvinen, T., Karjalainen, J.; Turpeinen, A.; Uusaro, A.; Halonen, P.; Hartikainen, J. & Hippelaeinen, M. (2006). Intravenous administration of metoprolol is more effective than oral administration in the prevention of atrial fibrillation after cardiac surgery. *Circulation*, Vol.114, pp. 1-4, ISSN 0009-7322

Halonen, J.; Halonen, P.; Jarvinen, O.; Taskinen, P.; Auvinen, T.; Tarkka, M.; Hippeläinen, M.; Juvonen, T.; Hartikainen, J. &

Hakala, T. (2007). Corticosteroids for the prevention of atrial fibrillation after cardiac surgery- a randomized controlled trial. *Journal of the American Medical Association*, Vol.297, pp. 1562-1567, ISSN 0098-7484

Halvorsen, P.; Raeder, J.; White, P.; White, P.; Almdahl, S.; Nordstrand, K.; Saatvedt, K. & Veel, T. (2003). The effect of dexamethasone on side effects after coronary revascularization procedures. *Anesthesia and Analgesia*, Vol.96, pp. 1578-1583, ISSN 0003-2999

Heidarsdottir, R.; Arnar, D.; Skuladottir, G.; Torfason, B.; Edvardsson, V.; Gottskalksson, G.; Palsson, R. &

Indridason, O. (2010). Does treatment with n-3 polyunsaturated fatty acids prevent atrial fibrillation after open heart surgery? *Europace: European Pacing, Arrhythmias, and Cardiac Electrophysiology: Journal Of The Working Groups On Cardiac Pacing, Arrhythmias, And Cardiac Cellular Electrophysiology Of The European Society Of Cardiology*, Vol.12, No.3, pp. 356-363, ISSN 1532-2092

Heidt, M.; Vician, M.; Stracke, K.; Grebe, M.; Boening, A.; Vogt, P. & Erdogan, A. (2009). Beneficial effects of intravenously administered N-3 fatty acids for the prevention of atrial fibrillation after coronary artery bypass surgery: a prospective randomized study. *The Journal of Thoracic and Cardiovascular Surgery*, Vol.57, pp. 276-280, ISSN 1097-685X

Henyan, N.; Gillespie, E.; White, C.; Kluger, J. & Coleman, C. (2005). Impact of intravenous magnesium on post-cardiothoracic surgery atrial fibrillation and length of hospital stay: a meta-analysis. *The Annals of Thoracic Surgery*, Vol.80, pp. 2402-2406, ISSN 0003-4975

Ho, K. & Tan, J. (2009). Benefits and risks of corticosteroid prophylaxis in adult cardiac surgery: a dose–response meta-analysis. *Circulation*, Vol.119, pp. 1853–1866, ISSN 0009-7322

Howard, P. & Barnes, B. (2008). Potential use of statins to prevent atrial fibrillation after coronary artery bypass surgery. *Annals of Pharmacotherapy*, Vol.42, pp. 253-258, ISSN 1060-0280

Ishii, T.; Schuessler, R.; Gaynor, S.; Yamada, K.; Fu, A.; Boineau, J. & Damiano, R. (2005). Inflammation of atrium after cardiac surgery is associated with in homogeneity of atrial conduction and atrial fibrillation. *Circulation*, Vol.111, No.22, pp. 2881-2888, ISSN 0009-7322

Janssen, J.; Loomans, L.; Harink, J.; Taams, M.; Brunninkhuis, L.; van der Starre, P. & Kootstra, G. (1986). Prevention and treatment of supraventricular tachycardia shortly after coronary artery bypass grafting: a randomized open trial. *Angiology*, Vol.37, No.1, pp. 601-609, ISSN 0003-3197

Ji, Q.; Mei, Y.; Wang, X.; Sun, Y.; Feng, J.; Cai, J.; Xie, S. & Chi, L. (2009). Effect of preoperative atorvastatin therapy on atrial fibrillation following off-pump coronary artery bypass grafting. *Circulation Journal: Official Journal Of The Japanese Circulation Society*, Vol.73, No.12, pp. 2244-2249, ISSN 1347-4839

Jideus, L.; Blomstrom, P.; Nilsson, L.; Stridsberg, M.; Hansell, P. & Blomström-Lundqvist, C. (2000). Tachyarrhythmias and triggering factors for atrial fibrillation after coronary artery bypass operations. *Annals of Thoracic Surgery*, Vol.69, pp. 1064-9, ISSN 0003-4975

Kaireviciute, D.; Aidietis, A. & Lip, G. (2009). Atrial fibrillation following cardiac surgery: clinical features and preventive strategies. *European Heart Journal*, Vol.30, pp. 410-425, ISSN 1522-9645

Kalman, J.; Munawar, M.; Howes, L.; Louis, W.; Buxton, B.; Gutteridge, G. & Tonkin, A. (1995). Atrial fibrillation after coronary artery bypass grafting is associated with sympathetic activation. *The Annals of Thoracic Surgery*, Vol.52, pp. 529-533, ISSN 0003-4975

Kerr, C. & Roy, D. Canadian Cardiovascular Society Consensus Conference: Atrial fibrillation 2004, Executive summary. Available at : http://www.ccs.ca/download/consensus_conference/consensus_conference_archives/2004_Atrial_Fib_full.pdf

Kim, Y.; Kattach, H.; Ratnatunga, C.; Pillai, R.; Channon, K. & Casadei, B. (2008). Association of atrial nicotinamide adenine dinucleotide phosphate oxidase activity with the development of atrial fibrillation after cardiac surgery. *Journal of the American College of Cardiology*, Vol.51, pp. 68-74, ISSN 1936-8798

Kim M.; Deeb G.; Morady, F.; Bruckman, D.; Hallock, L.; Smith, K.; Karavite, D.; Bolling, S.; Pagani, F.; Wahr, J.; Sonnad, S.; Kazanjian, P.; Watts, C.; Williams, M. & Eagle, K. (2001). Effect of postoperative atrial fibrillation on length of stay after cardiac surgery (The Postoperative Atrial Fibrillation in Cardiac Surgery Study [PACS]). *The American Journal of Cardiology*, Vol.87, pp. 881-885, ISSN 1879-1913

Kinoshita, T.; Asai, T.; Nishimura, O.; Hiramatsu, N.; Suzuki, T.; Kambara, A. & Matsubayashi, K. (2010). Statin for prevention of atrial fibrillation after off-pump coronary artery bypass grafting in Japanese patients. *Circulation Journal: Official Journal Of The Japanese Circulation Society*. 2010. Vol.74, No.9, pp. 1846-1851, ISSN 1347-4839

Klemperer, J.; Klein, I.; Gomez, M.; Helm, R.; Ojamaa, K.; Thomas, S.; Isom, O. & Krieger, K. (1995).Thyroid hormone treatment after coronary-artery bypass surgery. *The New England Journal of Medicine*, Vol.333, pp. 1522-1527, ISSN 0028-4793

Klemperer, J.; Klein, I.; Ojamaa, K.; Helm, R.; Gomez, M.; Isom, O. & Krieger; H. (1996). Triiodothyronine therapy lowers the incidence of atrial fibrillation after cardiac operations. *The Annals of Thoracic Surgery*, Vol.61, No.5, pp. 1323-1327, ISSN 0003-4975

Kohno, H.; Koyanagi, T.; Kasegawa, H. & Miyazaki, M. (2005). Three day magnesium administration prevents atrial fibrillation after coronary artery bypass grafting. *Annals of Thoracic Surgery*, Vol.79, pp. 117-126, ISSN 0003-4975

Korantzopoulos, P.; Kolettis, T.; Kountouris, E.; Dimitroula, V.; Karanikis, P.; Pappa, E.; Siogas, K.; Goudevenos, J. (2005). Oral vitamin C administration reduces early recurrences rates after electrical cardioversion of persistent atrial fibrillation and attenuates associated inflammation. *International Journal of Cardiology*, Vol.102, pp. 321-326, ISSN 0167-5273

Korantzopoulos, P.; Kolettis, T. & Goudevenos, J. (2006). Effects of N-3 fatty acids on postoperative atrial fibrillation following coronary artery bypass surgery. *Journal of the American College of Cardiology*, Vol.47, No.2, pp. 467(Letter), ISSN 1936-8798

Kourlioros, A.; DeSouza, A.; Roberts, N.; Marciniak, A.; Tsiouris, A.; Valencia, O.; Camm, J. & Jahangiri, M. (2008). Dose-related effects of statins on atrial fibrillation after cardiac surgery. *The Annals of Thoracic Surgery*, Vol.85, pp. 1515-1520, ISSN 0003-4975

Kris-Etherton, P.; Harris, W. & Appel, L. (2002). Fish Consumption, Fish Oil, Omega-3 Fatty Acids, and Cardiovascular Disease, *Arteriosclerosis, Thrombosis and Vascular Biology*, Vol.106, pp. 2747-2757, ISSN 1524-4636

Laikopoulos, O.; Choi, Y.; Haldenwang, P.; Strauch, J.; Wittwer, T.; Dörge, H.; Stamm, C.; Wassmer, G. & Wahlers, T. (2008). Impact of preoperative statin therapy on adverse postoperative outcomes in patients undergoing cardiac surgery: a meta-analysis of over 30000 patients. *European Heart Journal*, Vol.29, pp. 1548-1559, ISSN 1522-9645

Lamm, G.; Auer, J.; Weber, T.; Berent, R.; Ng, C. & Eber, B. (2006). Postoperative white blood cell count predicts atrial fibrillation after cardiac surgery. *Journal of Cardiothoracic and Vascular Anesthesia*, Vol.20, pp. 51-56, ISSN 1532-8422

Lertsburapa, K.; White, C.; Kluger, J.; Faheem, O.; Hammond, J. & Coleman, C. (2008). Preoperative statins for the prevention of atrial fibrillation after cardiothoracic surgery. *Journal of Thoracic and Cardiovascular Surgery*, Vol.135, pp. 405-411, ISSN 0022-5223

Lilleberg, J.; Nieminen, M.; Akkila, J.; Heikkilä, L.; Kuitunen, A.; Lehtonen, L.; Verkkala, K.; Mattila, S. & Salmenperä, M. (1998). Effects of a new calcium sensitizer, levosimendan, on haemodynamic, coornar blood flow, and myocardial substrate utilization early after coronary artery bypass grafting. *European Heart Journal* Vol.19, pp.660-668, ISSN 1522-9645

Maisel, W. & Epstein, A. (2005). The role of cardiac pacing. *Chest*, Vol.128, pp. 36S-38S, ISSN 1931-3543

Makkar, K.; Sanoski, C. & Spinler, S. (2009). Role of angiotensin-converting enzyme inhibitors, angiotensin II receptor blockers, and aldosterone antagonists in the prevention of atrial and ventricular arrhythmias. *Pharmacotherapy*, Vol.29, pp. 31-48, ISSN 0277-0008

Mariscalco, G.; Lorusso, R.; Klersy, C.; Ferrarese, S.; Tozzi, M.; Vanoli, D.; Domenico, B. & Sala, A. (2007). Observational study on the beneficial effect of preoperative statins in reducing atrial fibrillation after coronary surgery. *The Annals of Thoracic Surgery*, Vol.84, pp. 1158-1165,ISSN 0003-4975

Maslow, A.; Regan, M.; Heindle, S.; Panzica, P.; Cohn, W. & Johnson, R. (2000). Postoperative atrial tachyarrhythmias in patients undergoing coronary artery bypass graft surgery without cardiopulmonary bypass: a role for intraoperative magnesium supplementation. *Journal of Cardiothoracic and Vascular Anesthesia*, Vol.14, No.5, pp. 524-530, ISSN 1532-8422

Mathew, J.; Fontes, M.; Tudor, J.; Ramsay, J.; Duke, P.; Mazer, C.; Barash, P.; Hsu, P. & Mangano, D. (2004). A multicenter risk index for atrial fibrillation after cardiac surgery. *Journal of the American Medical Association*, Vol.291, pp. 1720-1729, ISSN 0098-7484

Miceli, A.; Fino, C.; Fiorani, B.; Yeatman, M.; Narayan, P.; Angelini, G. & Caputo, M. (2009a). Effects of preoperative statin treatment on the incidence of postoperative atrial fibrillation in patients undergoing coronary artery bypass grafting. *The Annals of Thoracic Surgery*, Vol.87, No.6, pp. 1853-1858, ISSN 0003-4975

Miceli, A.; Capoun, R.; Fino, C.; Narayan, P.; Bryan, A.; Angelini, G. & Caputo, M. (2009b). Effects of angiotensin-converting enzyme inhibitor therapy on clinical outcome in patients undergoing coronary artery bypass grafting. *Journal of the American College of Cardiology*, Vol.54, No.19, pp. 1778–84, ISSN 1936-8798

Miller, S.; Crystal, E.; Garfinkle, M.; Lau, C.; Lashevsky, I. & Connolly, S. (2005). Effects of magnesium on atrial fibrillation after cardiac surgery: a meta-analysis. *Heart*, Vol.91, pp. 618-623, ISSN 1355-6037

Mitchell, L.; Crystal, E.; Heilbron, B. & Page, P. (2005a). Atrial fibrillation following cardiac surgery. *The Canadian Journal of Cardiology*, Vol.21, Suppl B, pp. 45B-50B, ISSN 0828-282X

Mitchell, L.; Exner, D.; Wyse, D.; Connolly, C.; Prystai, G.; Bayes, A.; Kidd, W.; Kieser, T.; Burgess, J.; Ferland, A.; MacAdams, C. & Maitland, A. (2005b). Prophylactic oral amiodarone for the prevention of arrhythmias that begin early after revascularization, valve replacement, or repair. PAPABEAR: A randomized controlled trial. *Journal of the American Medical Association*, Vol.294, pp. 3093-3100, ISSN 0098-7484

Mithani, S.; Akbar, M.; Johnson, D.; Kuskowski, M.; Apple, K.; Bonawitz-Conlin, J.; Ward, H.; Kelly, R.; McFalls, E.; Bloomfield, H.; Li, J.; Adabag, S. (2009). Dose dependent effect of statins on postoperative atrial fibrillation after cardiac surgery among patients treated with beta blockers. *Journal of Cardiothoracic Surgery*, Vol.4, pp. 61-61, ISSN 1749-8090

Nisanoglu, V.; Erdil, N.; Aldemir, M.; Ozgur, B.; Berat Cihan, H.; Yologlu, S. & Battaloglu, B. (2007). Atrial fibrillation after coronary artery bypass grafting in elderly patients: incidence and risk factor analysis. *Journal of Thoracic and Cardiovascular Surgery*, Vol.55, pp. 32-38, ISSN 0022-5223

Nurozler, F.; Tokgozoglu, L.; Pasaoglu, I.; Boke, E.; Ersoy, U. & Bozer, A. (1996). Atrial fibrillation after coronary artery bypass surgery: predictors and the role of MgSO4 replacement. *Journal of Cardiothoracic and Vascular Anesthesia*, Vol.11, pp. 421-427, ISSN 1532-8422

Ozaydin, M.; Dogan, A.; Varol, E.; Kapan, S.; Tuzun, N.; Peker, O.; Aslan, S.; Altinbas, A.; Ocal, A. & Ibrisim, E (2007). Statin use before by-pass surgery decreases the incidence and shortens the duration of postoperative atrial fibrillation. *Cardiology*, Vol.107, pp. 117-121, ISSN 0008-6312

Ozaydin, M.; Dede, O.; Varol, E.; Kapan, S.; Turker, Y.; Peker, O.; Duver, H. & Ibrisim, E. (2008a). Effect of renin-angiotensin aldosterone system blockers on postoperative atrial fibrillation. *International Journal of Cardiology*, Vol.127, pp. 362-367, ISSN 0167-5273

Ozaydin, M.; Peker, O.; Erdogan, D.; Kapan, S.; Turker, Y.; Varol, E.; Ozguner, F.; Dogan, A. & Ibrisim, E. (2008b). N-acetylcysteine for the prevention of postoperative atrial fibrillation: a prospective, randomized, placebo-controlled pilot study. *EuropeanHeart Journal*, Vol.29, pp. 625-631, ISSN 1522-9645

Ozaydin M.; Varol, E.; Türker, Y.; Peker, O.; Erdoğan, D.; Doğan, A. & Ibrişim, E. (2010). Association between renin-angiotensin-aldosterone system blockers and postoperative atrial fibrillation in patients with mild and moderate left ventricular dysfunction. *Anadolu Kardiyoloji Dergisi: AKD = Anatolian Journal Of Cardiology*, Vol.10, No.2, pp. 137-142, ISSN 1308-0032

Paraskevas, K. (2008). Applications of statins in cardiothoracic surgery: more than just lipid lowering. *European Journal of Cardiothoracic Surgery*, Vol.33, pp. 377-390, ISSN 1010-7940

Park, Y.; Yoon, J.; Kim, K.; Lee, Y.; Kim, K.; Choi, S.; Lim, S.; Choi, D.; Park, K.; Choh, J.; Jang, H.; Kim, S.; Cho, B. & Lim, C. (2009). Subclinical hypothyroidism might increase the risk of transient atrial fibrillation after coronary artery bypass grafting. *The Annals of Thoracic Surgery*, Vol.87, pp. 1846-1852, ISSN 0003-4975

Patel, A. & Dunning, J. (2005). Is sotalol more effective than standard beta-blockers for prophylaxis of atrial fibrillation during cardiac surgery? *Interactive Cardiovascular and Thoracic Surgery*, Vol.4, pp.147-150, ISSN 1569-9285

Patel, A.; White, C.; Gillespie, E.; Kluger, J. & Coleman, C. (2006). Safety of amiodarone in prevention of postoperative atrial fibrillation: a meta-analysis. *The American Journal of Health-System Pharmacy*, Vol.63, pp. 829-839, ISSN 1079-2082

Patel, A.; White, C.; Shah, S.; Dale, K.; Kluker, J. & Coleman, C. (2007). The relationship between statin use and atrial fibrillation. *Current Medical Research and Opinion*, Vol.23, pp. 1177-1185, ISSN 0300-7995

Patti, G.; Chello, M.; Candura, D.; Pasceri, V.; D'Ambrosio, A.; Covino, E. & Di Sciascio, G. (2006). Randomized trial of atorvastatin for reduction of postoperative atrial fibrillation in patients undergoing cardiac surgery- results of the ARMYDA-3 (Atorvastatin for Reduction of MYocardial Dysrhythmia After cardiac surgery) Study. *Circulation*, Vol.114, pp. 1455-1461, ISSN 0009-7322

Prasongsukarn, K.; Abel, J.; Jamieson, E.; Cheung, A.; Russell, J.; Walley, K. & Lichtenstein, S. (2005). The effects of steroids on the occurrence of postoperative atrial fibrillation after coronary artery bypass grafting surgery: a prospective randomized trial. *Journal of Thoracic and Cardiovascular Surgery*, Vol.130, pp. 193-198, ISSN 0022-5223

Quan, K.; Lee, J.; Van Hare, G.; Biblo, L.; Mackall, J. & Carlson, M. (2001). Identification and characterization of atrioventricular parasympathetic innervation in humans. *Journal of Cardiovascular Electrophysiology*, Vol.13, No.8, pp. 737-739, ISSN 1540-8167

Rader, F.; Van Wagoner, D.; Gillinov, A. & Blackstone, E. (2010). Preoperative angiotensin-blocking drug therapy is not associated with atrial fibrillation after cardiac surgery. *American Heart Journal,* Vol.160, No.2, pp. 329-336.e1, ISSN 0002-8703

Rahimi, K.; Martin, J.; Emberson, J.; McGale, P.; Majoni, W.; Merhi, A.; Asselbergs, F.; Krane, V. & Macfarlane, P. (2011). Effect of statins on atrial fibrillation: collaborative meta-analysis of published and unpublished evidence from randomized controlled trials. *British Medical Journal,* Vol.342,d1250, pp. 1-11, ISSN 0267-0623

Ramlawi, B.; Out, H.; Mieno, S.; Boodhwani, M.; Sodha, N.; Clements, R.; Bianchi, C. & Sellke, F. (2007). Oxidative stress and atrial fibrillation after cardiac surgery: a case control study. *The Annals of Thoracic Surgery,* Vol.84, pp. 1166-1173, ISSN 0003-4975

Reichert, M. & Verzino, K. (2001). Triiodothyronine supplementation in patients undergoing cardiopulmonary bypass. *Pharmacotherapy,* Vol.21, No.11, pp. 1368-1374, ISSN 0277-0008

Ricote, M.; Li, A.; Willson, T.; Kelly, C. & Glass, C. (1998). The peroxisome proliferators-activated receptor-gamma is a negative regulator of macrophage activation. *Nature,* Vol.391, pp. 79-82, ISSN 0028-0836

Rodrigo, R.; Cereceda, M.; Castillo, R.; Asenjo, R.; Zamorano, J.; Araya, J.; Castillo-Koch, R.; Espinoza, J. & Larraín, E. (2008). Prevention of atrial fibrillation following cardiac surgery: basis for a novel therapeutic strategy based on non-hypoxic myocardial preconditioning. *Pharmacology and Therapeutics,* Vol.118, pp. 104-127, ISSN 0163-7258

Salamon, T.; Michler, R.; Knott, K. & Brown, D. (2003). Off pump coronary artery bypass grafting does not decrease the incidence of atrial fibrillation . *The Annals of Thoracic Surgery,* Vol.73, pp. 505-507, ISSN 0003-4975

Sano, T.; Morita, S.; Masuda, M. & Yasui, H. (2006). Minor infection encouraged by steroid administration during cardiac surgery. *Asian Cardiovascular Thoracic Annals,* Vol.14, pp. 505-510, ISSN 1816-5370

Saravanan, P.; Bridgewater, B.; West, O'Neill, S.; Calder, P. & Davidson, N. (2010). Omega-3 fatty acid supplementation does not reduce risk of atrial fibrillation after coronary artery bypass surgery: a randomized, double-blind, placebo-controlled clinical trial. *Circulation. Arrhythmia and Electrophysiology,* Vol.3, No.1, pp. 46-53, ISSN 1941-3084

Serafimovski, N.; Burke, P.; Khawaja, O.; Sekulic, M. & Machado, C. (2008). Usefulness of dofetilide for the prevention of atrial tachyarrhythmias (atrial fibrillation or flutter) after coronary artery bypass grafting. *The American Journal of Cardiology,* Vol.101, pp.1574-1579, ISSN 1879-1913

Shakerinia, T.; Ali, I. & Sullivan, J. (1996). Magnesium in cardioplegia: is it necessary? *Canadian Journal of Surgery,* Vol.39, No.5, pp. 397-400, ISSN 1488-2310

Shepherd, J.; Jones, J.; Framptom, G.; Tanajewske, L.; Turner, D. & Price, A. (2008). Intravenous magnesium sulphate and sotalol for prevention of atrial fibrillation after coronary artery bypass surgery: a systemic review and economic evaluation. *International Journal of Technology Assessment in Health Care,* Vol.12, No.28, pp. 1-95, ISSN 1471-6348

Shiga, T.; Wajima, Z.; Inoue, T. & Ogawa, R. (2004). Magnesium prophylaxis for arrhythmias after cardiac surgery: a meta-analysis of randomized controlled trials. *The American Journal of Medicine,* Vol.117, pp. 325-333, ISSN 0002-9343

Singh, S.; Johnson, P.; Lee, R.; Orfei, E.; Lonchyna, V.; Sullivan, H.; Montoya, A.; Tran, H.; Wehrmacher, W. & Wurster, R. (1996). Topography of cardiac ganglia in the adult human heart. *The Journal of Thoracic and Cardiovascular Surgery*, Vol.112, pp. 943-953, ISSN 0022-5223

Solomon, A.; Berger, A.; Trivedi, K.; Hannan, R. & Katz, N. (2000). The combination of propranolol and magnesium does not prevent postoperative atrial fibrillation. *The Annals of Thoracic Surgery*, Vol.69. pp. 126-129, ISSN 0003-4975

Song, Y.; On, Y.; Kim, J.; Shin, D.; Kim, J.; Sung, J.; Lee, S.; Kim, W. & Lee, Y. (2008). The effects of atorvastatin on the occurrence of postoperative atrial fibrillation after off-pump coronary artery bypass grafting surgery. *American Heart Journal*, Vol.156, pp. 373e379-373e316, ISSN 0002-8703

Subramaniam, K.; Koch, C. & Allen, B. (2005). Preoperative statin use is associated with a reduction in postoperative atrial arrhythmias in isolated coronary artery bypass grafting. *Anesthesia and Analgesia*, Vol.100, SCA1-116 (Abstract SCA110), ISSN 0003-2999

Surgical Care Improvement Project (SCIP) National Hospital Inpatient Quality Measures. (2009) Version 3.0a. Set Measure ID#: SCIP-Card-2. Specifications Manual for National Hospital Inpatient Quality Measures. Available from qualitynet.org

Suttorp, M.; Kingma, Koomen, E.; Tijssen, G.; van Hemel, N.; Defauw, J. & Ernst, S. (1991). Effectiveness of sotalol in preventing supraventricular tachyarrhythmias shortly after coronary artery byp J.; Peels, H.; ass grafting. *The American Journal of Cardiology*, Vol.68, pp.1163-1169, ISSN 1879-1913

Tamura, K.; Ito, F. & Ushiyama, T. (2010). Pravastatin treatment before coronary artery bypass grafting for reduction of postoperative atrial fibrillation. *General Thoracic and Cardiovsacular Surgery*, Vol.58, pp. 120-125, ISSN 1863-6713

Thielmann, M.; Neuhauser, M.; Marr, A.; Jaeger, B.; Wendt, D.; Schuetze, B.; Kamler, M.; Massoudy, P.; Erbel, R. & Jakob, H. (2007). Lipid-lowering effect of preoperative statin therapy on postoperative major adverse cardiac events after coronary artery bypass surgery. *Journal of Thoracic and Cardiovascular Surgery*, Vol.134, pp. 1143-1149, ISSN 0022-5223

Tokmakoglu, H.; Kandemir, O.; Gunaydin, S.; Catav, Z.; Yorgancioglu, C. & Zorlutuna, Y. (2002). Amiodarone versus digoxin and metoprolol combination for the prevention for post coronary bypass atrial fibrillation. *European Journal of Cardio-Thoracic Surgery*, Vol.21, pp. 401-405, ISSN 1873-734X

Treggiari-Venzi, M.; Waeber, J.; Perneger, T.; Suter, P.; Adamec, R. & Romand, J. (2000). Intravenous amiodarone or magnesium sulphate is not cost-beneficial prophylaxis for atrial fibrillation after coronary artery bypass surgery. *British Journal of Anaesthesia*, Vol.85, pp. 690-695, ISSN 0007-0912

Tsai, C.; Lai,I.; & Lin, J. (2004). Renin-angiotensin system gene polymorphisms and atrial fibrillation. *Circulation*, Vol.109, pp. 1640-1646, ISSN 0009-7322

Tselentakis, E.; Woodford, E.; Chandy, J.; Gaudette, G. & Saltman, A. (2006). Inflammation effects on the electrical properties of atrial tissue and inducibility of postoperative atrial fibrillation. *Journal of Surgical Research*, Vol.135, No.1, pp. 68-75, ISSN1095-8673

Wang, G.; Bainbridge, D.; Martin, J. & Cheng, D. N-acetylcysteine in cardiac surgery: do the benefits outweight the risks? A meta-analytic reappraisal. (2011). *Journal of Cardiothoracic and Vascular Anesthesia,* Vol.25, No.2, pp. 268-275, ISSN 1532-8422

Weber, U.; Osswald, S.; Huber, M.; Buser, P.; Skarvan, K.; Stulz, P.; Schmidhauser, C. & Pfisterer, M. (1998). Selective versus non-selective antiarrhythmic approach for prevention of atrial fibrillation after coronary surgery: is there a need for pre-operative risk stratification? *European Heart Journal,* Vol.19, pp.794-800, ISSN 1522-9645

Wenke, K.; Parsa, M.; Imhof, M. & Kemkes, B. (1999). Efficacy of metoprolol in prevention of supraventricular arrhythmias after coronary artery bypass grafting. *Zeitschrift für Kardiologie*, Vol.88, pp. 647-652, ISSN 1861-0692

White, C.; Caron, M.; Kalus, J.; Rose, H.; Song, J.; Reddy, P.; Gallagher, R. & Kluger, J. (2003). Intravenous plus oral amiodarone, atrial septal pacing, or both strategies to prevent post-cardiothoracis surgery atrial fibrillation: The Atrial Fibrillation Suppression Trial II (AFIST II). *Circulation*, Vol.108, Suppl II, pp. II200-II206, ISSN 0009-7322

White, C.; Kluger, J.; Lertsburapa, K.; Faheem, O. & Coleman, C. (2007a). Effect of preoperative angiotensin converting enzyme inhibitor or angiotensin receptor blocker use on the frequency of atrial fibrillation after cardiac surgery: a cohort study from the atrial fibrillation suppression trials II and III. *European Journal of Cardiothoracic Surgery*, Vol.31, pp. 817-820, ISSN 1010-7940

White, C.; Sander, S.; Coleman, C.; Gallagher, R.; Takata, H.; Humphrey, C.; Henyan, N.; Gillespie, E. & Kluger, J. (2007b). Impact of epicardial anterior fat pad retention on post-cardiothoracic surgery atrial fibrillation incidence: the atrial fibrillation suppression trial III. *Journal of the American College of Cardiology*, Vol.49, pp. 298-303, ISSN 1936-8798

White, D.; Giri, S.; Tsikouris, J.; Dunn, A.; Felton, K.; Reddy, P, & Kluger, J. (2002). A comparison of two individual amiodarone regimens to placebo in open heart patients. *The Annals of Thoracic Surgery*, Vol.74, pp. 69-74, ISSN 0003-4975

Whitlock, R.; Chan, S.; Devereaux, P.; Sun, J.; Rubens, F.; Thorlund, K. & Teoh, K. (2008). Clinical benefit of steroid use in patients undergoing cardiopulmonarybypass: a meta-analysis of randomized trials. *European Heart Journal*, Vol.29, pp. 2952-2960, ISSN 1522-9645

Wijeysundera, D.; Beattie, W.; Rao, V. & Karski, J. (2003).Calcium antagonists reduce cardiovascular complications after cardiac surgery. *Journal of the American College of Cardiology*, Vol.41, pp. 1496-1505, ISSN 1936-8798

Wilkes, N.; Mallett, S.; Peachey, T.; DiSalvo, C. & Walesby, R. (2002). Correction of ionized plasma magnesium during cardiopulmonary bypass reduces the risk of postoperative cardiac arrhythmia. *Anesthesia & Analgesia*, Vol.95, pp. 828-834, ISSN 1526-7598Yazigi, A.; Rahbani, P.; Zeid, H.; Madi-Jebara, S.; Haddad, F. & Hayek, G. (2002). Postoperative oral amiodarone as prophylaxis against atrial fibrillation after coronary artery surgery. *Journal of Cardiothoracic and Vascular Anesthesia,* Vol.16, pp. 603-606, ISSN 1532-8422

Woodend, A.; Nichol, G.; Carey, C. & Tang, L. (1998). Sotalol confers no additional benefit over beta-blockers in post-coronary artery bypass atrial fibrillation. *Journal of the American College of Cardiology*, Vol.31, p. 383 (Abstract), ISSN 1936-8798

Zangrillo, A.; Londoni, G.; Sparicio, D.; Pappalardo, F.; Bove, T.; Cerchierini, E.; Sottocoma, O.; Aletti, G. & Crescenzi, G. (2005). Perioperative magnesium supplementation to prevent atrial fibrillation after off-pump coronary artery surgery: a randomized controlled study. *Journal of Cardiothoracic and Vascular Anesthesia,* Vol.19, No.6, pp. 723-728, ISSN 1532-8422

Zebis, L.; Christensen, T.; Thomsen, H.; Mikkelsen, M.; Folkersen, L.; Sørensen, H. & Hjortdal, V. (2007). Practical regimen for amiodarone use in preventing postoperative atrial fibrillation. *The Annals of Thoracic Surgery*, Vol.83, pp. 1326-1331, ISSN 0003-4975

Zimmer, J.; Pezzullo, J.; Choucair, W.; Southard, J.; Kokkinos, P.; Karasik, P.; Greenberg, M. & Singh S. (2003). Meta-analysis of antiarrhythmic therapy in the prevention of postoperative atrial fibrillation and the effect on hospital length of stay, costs, cerebrovascular accidents, and mortality in patients undergoing cardiac surgery. *The American Journal of Cardiology*, Vol.91, pp. 1137-1140, ISSN 1879-1913

10

Post Operative Arrhythmias

Rama Dilip Gajulapalli and Florian Rader
Case Western Reserve University
USA

1. Introduction

Heart rhythm disturbances are being increasingly recognized during the postoperative period. While many are transient and short lived without altering the recovery phase after cardiac or non-cardiac surgery, they do have the potential to pose a threat to patient's health, prolong hospital stay, and in a minority of patients may even cause death. Continuous monitoring is becoming the standard of care after surgery and therefore rhythm disturbances are being more frequently diagnosed during the postoperative recovery period. While cardiology consultation may be required, surgeons and anesthesiologists are often the first responders and are expected to be able to recognize the rhythm disturbance and treat them appropriately.

2. Normal physiology

Normal sinus rhythm is when the heart beats in an orderly predetermined sequence. The atria contract initially in response to the firing of an impulse by the Sino-Atrial (SA) node located at the junction of the superior vena cava and the right atrium. The SA node contains specialized tissue with 'pacemaker cells', which can initiate repetitive rhythmic action potentials. These potentials then travel via internodal atrial pathways to the AtrioVentricular (AV) node located at the right posterior portion of the interatrial septum. The AV node slows conduction into the bundle of HIS which then leads to its right and left branches. The left bundle branch further divides into anterior and posterior fascicles. The final pathway of conduction is the Purkinje system, which consists of a network of fibers that transmit the electrical impulse to the myocardium near the apex of the heart. (1)

The Electrocardiogram (ECG) is a reliable and practical way to document the underlying cardiac rhythm. It essentially consists of a recording obtained by 12 surface leads which trace the electrical activity of the heart from different directions. The 12 leads include 6 limb and 6 precordial leads. The limb leads include 3 bipolar leads (I, II, III) meaning they have 2 electrodes of opposite polarity. The other limb leads are aVR, aVL, aVF which are the unipolar leads meaning they have only one electrode connecting to a central terminal. The precordial leads are all unipolar and include V1-V6.

The limb leads are the frontal plane leads representing electrical current along the coronal plane of the heart, i.e. right/left and superior/inferior. The precordial leads represent the horizontal plane of the heart measuring transverse currents, i.e. right/left and anterior/posterior. Lead I traces currents from right shoulder to left shoulder, lead II from right shoulder to left leg, and lead III from left arm to left leg. Lead aVF traces from central terminal, which corresponds to zero potential to the left leg, aVL from centre to left arm and aVR from centre to right arm. The precordial leads work in a similar fashion in that leads V1 - V6 trace their axis center out from right to left respectively, so that V1 represents right of the interventricular septum, V2 and V3 the interventricular septum (anterior wall), V4 the apex (anterolateral), V5 and V6 the lateral ventricular wall. Any current flowing towards the lead causes a positive deflection and current flowing away from the lead causes a negative deflection and vice versa. The strength of the deflection depends on the amount of potential recorded and is affected by cardiac and extracardiac structures. To understand the electrophysiological basis of the 12-lead tracings on an ECG is important, because it gives clues about the origin of an arrhythmia and sometimes guides their therapies.

The first deflection on an ECG is the P wave which represents atrial depolarization. In sinus rhythm without any discernable atrial pathology, P wave is an upright, smooth, rounded wave with relatively low voltage. The PR interval consists of the P wave and the normally isoelectric segment up to the initial deflection of the QRS complex. The PR interval represents the conduction through atria, AV node, bundle branches and Purkinje system. The QRS complex follows the PR segment. The initial negative deflection is the Q wave, a positive deflection which can occur either initially or after the Q is the R wave while any negative deflection which follows the R is the S wave. QRS complex represents intraventricular conduction and depolarization. The J point represents the junction between QRS and the ST segment. The ST segment corresponds with the end of ventricular depolarization and start of the ventricular repolarization. The T wave, which follows the ST segment, represents ventricular repolarization. As such the QT interval represents the complete ventricular depolarization and repolarization period. Occasionally a small hump-like U wave follows the T wave, and is felt to be due to repolarization of the purkinje system. (2,3)

The bedside monitors which are routinely used for continuous cardiac monitoring are typically wireless, i.e. telemetry systems. These can be either 5 lead wire or 3 lead wire systems. The 5 lead wire system allows for monitoring all of the limb leads or the precordial leads while the 3 lead wire system allows monitoring one lead at a time, usually lead II, because the P wave is best visible in this lead. Depending on the monitoring system available it is essential for health care providers to be able to recognize the cardiac rhythm changes based only on a few select leads seen on the monitor as there may be no time to record a 12 lead ECG.

3. Recognition of arrhythmias

Postoperative arrhythmias though transient are usually sudden in onset. It is essential to recognize a rhythm disturbance and institute treatment as quickly as possible in most cases. A 12 lead ECG is recommended but may be impractical if the rhythm disturbance is an immediate threat to the patient's life. The wave forms visible on the telemonitor or a rhythm strip in one lead tracing may be the only available clue.

It is worthwhile to note some salient points early. Is the patient stable as assessed by the blood pressure, oxygen saturation or mental status? If deemed unstable then more aggressive steps are warranted.

A rapid and accurate interpretation of the ECG can be tricky and readers are advised to develop a personal strategy to identify any given cardiac tracing so that a quick diagnosis can be made. One approach is to identify and describe 5 basic features of the electrocardiogram (2):

Step 1. Determine the ventricular rate – tachycardia is >100 / Bradycardia is < 60
Step 2. Measure the QRS complex – Narrow is < 0.12ms / Broad is > 0.12 ms
Step 3. Determine the regularity of the QRS complex – Regular/irregular
Step 4. Identify the P waves – upright in lead II and III and negative in aVR usually identifies sinus rhythm, P waves are absent in atrial fibrillation, saw tooth appearance at an atrial rate of 300 bpm may indicate atrial flutter
Step 5: Measure the PR interval – helps identify AV delay

The above steps should help one to identify the salient features of any rhythm and place it in one of the following mentioned categories. (Figure 1) We would like to point out that this scheme is only one of many and sometimes more than one arrhythmia can be present in a patient. This scheme also, at times over simplifies natural heart rhythms. For example, a heart rate of 40 beats per minute (bpm) during sleep or in an athletic patient can be normal, while patients with an abnormal conduction system can have supraventricular arrhythmias with heart rates less than 100 bpm.

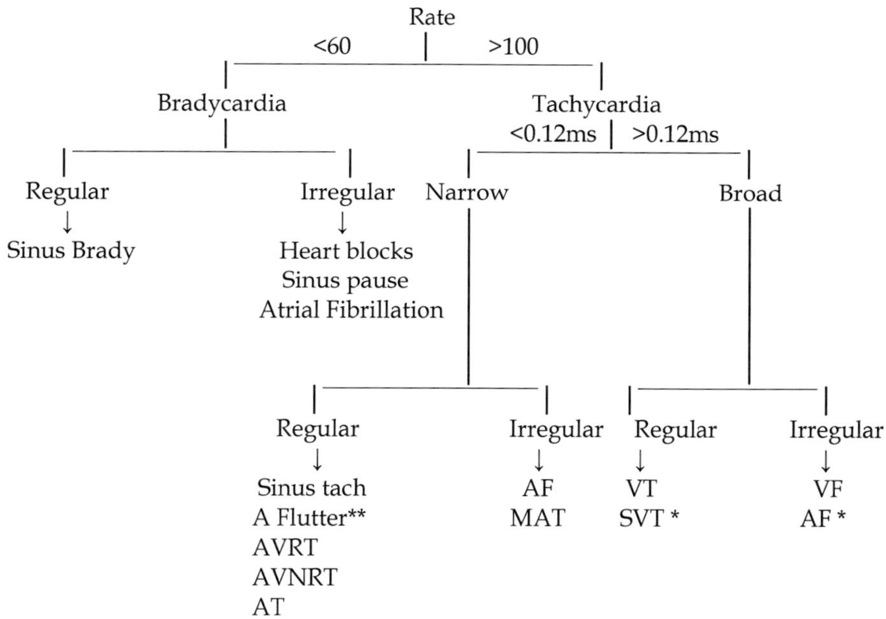

(AF – Atrial Fibrillation, AT – Atrial tachycardia, MAT – Multifocal atria tachycardia, SVT – Supra ventricular tachycardia, VF – Ventricular Fibrillation, VT – Ventricular tachycardia)

*With Aberrancy

** Flutter can be irregular occasionally when the AV block is variable

Fig. 1. Various cardiac rhythm disturbances noted in clinical practice

The Brugada criteria can be used to identify any broad complex tachycardia (4)
Step 1. Are there RS complexes in any of the chest leads?
Step 2. Is the onset of the R wave to the nadir of S > 100 ms?
Step 3. Is there any AV dissociation?
Step 4. Is there any typical bundle branch morphology in leads V1 or V6?

If the answer to any of questions 1-3 is yes or to question 4 is no, the rhythm is probably ventricular tachycardia. There are several additional ways to distinguish between supra ventricular and ventricular arrhythmias, which exceed the objectives of this review.

4. Types of arrhythmias

The conduction system of the heart has to be intact anatomically and physiologically for synchronized contraction of the heart in a regular and coordinated fashion. Arrhythmias are caused when there is disturbance in the working of the conduction system for any reason. The accepted mechanisms include abnormality of conduction (i.e. blocking or Re-entry of the impulse), abnormality of impulse initiation (i.e. altered automaticity or triggered activity). The underlying causes can include ischemia, electrolyte imbalances, scarring or fibrosis of atrial and ventricular tissue, increased or decreased excitability for various reasons including changes in autonomic nervous system, action of drugs and others.

Disturbances of the normal cardiac rhythm can be of many types. A universal hierarchical classification which can encompass all the salient arrhythmias is difficult to conceive. Arrhythmias are usually classified based on morphology, rate or origin. They can be divided into fast or slow based on the rate- Tachyarrhythmias when heart rate is faster than 100 bpm and bradyarrhythmias when rate is slower than 60 bpm. The QRS duration which defines the ventricular depolarization is usually less than 0.12 seconds (or 3 small boxes on the ECG at 25 mm/sec paper speed). If it is more than 0.12 seconds it represents delayed depolarization and can be used as a feature to divide the tachyarrhythmias into narrow complex and wide complex tachycardia. Another classification of arrhythmias describes regular versus irregular rhythms. Finally arrhythmias can generally be classified based on various anatomical substrates of the heart, which initiate these rhythm changes like atrial (or supraventricular) or ventricular arrhythmias. As mentioned above these classifications are an attempt, far from perfect, to distinguish normal from abnormal and define categories with different underlying pathophysiology and treatment options.

The following chapter will discuss Atrial Fibrillation (AF) after cardiac surgery initially as this seems to be the most common and most extensively studied arrhythmia.

5. Postoperative AF

Incidence:

The incidence of any arrhythmia postoperatively can be up to 85% (5). The Multi center anesthesia outcomes study quotes that postoperative arrhythmias can complicate about 70% of the operations. (6) AF seems to be the most common arrhythmia in the post operative period (7). Goldman concluded as early as 1978 utilizing a prospective registry that the incidence of postoperative AF was nearly 3% after non-cardiac surgeries. (8) While AF is certainly more frequent after cardiac surgery, incidence varies between studies. Reasons for these variations seem to be different ascertainment methods between studies (12 lead ECG vs. continuous telemetry monitoring etc). Mathew et al document an incidence of up to 34% with similar incidences in North America and Europe but lower incidence in Asia at 16 %. (13) The incidence also varies depending on the type of cardiac surgery undertaken. AF seems to occur 60% of the time post mitral valve surgery, 36% of the time post aortic valve surgery, (10) and 25% post cardiac transplants. (11) The combination of coronary artery bypass graft surgery (CABG) with valve surgery seems to increase the risk for AF as well. (12) Often times the definition for postoperative AF includes the need of medical treatment or electrical cardioversion (14) or confirmation on a 12 lead ECG (13) altering the incidence rates further. The peak incidence of postoperative AF (POAF) has been consistently described on day 2 and 3 after surgery. (10) It usually is transient with 80% of the patients converting to sinus rhythm within 24 hours. The recurrence rate has been quoted to be as much as 50% but still only 10% of patients are still in AF at 6 weeks post operation. (13) Late Postoperative AF is less frequent but was seen in nearly 5% of the postoperative patients after discharge from the hospital. This was found when patients were being followed for cardiac rehabilitation and documented in the ISYDE and ICAROS registries in Italy. (15) Despite better coordinated postoperative care and advances in cardiothoracic surgical and anesthetic practices, the incidence of AF seems stable with no reduction over the last 2 decades.

Pathophysiology of Postoperative AF:

AF is generally due to reentry of multiple wavelets circling the atria. It is likely that a pre-existing substrate is needed to allow peri-operative triggers to initiate AF. It is thus a specific interaction of preexisting and perioperative risk factors which can lead to AF.

Preexisting factors:

Age is the most consistent risk factor seen in past studies. Advancing age increases the risk with each decade. The incidence of POAF is around 6% when less than 40y of age, 18% in less than 60y olds and increasing to as much as 50% in patients older than 80 years. (13,14,16) Other risk factors include male gender, history of prior AF, heart valve disease (especially if the mitral valve is affected), prior cardiac surgery, prior cardiac structural changes like increased left atrial size and left ventricular hypertrophy. Preexisting medical conditions like obesity, chronic lung disease, peripheral vascular disease, hypertension, prior stroke are associated with increased incidence of POAF. However certain other morbid factors like preexisting diabetes, chronic kidney disease, hyperlipidemia, smoking have not been shown to be individual risk factors for POAF in some studies. (17) Pericarditis which is usually a consequence of the cardiac surgery itself is mechanistically involved. Other unique factors such as preoperative use of Digoxin or Dopamine, raised Brain natriuretic peptide (BNP) and right-sided coronary artery disease have been associated as well. ECG features like increased P wave duration of more than 140 ms, which is suggestive of atrial conduction delay can increase the susceptibility to AF. (18) Withdrawal of preoperative Angiotensin converting enzyme inhibitor (ACE I) or Beta blocker therapy is also contributory if not immediately initiated after the surgery. (13)

Intraoperative factors:

Certain operative features like aortic cross clamping, pulmonary venting, bicaval venous cannulation, increased length of cardiopulmonary bypass time and mitral valve surgery can increase the propensity for POAF. It has also been noted that at times cardioplegia via coronary sinus does not stun the atria completely and may be associated with occurrence of POAF(19) Direct cardiac injury due to operative techniques causing inflammation is perceived as plausible cause as well.

Postoperative features:

The postoperative period is a critical stage as the body is yet to recover from the operative stress completely. Many proarrhythmic features such as pericardial inflammation, acute blood pressure or volume changes, acute cardiac ischemia, electrolyte imbalances, hypothyroidism are present at this juncture. (20, 21, 22) Increased sympathetic activation causing exaggerated adrenergic responses could be a factor as well. (23)

The assumption is that non-uniform disruption of the electric conduction properties leads to changes in the resistance between adjacent cells in the atria. This causes decreased atrial conduction and creation of micro reentry loops causing AF. (24) Various factors mentioned above change the atrial refractoriness/transmembrane potentials causing increased local reentry and subsequent AF. (25) The suggestion that expression of connexin 40, a gap junction protein in the atria is altered during the postoperative period lends credence to the theory that the gap junction function in the atria is altered. (26)

Clinical Significance:

POAF is usually transient as the underlying mechanical and metabolic changes are usually reversible and not long lasting. However it is associated with significant morbidity and mortality even when it occurs briefly. POAF can increase the risk of stroke by 3-4 folds. (27) Cresswell et al noted that the occurrence of stroke postoperatively with AF was at 3.3 vs.1.2% without AF. (12) However, other features such as increased age, prior stroke, length of cardiac bypass time seem to be playing additional role in the additive risk of stroke postoperatively.

AF has been shown to increase overall health care cost. The hospitalization time is increased by an average of 2 to 5 days. (13, 14) The costs were higher by as much as $10,000 per patient if AF occurred postoperatively. The chances that the patient will suffer infection, renal failure, and mechanical ventilation also seem to be higher when AF is present. There has been suspicion that cognition of the patients can be affected as evidenced by a fall in the Mini Mental Score postoperatively when AF occurred. (10, 17, 28)

AF remains the leading cause for readmission after hospital discharge following cardiac surgery. It is estimated that AF contributed to nearly 23% of readmissions in one series. (9) So it would seem AF is a problem even after discharge and it would argue for continued monitoring of the patient as an outpatient preferably in a cardiac rehabilitation program.

AF seems to be associated with increased mortality both early and late after operation even after correction for many important confounding variables. It is estimated that the mortality associated with postoperative AF is around 5% compared to around 2% without AF. (13)

Management:

Given the morbidity and mortality associated with POAF it has long been a target for preventive as well as suppressive therapy. A variety of interventions have been studied and validated. We would like to clarify that our list does not claim to be complete, but only gives an overview of some of the most important therapies available. In most cases consultation with a Cardiologist is recommended. Multiple studies (29) have shown that AF can be suppressed in the postoperative period and various meta analyses confirmed their findings. Incidence of AF was reduced by as much as 50%. (30, 31) We categorize preventative measures into preoperative, operative and postoperative measures.

Preoperative measures:

The main thrust has been to reduce the sympathetic drive and Beta blockers seem to be the mainstay of this preventive approach. The 2004 ACC/AHA guidelines give a class I recommendation for preoperative and early postoperative beta blockade to prevent POAF. (32)

Amiodarone which blocks Potassium and Calcium ion channels, and has both alpha and beta blockade properties has been assessed in various trials such as AFIST, ARCH, AFIST 2, GAP and PapaBear for prevention of POAF and has been summarized in a meta analysis

(33). It can reduce postoperative AF by 50% - 70% and evidence suggests that ventricular arrhythmias are also reduced. However, there is concern about possible complications including proarrhythmia, sudden respiratory distress or bradycardia requiring pacing following Amiodarone prophylaxis or treatment. Therefore, Amiodarone therapy needs to be closely monitored.

Digoxin has also been studied but seems to be better only when used along with beta blockers and is currently not recommended. (34)

Magnesium has been studied as a preventive strategy and while hypomagnesaemia does definitely portend arrhythmias (20) supplementation does not seem to be helpful in reducing rhythm disturbances. One meta analysis (35) has shown a positive outcome but another study (36) has cast a doubt on the utility of Magnesium supplementation in preventing POAF.

Sotalol which has beta blocker as well as potassium channel blocking properties has been shown in certain studies (37) to be useful in preventing AF with relative risk reduction of up to 90%. However, studies generally involved small sample sizes. (29) There may not be an incremental effect of Sotalol along with Beta blocker therapy to prevent POAF.

Angiotensin Converting Enzyme inhibitor (ACE I) therapy did not consistently reduce POAF, but incidence may be increased if the ACE inhibitor therapy is withdrawn in patients who were receiving it before surgery.

Statins appear to have a beneficial effect in preventing AF. The ARMYDA 3 trial showed that taking a statin two weeks prior to surgery significantly reduces the incidence of POAF, although there were concerns about the relatively high incidence of AF in the control group. (38)

Various other agents like Non steroidal anti inflammatory agents (NSAID), Ascorbic acid, N-acetyl cysteine, Nitroprusside, Glucocorticoids, Fish oil have been tried on the premise that they reduce the oxidative stress and help modify the inflammatory process that seems to be present postoperatively and thereby contributing to lower the risk of POAF. However despite positive results in small trials, larger randomized controlled trials are necessary to ascertain any true benefit. (39)

Pacing via epicardial wires introduced at the time of the surgery has been recognized as an effective method in controlling AF in as much as 63% of the cases. (40) Pacing is done either at the sinus rate or faster with overdrive pacing. Studies have showed that bi atrial pacing (BAP) seems to be better than pacing in only one atrium. The American College of Chest Physicians (ACCP) guide recommends BAP over either right or left single atrial pacing. (41) Beta blockers seem to provide additive benefits along with pacing in preventing POAF.

The odds ratios of various agents used in POAF prevention are given below: (21)

Beta blockers - 0.35
Sotalol - 0.36
Amiodarone - 0.54
Pacing - 0.57
Potassium - 0.53
NSAID - 0.49
ACE inhibition - 0.62

The ACC/AHA/ESC 2006 guidelines recommend using a beta blocker routinely to prevent POAF and using Amiodarone or pacing only if the patient is intolerant of beta blockers or in high risk cases such as when the patient is undergoing mitral valve surgery or if they have had prior history of AF. (32)

Intraoperative measures:

Certain operative practices and techniques have shown to be of some benefit in reducing the incidence of POAF. Off pump surgery may decrease occurrence of AF, even when taking age into account. (42, 43) The anterior fat pad present in the mediastinum is considered to have parasympathetic nerves, which may play a role in initiating POAF. One study showed that preservation of the fat pad was protective but it could not be replicated in other studies. (44,45) Other factors include inducing hypothermia during Cardio Pulmonary Bypass (CPB), using posterior pericardiotomy and Heparin coated CPB circuit etc. (27)

Postoperative measures:

The only postoperative preventative measure may be early reinitiation of beta blockers and ACE-inhibitors. (13) There was a suggestion in a recent study that early statin use post operatively may be beneficial in preventing POAF after cardiac surgery as well. (46)

If AF does occur and is persistent despite the prophylactic measures, treatment should be initiated. There are two general approaches to AF treatment, Rate control or Rhythm control with both being acceptable as to preferred outcomes. (47) Whatever approach is taken, initial efforts need to be made to try and correct any obvious precipitating or co-existent mitigating factors. Meticulous attention needs to be paid to pain control, volume status, electrolyte balance, correcting anemia and hypoxia. Anticoagulation needs to be initiated as well if the AF is persistent for more than 48 hours.

Rhythm control where in AF is converted to sinus rhythm is preferred when the patient is deemed unstable such as if there is hypotension, ongoing ischemia, co-existing heart failure, if pre excitation is suspected or if the patient is very symptomatic. It is also preferred if anticoagulation is not an option for any reason. Rhythm control can be achieved either with pharmacological cardioversion or electrical cardioversion. Various anti arrhythmic agents can be used to convert AF, Amiodarone is typically preferred, because it can be transitioned to oral route, has comparatively lower proarrhythmic potential and may be better at ventricular rate control. Also as most patients have some underlying left ventricular dysfunction or coronary artery disease, Amiodarone is a safer choice in such patients. It is usually given as an initial bolus at 5 mg/Kg body weight over 30 minutes and then continued as an infusion at a dose of 25 mg /Hr. Various other pharmacological rhythm control agents used include Disopyramide, Procainamide, Flecainide, Ibutilide and Dofetilide. (10)

Direct current (DC) cardioversion is a quick and safe way to attempt rhythm control. Initial shock is attempted at 100 - 200 joules with synchronization when monophasic waveforms are used and 50 – 100 joules when biphasic waveforms are used. As usually the POAF has been present only for a short time DC cardioversion can successfully convert the AF to sinus in up to 95% of the cases. If it is not successful, intra venous Ibutilide can be given before repeat electrical cardioversion. However, significant pauses and risk for Torsades make Ibutilide less attractive for most practitioners. The transvenous electrodes or epicardial wires placed during surgery can be used for cardioversion or patient can be shocked by two pairs of external patch electrodes.

Rate control can be achieved with a variety of agents such as beta blockers including Metoprolol, Esmolol, Atenolol or Calcium channel antagonists like Diltiazem. Digoxin, Amiodarone or the newer agent Dronedarone are also popular choices at rate control. (48) Anticoagulation with warfarin is recommended if the AF is persisting for more than 48 hours. (32, 48) Heparin bridging is not recommended unless high risk features are present such as Mitral valve disease, prior stroke. (49) The criteria for anti coagulation per ESC are based on the CHADS2 - VASc score. Risk factors including increased Age > 75y and prior

Stroke, transient ischemic attack (TIA) or thrombo embolism are given 2 points each. Factors including Hypertension, Congestive heart failure, Diabetes, Ages 65-74y, female Sex and co existent Vascular disease are scored 1 point each. Anticoagulation is indicated if the combined score is $\geq$ 2. (48) Newer agents like Dabigatran are available on the market but studies will need to be done to assess its value specifically in the postoperative period.

Not much significant data is available as to the management of patients after discharge. They are usually reassessed 4-6 weeks after discharge and often times Holter monitoring is employed. Most of the patients can stop their anti arrhythmic medications and anti coagulation if they are deemed to be in sinus rhythm without intermittent AF, 3-6 months after hospital discharge.

In spite of all studies and evidence regarding preventing and treating POAF, doubts still exist whether any real benefit is obtained. Some evidence suggests that AF prevention does not or only minimally reduces the length of stay or the overall cost. (50) It is also noted that there is no actual decrease in the stroke incidence post operatively even if the AF is suppressed. It is unclear if the mortality and morbidity are improved if the AF is indeed suppressed. (51) It seems that stroke may be an epiphenomenon and not directly related to the occurrence of POAF. However a large Meta analysis does seem to suggest some overall benefit with prophylaxis measures and prevention of POAF. (52)

6. Post cardiac surgery ventricular arrhythmias

These include the more common benign isolated ectopic beats or Non sustained ventricular tachycardia (NSVT) and the more dangerous ventricular tachycardia or ventricular fibrillation (VT/VF) which fortunately are less common. The incidence of sustained ventricular arrhythmias has been quoted at around 0.4 - 1.4% (53) to 0.7 - 3% (54). The benign rhythm changes including ectopic ventricular beats and NSVT can occur in up to 60% of patients (55) but are not known to portend the more malignant rhythms like VT/VF (56) nor do they portend any rise in mortality risk (55, 57) if no underlying structural heart disease is suspected. The mortality of sustained VT is high at around 50% in hospital and a further 10% die within 2 years. (53)

The risk factors for the occurrence of VT/VF seem to correlate with factors associated in general cardiology practice. Any underlying structural heart disease, prior myocardial infarction, reduced left ventricular ejection fraction or congestive heart failure increase the risk of life threatening ventricular arrhythmias. Immediate postoperative features which set off the rhythm disturbance include any hemodynamic instability, electrolyte or acid base disturbances, hypoxia, anemia, new onset ischemia etc. An occasional cause can be acute graft closure after bypass grafting. Any inotropes used in the postoperative phase can also be pro arrhythmic.

Treatment:

Even though frequent ectopics and NSVT are considered benign it would be prudent to look for any reversible factors mentioned before in the acute phase. Lidocaine and pacing have been studied to suppress these rhythm disturbances but no actual benefit was observed. (53, 58) Sustained Ventricular arrhythmia is invariably quite unstable and quick remedial measures need to be instituted to treat the patient. Electrical cardioversion with 200 - 360 Joules is usually the first line option to convert the arrhythmia. If Direct Current cardioversion is not an option or if medications are preferred as per the clinical situation, various drugs like Lidocaine, Amiodarone, Procainamide can be considered. Emergency pacing via epicardial leads placed during surgery can be used sometimes to provide overdrive pacing to get the heart out of the arrhythmia. Emergency bypass surgery can be considered in some situations. (59) Readers are also referred to the American Heart Association (AHA) 2010 guidelines on advanced cardiovascular life support (ACLS) for dealing with unstable tachycardia. (75)

If the patient does survive and is back in sinus it is prudent to initiate them on long term beta blocker and ACE inhibitor therapy according to current ACC guidelines. For those who sustained VT/VF and have recovered, if there are no underlying risk factors mentioned prior, a cardiac electrophysiological study can be considered and an implantable cardiac defibrillator (ICD) is advised if there is any inducible VT or VF. If the patient is deemed to have an underlying heart disease that is unlikely to respond to medical therapy, an ICD may be indicated without electrophysiological study.

7. Bradyarrhythmias after cardiac surgery

Bradyarrhythmias include sinus pauses, sinus bradycardia and various blocks depending on the site of abnormal conduction including SA node, AV node or parts of HIS bundle. Bundle branch blocks are common and are not only transient but also harmless in most cases. Various bundle branch blocks can occur in up to 50 - 60% of cases after CABG but are usually transient. (60, 61, 62, 63) Symptomatic blocks needing permanent pacemaker (PPM) insertion complicate 0.8 - 3.4% of CABG operations and up to 2 - 4% of valve surgeries. (64, 65) The incidence of symptomatic bradyarrhythmias is higher after aortic or tricuspid valve surgeries. Repeat surgeries are complicated by blocks needing pacing more often. (65) Heart transplantation is complicated by sinus node dysfunction needing a pacemaker in 21% of cases while AV node blocks needing pacemaker can happen in 4-5% of cases. (53)

Risk factors include increased age, prior Left bundle branch block (LBBB), valve calcification, left main coronary blockage, longer cardiopulmonary bypass time, higher number of bypassed arteries during surgery, associated Left Ventricular aneurysmectomy etc. Valve surgeries seem to be more of a risk than CABG. Increased vagal tone due to surgery, the type of anesthesia used or occurrence of postoperative pain seem to be important underlying factor as well.

Specific factors involved in increasing the risk of bradyarrhythmias after heart transplantation include Biatrial rather than bicaval transplant, older donor age, longer donor ischemic time, longer aortic cross clamp time.

Treatment:

It is prudent to stop all unnecessary medications that can cause increased AV block like beta blockers or calcium channel blockers. Atropine can reverse symptomatic bradycardia. Aminophylline and Theophylline can be used to increase the heart rate during sinus node dysfunction or high grade AV blocks. (66, 67) Readers are also referred to the AHA 2010 guidelines on advanced ACLS for dealing with unstable bradycardia. (75)

Patients with complete heart block, symptomatic AV block or sinus node dysfunction need to have a temporary pacer inserted. It is advisable to wait for 5 - 7 days post op so that any possible edema of the conduction system of the heart resolves before a permanent pacemaker is inserted if still indicated. (68)

Patients who already have a permanent pacemaker or ICD prior to surgery pose a challenge for the surgeons and anesthetists. Electrocautery-induced electromagnetic interference can cause problems during the surgery. The cautery can inhibit the pacer and may cause inappropriate discharge of the ICD if the sensing function is not disabled. A comprehensive evaluation of the patient prior to surgery by an electrophysiologist is indicated. A magnet can be placed on top to disable the devices during the surgery so as to not cause any interference. Another option is to switch the pacer/ICD to asynchronous mode so that the cautery does not influence its function. However, patients need to be continuously monitored while the devices are in asynchronous mode as any malignant arrhythmias need to be treated via external defibrillator. (76)

8. Postoperative arrhythmias after non cardiac surgery

Arrhythmias complicate postoperative period after non cardiac surgery in up to 5 -20 % of the times. (69) Again, AF seems to be the most common arrhythmia making up about 68% of the documented arrhythmias. (8) Benign ventricular rhythms like ectopics or NSVT occur in up to 5 -25% of the patients and sustained VT is rather rare occurring in less than 1% of the cases. (70)

The rate of incidence after non-cardiac surgery also seems to depend on the type of surgery. Non vascular abdominal surgery, especially colorectal surgery seems more prone with rates of around 20%. The incidence seems increased after any instance of thoracotomy (10%) as well. In other instances the rate is around 0.01% after ophthalmologic surgery and 4% after orthopedic surgery.

The risk factors seem to be similar to those implicated in post cardiac surgery including male sex, increased age > 70y, heart valve disease, prior history of arrhythmia, co existing asthma, congestive heart failure, and hypertension. (71) Post operative causes include electrolyte imbalances, hypoxia, and hypercarbia. (72) Sepsis seems to be a recurring factor implicated as a causative factor of arrhythmias. In fact all kinds of stress inducing causes like stroke, Gastrointestinal bleed, Pulmonary Embolism, Myocardial Infarction, pulmonary edema and others have been implicated. Some specific factors noted to cause postoperative arrhythmias also include anastomotic leak (77) or acute alcohol withdrawal. (69) Increased vagal tone due to anesthetic practices like laryngoscopy is also a risk factor for any bradyarrhythmia.

Apart from associated morbidity similar to post cardiac surgery arrhythmias, post non-cardiac surgery arrhythmias can also cause mortality of around 12 – 50%. (72, 73, 74)

Management:

No large scale randomized trials validating the treatment of post non-cardiac surgery arrhythmias are available. However the management can be closely extrapolated from both post cardiac surgery treatment and non-surgical related general cardiology treatment protocols. Initial priority is to assess the physiological impact and stabilize the patient hemodynamically while searching for the specific causes that initiated the rhythm disturbance. One needs to rectify these issues while simultaneously initiating specific therapy to halt the arrhythmia. Specific treatment methods for individual rhythms are similar to the approach already explained for post cardiac surgery arrhythmias.

In conclusion, postoperative arrhythmias, especially AF are common and are associated with significant morbidity and mortality but can be prevented to some extent. Further research is required to completely understand causes of such arrhythmias and to improve their prevention and treatment.

9. Abbreviations

Postoperative Atrial Fibrillation (POAF), Coronary artery bypass graft (CABG), SinoAtrial (SA) node, AtrioVentricular (AV) node, Electrocardiogram (ECG), Ventricular tachycardia (VT), Ventricular fibrillation (VF), Angiotensin converting enzyme inhibitor (ACE I), Cardio Pulmonary Bypass (CPB), Implantable cardiac defibrillator (ICD), Permanent Pacemaker (PPM), American college of Cardiology (ACC), American Heart Association (AHA), European society of Cardiology (ESC), Advanced cardiovascular life support (ACLS).

10. References

[1] Ganong WF. Review of Medical Physiology. 22nd Edition.

[2] Huff J. ECG work out. 5th Edition.

[3] Conover MB. Understanding Electrocardiography. 8th Edition.

[4] Brugada P, Brugada J, Mont L, Smeets J, Andries EW. A new approach to the differential diagnosis of a regular tachycardia with a wide QRS complex. Circulation. 1991 May; 83(5):1649-59.

[5] Sloan SB, Weitz HH. Postoperative arrhythmias and conduction disorders. Med Clin North Am. 2001 Sep; 85(5):1171-89

[6] Forrest JB, Cahalan MK, Rehder K, Goldsmith CH, Levy WJ, Strunin L, Bota W, Boucek CD, Cucchiara RF, Dhamee S, et al. Multicenter study of general anesthesia. II. Results. Anesthesiology. 1990 Feb; 72(2):262-8.

[7] Lauer MS, Eagle KA, Buckley MJ, DeSanctis RW. Atrial fibrillation following coronary artery bypass surgery. Prog Cardiovasc Dis. 1989 Mar-Apr; 31(5):367-78.

[8] Goldman L. Supraventricular tachyarrhythmias in hospitalized adults after surgery. Clinical correlates in patients over 40 years of age after major noncardiac surgery. Chest. 1978 Apr; 73(4):450-4.

[9] Lahey SJ, Campos CT, Jennings B, Pawlow P, Stokes T, Levitsky S. Hospital readmission after cardiac surgery. Does "fast track" cardiac surgery result in cost saving or cost shifting? Circulation. 1998 Nov 10; 98(19 Suppl):II35-40.

[10] Maisel WH, Rawn JD, Stevenson WG; Atrial fibrillation after cardiac surgery; Ann Intern Med. 2001 Dec 18; 135(12):1061-73

[11] Pavri BB, O'Nunain SS, Newell JB, Ruskin JN, William G. Prevalence and prognostic significance of atrial arrhythmias after orthotopic cardiac transplantation. J Am Coll Cardiol. 1995 Jun; 25(7):1673-80

[12] Creswell LL, Schuessler RB, Rosenbloom M, Cox JL. Hazards of postoperative atrial arrhythmias. Ann Thorac Surg. 1993 Sep; 56(3):539-49

[13] Mathew JP, Fontes ML, Tudor IC, Ramsay J, Duke P, Mazer CD, Barash PG, Hsu PH, Mangano DT; Investigators of the Ischemia Research and Education Foundation; Multicenter Study of Perioperative Ischemia Research Group. A multicenter risk index for atrial fibrillation after cardiac surgery. JAMA. 2004 Apr 14; 291(14):1720-9

[14] Aranki SF, Shaw DP, Adams DH, Rizzo RJ, Couper GS, VanderVliet M, Collins JJ Jr, Cohn LH, Burstin HR. Predictors of atrial fibrillation after coronary artery surgery. Current trends and impact on hospital resources. Circulation. 1996 Aug 1; 94(3):390-7

[15] Ambrosetti M, Tramarin R, Griffo R, De Feo S, Fattirolli F, Vestri A, Riccio C, Temporelli PL; on behalf of the ISYDE and ICAROS investigators of the Italian Society for Cardiovascular Prevention, Rehabilitation and Epidemiology (IACPR-GICR). Late postoperative atrial fibrillation after cardiac surgery: a national survey within the cardiac rehabilitation setting. J Cardiovasc Med (Hagerstown). 2011 Jun; 12(6):390-395

[16] Fuster V, Rydén LE, Cannom DS, Crijns HJ, et al; ACC/AHA/ESC 2006 Guidelines for the Management of Patients with Atrial Fibrillation. Circulation. 2006 Aug 15; 114(7):e257-354.
[17] Villareal RP, Hariharan R, Liu BC, Kar B, Lee VV, Elayda M, Lopez JA, Rasekh A, Wilson JM, Massumi A. Postoperative atrial fibrillation and mortality after coronary artery bypass surgery. J Am Coll Cardiol. 2004 Mar 3; 43(5):742-8
[18] Steinberg JS, Zelenkofske S, Wong SC, Gelernt M, Sciacca R, Menchavez E. Value of the P-wave signal-averaged ECG for predicting atrial fibrillation after cardiac surgery. Circulation. 1993 Dec; 88(6):2618-22
[19] Tchervenkov CI, Wynands JE, Symes JF, Malcolm ID, Dobell AR, Morin JE. Persistent atrial activity during cardioplegic arrest: a possible factor in the etiology of postoperative supraventricular tachyarrhythmias.Ann Thor Surg.1983 Oct; 36(4):437-43
[20] Aglio LS, Stanford GG, Maddi R, Boyd JL 3rd, Nussbaum S, Chernow B. Hypomagnesemia is common following cardiac surgery. J Cardiothorac Vasc Anesth. 1991 Jun; 5(3): 201-8
[21] Hogue CW Jr, Creswell LL, Gutterman DD, Fleisher LA; American College of Chest Physicians. Epidemiology, mechanisms, and risks: American College of Chest Physicians guidelines for the prevention and management of postoperative atrial fibrillation after cardiac surgery. Chest. 2005 Aug; 128(2 Suppl):9S-16S
[22] Wahr JA, Parks R, Boisvert D, Comunale M, Fabian J, Ramsay J, Mangano DT. Preoperative serum potassium levels and perioperative outcomes in cardiac surgery patients. Multicenter Study of Perioperative Ischemia Research Group. JAMA. 1999 Jun 16; 281(23):2203-10
[23] Kalman JM, Munawar M, Howes LG, Louis WJ, Buxton BF, Gutteridge G, Tonkin AM. Atrial fibrillation after coronary artery bypass grafting is associated with sympathetic activation. Ann Thorac Surg. 1995 Dec; 60(6):1709-15
[24] Zaman AG, Archbold RA, Helft G, Paul EA, Curzen NP, Mills PG. Atrial fibrillation after coronary artery bypass surgery: a model for preoperative risk stratification. Circulation. 2000 Mar 28; 101(12):1403-8
[25] Cox JL. A perspective of postoperative atrial fibrillation in cardiac operations. Ann Thorac Surg. 1993 Sep; 56(3):405-9
[26] Dupont E, Ko Y, Rothery S, Coppen SR, Baghai M, Haw M, Severs NJ. The gap-junctional protein connexin40 is elevated in patients susceptible to postoperative atrial fibrillation. Circulation. 2001 Feb 13; 103(6):842-9
[27] McKeown PP; Introduction: American College of Chest Physicians guidelines for the prevention and management of postoperative atrial fibrillation after cardiac surgery. Chest. 2005 Aug; 128(2 Suppl):6S-8S
[28] Ommen SR, Odell JA, Stanton MS. Atrial arrhythmias after cardiothoracic surgery. N Engl J Med. 1997 May 15; 336(20):1429-34. Review. Erratum in: N Engl J Med 1997 Jul 17; 337(3):209
[29] Bradley D, Creswell LL, Hogue CW Jr, Epstein AE, Prystowsky EN, Daoud EG; American College of Chest Physicians. Pharmacologic prophylaxis: American College of Chest Physicians guidelines for the prevention and management of postoperative atrial fibrillation after cardiac surgery. Chest. 2005 Aug; 128(2 Suppl):39S-47S
[30] Burgess DC, Kilborn MJ, Keech AC. Interventions for prevention of post-operative atrial fibrillation and its complications after cardiac surgery: a meta-analysis. Eur Heart J. 2006 Dec; 27(23):2846-57

[31] Crystal E, Connolly SJ, Sleik K, Ginger TJ, Yusuf S. Interventions on prevention of postoperative atrial fibrillation in patients undergoing heart surgery: a meta-analysis. Circulation. 2002 Jul 2; 106(1):75-80

[32] Eagle KA, Guyton RA, Davidoff R, Edwards FH et al. ACC/AHA 2004 guideline update for coronary artery bypass graft surgery: Summary article. A report of the American College of Cardiology/American Heart Association Task Force on Practice Guidelines (Committee to Update the 1999 Guidelines for Coronary Artery Bypass Graft Surgery). J Am Coll Cardiol. 2004 Sep1; 44(5):e213-310

[33] Aasbo JD, Lawrence AT, Krishnan K, Kim MH, Trohman RG. Amiodarone prophylaxis reduces major cardiovascular morbidity and length of stay after cardiac surgery: a meta-analysis. Ann Intern Med. 2005 Sep 6; 143(5):327-36

[34] Kowey PR, Taylor JE, Rials SJ, Marinchak RA. Meta-analysis of the effectiveness of prophylactic drug therapy in preventing supraventricular arrhythmia early after coronary artery bypass grafting. Am J Cardiol. 1992 Apr 1; 69(9):963-5

[35] Shiga T, Wajima Z, Inoue T, Ogawa R. Magnesium prophylaxis for arrhythmias after cardiac surgery: a meta-analysis of randomized controlled trials. Am J Med. 2004 Sep 1; 117(5):325-33

[36] Hazelrigg SR, Boley TM, Cetindag IB, Moulton KP, Trammell GL, Polancic JE, Shawgo TS, Quin JA, Verhulst S. The efficacy of supplemental magnesium in reducing atrial fibrillation after coronary artery bypass grafting. Ann Thorac Surg. 2004 Mar; 77(3):824-30

[37] Gomes JA, Ip J, Santoni-Rugiu F, Mehta D, Ergin A, Lansman S, Pe E, Newhouse TT, Chao S. Oral d, l Sotalol reduces the incidence of postoperative atrial fibrillation in coronary artery bypass surgery patients: a randomized, double-blind, placebo-controlled study. J Am Coll Cardiol. 1999 Aug; 34(2):334-9

[38] Patti G, Chello M, Candura D, Pasceri V, D'Ambrosio A, Covino E, Di Sciascio G. Randomized trial of atorvastatin for reduction of postoperative atrial fibrillation in patients undergoing cardiac surgery: results of the ARMYDA-3 (Atorvastatin for Reduction of Myocardial Dysrhythmia After cardiac surgery) study. Circulation. 2006 Oct 3; 114(14):1455-61

[39] Davis EM, Packard KA, Hilleman DE. Pharmacologic prophylaxis of postoperative atrial fibrillation in patients undergoing cardiac surgery: beyond beta-blockers. Pharmacotherapy. 2010 Jul; 30(7):749, 274e-318e.

[40] Blommaert D, Gonzalez M, Mucumbitsi J, Gurné O, Evrard P, Buche M, Louagie Y, Eucher P, Jamart J, Installé E, De Roy L. Effective prevention of atrial fibrillation by continuous atrial overdrive pacing after coronary artery bypass surgery. J Am Coll Cardiol. 2000 May; 35(6):1411-5

[41] Maisel WH, Epstein AE; American College of Chest Physicians. The role of cardiac pacing: American College of Chest Physicians guidelines for the prevention and management of postoperative atrial fibrillation after cardiac surgery. Chest. 2005 Aug; 128(2 Suppl):36S-38S.

[42] Athanasiou T, Aziz O, Mangoush O, Weerasinghe A, Al-Ruzzeh S, Purkayastha S, Pepper J, Amrani M, Glenville B, Casula R. Do off-pump techniques reduce the incidence of postoperative atrial fibrillation in elderly patients undergoing coronary artery bypass grafting? Ann Thorac Surg. 2004 May; 77(5):1567-74

[43] Wijeysundera DN, Beattie WS, Djaiani G, Rao V, Borger MA, Karkouti K, Cusimano RJ. Off-pump coronary artery surgery for reducing mortality and morbidity: meta-analysis of randomized and observational studies. J Am Coll Cardiol. 2005 Sep 6;46(5):872-82

[44] Cummings JE, Gill I, Akhrass R, Dery M, Biblo LA, Quan KJ. Preservation of the anterior fat pad paradoxically decreases the incidence of postoperative atrial fibrillation in humans. J Am Coll Cardiol. 2004 Mar 17; 43(6):994-1000.
[45] White CM, Sander S, Coleman CI, Gallagher R, Takata H, Humphrey C, Henyan N, Gillespie EL, Kluger J. Impact of epicardial anterior fat pad retention on post cardiothoracic surgery atrial fibrillation incidence: the AFIST-III Study. J Am Coll Cardiol. 2007 Jan 23; 49(3):298-303.
[46] Rader F, Gajulapalli RD, Pasala T, Einstadter D. Effect of Early Statin Therapy on Risk of Atrial Fibrillation After Coronary Artery Bypass Grafting With or Without Concomitant Valve Surgery. Am J Cardiol. 2011 May 3.
[47] Lee JK, Klein GJ, Krahn AD, Yee R, Zarnke K, Simpson C, Skanes A, Spindler B. Rate-control versus conversion strategy in postoperative atrial fibrillation: a prospective, randomized pilot study. Am Heart J. 2000 Dec; 140(6):871-7
[48] Camm AJ, Kirchhof P, Lip GY, Schotten U, et al. Guidelines for the management of atrial fibrillation: the Task Force for the Management of Atrial Fibrillation of the European Society of Cardiology (ESC). Eur Heart J. 2010 Oct; 31(19):2369-429.
[49] Kollar A, Lick SD, Vasquez KN, Conti VR. Relationship of atrial fibrillation and stroke after coronary artery bypass graft surgery: when is anticoagulation indicated? Ann Thorac Surg. 2006 Aug; 82(2):515-23
[50] Reddy P. Does prophylaxis against atrial fibrillation after cardiac surgery reduce length of stay or hospital costs? Pharmacotherapy. 2001 Mar; 21(3):338-44
[51] Zimmer J, Pezzullo J, Choucair W, Southard J, Kokkinos P, Karasik P, Greenberg MD, Singh SN. Meta-analysis of antiarrhythmic therapy in the prevention of postoperative atrial fibrillation and the effect on hospital length of stay, costs, cerebrovascular accidents, and mortality in patients undergoing cardiac surgery. Am J Cardiol. 2003 May 1; 91(9):1137-40
[52] Crystal E, Garfinkle MS, Connolly SS, Ginger TT, Sleik K, Yusuf SS. Interventions for preventing post-operative atrial fibrillation in patients undergoing heart surgery. Cochrane Database Syst Rev. 2004 Oct 18; (4):CD003611
[53] Chung MK. Cardiac surgery: postoperative arrhythmias. Crit Care Med. 2000 Oct; 28(10 Suppl):N136-44
[54] Chung E, Martin D. Management of post operative arrhythmias, Surgical Intensive care Medicine 2010
[55] Smith RC, Leung JM, Keith FM, Merrick S, Mangano DT. Ventricular dysrhythmias in patients undergoing coronary artery bypass graft surgery: incidence, characteristics, and prognostic importance. Study of Perioperative Ischemia (SPI) Research Group. Am Heart J. 1992 Jan; 123(1):73-81.
[56] Rho RW, Bridges CR, Kocovic D. Management of postoperative arrhythmias. Semin Thorac Cardiovasc Surg. 2000 Oct; 12(4):349-61
[57] Pinto RP, Romerill DB, Nasser WK, Schier JJ, Surawicz B. Prognosis of patients with frequent premature ventricular complexes and nonsustained ventricular tachycardia after coronary artery bypass graft surgery. Clin Cardiol. 1996 Apr; 19(4):321-4
[58] King FG, Addetia AM, Peters SD, Peachey GO. Prophylactic lidocaine for postoperative coronary artery bypass patients, a double-blind, randomized trial. Can J Anaesth. 1990 Apr; 37(3):363-8
[59] Rousou JA, Engelman RM, Flack JE 3rd, Deaton DW, Owen SG. Emergency cardiopulmonary bypass in the cardiac surgical unit can be a lifesaving measure in postoperative cardiac arrest. Circulation. 1994 Nov; 90(5 Pt 2):II280-4

[60] Baerman JM, Kirsh MM, de Buitleir M, Hyatt L, Juni JE, Pitt B, Morady F. Natural history and determinants of conduction defects following coronary artery bypass surgery. Ann Thorac Surg. 1987 Aug; 44(2):150-3
[61] Chu A, Califf RM, Pryor DB, McKinnis RA, Harrell FE Jr, Lee KL, Curtis SE, Oldham HN Jr, Wagner GS. Prognostic effect of bundle branch block related to coronary artery bypass grafting. Am J Cardiol. 1987 Apr 1; 59(8):798-803
[62] Emlein G, Huang SK, Pires LA, Rofino K, Okike ON, Vander Salm TJ. Prolonged bradyarrhythmias after isolated coronary artery bypass graft surgery. Am Heart J. 1993 Nov; 126(5):1084-90
[63] Wexelman W, Lichstein E, Cunningham JN, Hollander G, Greengart A, Shani J. Etiology and clinical significance of new fascicular conduction defects following coronary bypass surgery. Am Heart J. 1986 May; 111(5):923-7
[64] Brodell GK, Cosgrove D, Schiavone W, Underwood DA, Loop FD. Cardiac rhythm and conduction disturbances in patients undergoing mitral valve surgery. Cleve Clin J Med. 1991 Sep-Oct; 58(5):397-9
[65] Jaeger FJ, Trohman RG, Brener S, Loop F. Permanent pacing following repeat cardiac valve surgery. Am J Cardiol. 1994 Sep 1; 74(5):505-7
[66] Haught WH, Bertolet BD, Conti JB, Curtis AB, Mills RM Jr. Theophylline reverses high-grade atrioventricular block resulting from cardiac transplant rejection. Am Heart J. 1994 Dec; 128(6 Pt 1):1255-7.
[67] Heinz G, Kratochwill C, Buxbaum P, Laufer G, Kreiner G, Siostrzonek P, Gasic S, Derfler K, Gössinger H. Immediate normalization of profound sinus node dysfunction by aminophylline after cardiac transplantation. Am J Cardiol. 1993 Feb 1; 71(4):346-9
[68] Gregoratos G, Abrams J, Epstein AE, Freedman RA, et al. ACC/AHA/NASPE 2002 guideline update for implantation of cardiac pacemakers and antiarrhythmia devices. Circulation. 2002 Oct 15; 106(16):2145-61
[69] Walsh SR, Tang T, Wijewardena C, Yarham SI, Boyle JR, Gaunt ME. Postoperative arrhythmias in general surgical patients. Ann R Coll Surg Engl. 2007 Mar; 89(2):91-5
[70] Amar D, Zhang H, Roistacher N. The incidence and outcome of ventricular arrhythmias after noncardiac thoracic surgery. Anesth Analg. 2002 Sep; 95(3):537-43
[71] Polanczyk CA, Goldman L, Marcantonio ER, Orav EJ, Lee TH. Supraventricular arrhythmia in patients having noncardiac surgery: clinical correlates and effect on length of stay. Ann Intern Med. 1998 Aug 15; 129(4):279-85
[72] Christians KK, Wu B, Quebbeman EJ, Brasel KJ. Postoperative atrial fibrillation in oncardiothoracic surgical patients. Am J Surg. 2001 Dec; 182(6):713-5
[73] Bender JS. Supraventricular tachyarrhythmias in the surgical intensive care Unit: an under-recognized event. Am Surg. 1996 Jan; 62(1):73-5.
[74] Brathwaite D, Weissman C. The new onset of atrial arrhythmias following major noncardiothoracic surgery is associated with increased mortality. Chest. 1998 Aug; 114(2):462-8.
[75] Neumar, R. W. et al. Circulation 2010; 122: S729-S767
[76] American Society of Anaesthesiologists Task Force on Perioperative Management of Patients with Cardiac Rhythm Management Devices. Practice advisory for the perioperative management of patients with cardiac rhythm management devices, pacemakers and implantable cardioverter-defibrillators: a report by the American Society of Anaesthesiologists Task Force on Perioperative Management of Patients with Cardiac Rhythm Management Devices. Anaesthesiology. 2005 Jul;103(1):186-98
[77] Kirkpatrick JR, Heilbrunn A, Sankaran S. Cardiac arrhythmias: an early sign of sepsis. Am Surg. 1973 Jul;39(7):380-2

Surgery for Atrial Fibrillation

Hunaid A. Vohra, Zaheer A. Tahir and Sunil K. Ohri
Wessex Cardiothoracic Centre, Southampton
UK

1. Introduction

Atrial Fibrillation (AF) is characterised by rapid and disorganised depolarisation of the atria resulting in uncoordinated atrial contraction. It is the most common cardiac arrhythmia encountered in clinical practice increasing in prevalence with age and the presence of heart disease[1] It is estimated that it affects 2.5 million people in the United States and 4.5 million in the European Union.[2,3] The actual incidence of the arrhythmia may be much higher owing to undetected or asymptomatic patients within the population. Since it is an age-associated arrhythmia its incidence has steadily risen over the past decade and will continue to increase due to a growing population of the elderly in the western world. Contributing risk factors include hypertension, diabetes, coronary artery disease, valvular disease, electrolyte imbalance.[4] Patients with atrial fibrillation have a higher risk for stroke, heart failure and death.[5]Given the significant morbidity and mortality associated with AF and its associated economic burden, it is not surprising that there has been great interest in developing effective treatments for it.

Atrial fibrillation is a supraventricular arrhythmia where uncoordinated rapid atrial contractions produce an irregular ventricular response. The atria may discharge between 300-600 beats per minute but not all these impulses are conducted by the AV node. Ventricular response can be between 100-160 beats per minute in untreated patients with normal AV conduction. This chaotic rhythm disrupts normal movement of blood through the heart reducing cardiac output and increasing the risk for thromboembolism such as stroke as a consequence of stasis of blood in the atria.[6]

The serious morbidity and mortality associated with AF are attributed to three detrimental consequences:

- Palpitations causing significant patient discomfort and anxiety
- Loss of the coordinated atrioventricular contraction and "atrial kick" compromising cardiac haemodynamics and can lead to varying levels of ventricular dysfunction
- Stasis and pooling of stagnant blood that can lead to intra-atrial thrombus formation and resulting in increased risk of thromboembolism

Medical therapy remains the most common and first line treatment for patients with AF but frequently ineffective at restoring sinus rhythm leaving the patient susceptible to cardiovascular morbidity and mortality. Therefore, the goal of pharmacological therapy is often shifted from rhythm control (maintenance of sinus rhythm) to rate control (slowing the ventricular response to AF).[7]

The Atrial Fibrillation Follow-Up Investigation of Rhythm Management (AFFIRM) trial demonstrated no survival benefit of rhythm control strategy over a rate control strategy.

Although rate control slows the ventricular response to AF, preventing tachycardia induced cardiomyopathy, it does not reduce the rates of thromboembolism or congestive heart failure. The atria are still in fibrillation and there is loss of the atrial "kick" resulting in worsening of congestive heart failure and requires indefinite anticoagulation with warfarin to counter the risk for developing thromboembolism. Although warfarin reduces the annual risk of ischaemic stroke and systemic thromboembolism to approximately 2%, its use is associated with significant morbidity with a 2% annual risk of drug associated haemorrhage.[8,9,10] Anticoagulation may reduce lifetime relative risk of stroke by 60% but does not eliminate it[11]

Although the results of the AFFIRM trial demonstrated no long-term benefit of rhythm versus rate control, some patients may still have advantages of being in sinus rhythm. These include freedom from palpitations, increased exercise tolerance and prevention of atrial remodelling. [12,13]

Ineffective results with rate and rhythm control strategies have helped to encourage the development of new interventional catheter and surgical treatments. Although catheter ablation is an established therapeutic option, the highest success rates are typically seen in patients with paroxysmal AF and minimal structural heart disease.[14]

Therefore it is limited to a small number of patients treated by highly skilled electrophysiologists. On the other hand, almost all cardiac surgeons are capable of performing surgical ablation of AF.

2. Classification of atrial fibrillation

The terms used to classify and describe AF categorise it as paroxysmal, persistent, longstanding or permanent (figure 1). Paroxysmal AF is defined as at least two episodes of AF that terminate spontaneously within 7 days. If this is sustained beyond 7 days it is described as persistent. Another category of persistent AF includes longstanding AF, defined by duration of greater than one year. This usually leads to permanent atrial fibrillation in whom cardioversion has either failed or abandoned.[15]

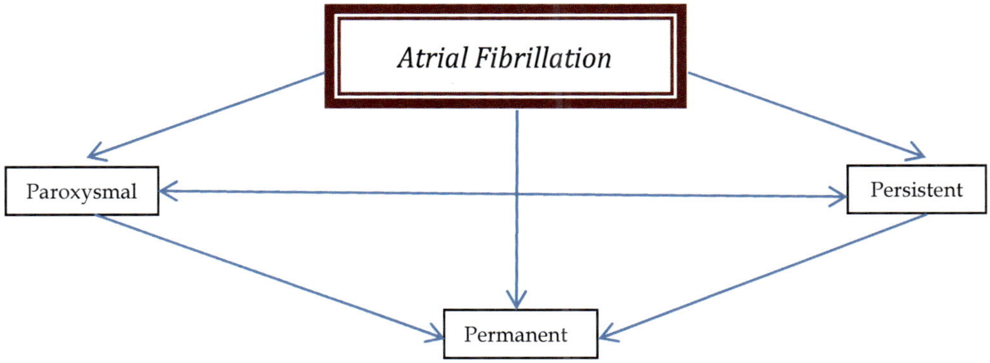

Fig. 1. Classification of Atrial Fibrillation

3. Electrophysiology of AF

In recent years there has been considerable progress in understanding the pathophysiology of AF. It was initially thought that AF was caused by random, multiple wavelets generated throughout the atria that propagated new wavelets to cause re-entry mechanism. In the 1980s, several procedures were developed aimed at curing atrial fibrillation. However, most of these were abandoned due to their inability to address all three detrimental sequelae of atrial fibrillation. It was discovered that electrical impulses were incapable of crossing areas of the heart that had been incised and sutured.[16,17]

This fostered the development of the Maze procedure, designed and first reported by Cox and colleagues in which multiple incisions were made and sutured in a manner that blocked the aberrant impulses within the atrium (figure 2). These incisions directed the SA node impulse to initiate and propagate throughout the atria to the AV node along a specified route created by the Maze incisional lesions[18]. However, recently studies have demonstrated that the initiation of paroxysmal but not necessarily persistent or permanent AF are generated by electrical waves from focal sources, particularly near the pulmonary veins. Haissaguerre et al.[19] mapped the triggers of paroxysmal AF to originate around the orifices of the pulmonary veins in 94% of patients with atrial diameters of less than 5cm. These findings have directed the development of more precisely targeted procedures that can be performed less invasively with less destruction of normal tissue.

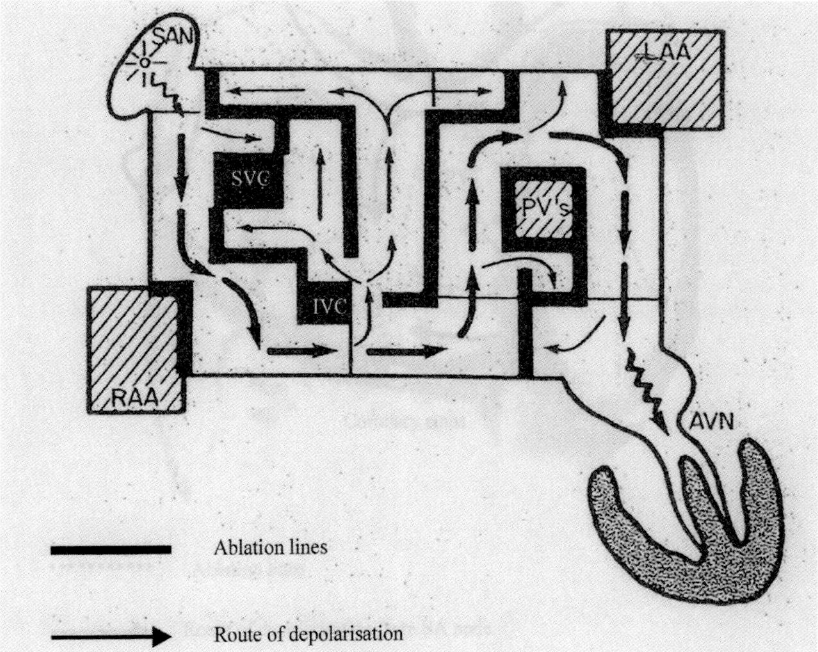

Fig. 2. The pathway taken in the atria by the aberrant impulses in atrialfibrillation (arrows). The thick lines are the ablation lesions used in the Maze procedure. Key- SAN: sino-atrial node, AVN: atrio-ventricular node, RAA: right atrial appendage, LAA: left atrial appendage, SVC: superior vena cava, IVC: inferior vena cava, PVs: pulmonary veins.

A key concept in understanding the development of persistent atrial fibrillation is that the atria undergo electrical remodelling. Atrial electrical remodelling results in shortening of the atrial refractory period, myocyte calcium overload, decreased conduction velocity, dispersion of conduction and increased sensitivity to catecholamines[4,20,21,22]. This phenomenon may be reversed after maintenance of sinus rhythm[23]. The more a patient experiences AF, the more susceptible they are to continue fibrillating as a result of remodelling. Therefore AF can become a self-sustaining arrhythmia once atrial remodelling has occurred. Micro-reentrant triggers are then no longer necessary and limited to pulmonary venous impulse-triggering sites.[24] Therefore, treatment for persistent or longstanding AF directed at the pulmonary veins only is likely to be unsuccessful.

4. Non pharmacological therapy

When pharmacological intervention is unsuccessful or contraindicated in patients, non-pharmacological therapy may be attempted. These include synchronised electrical cardioversion, catheter based ablation techniques or surgical intervention.[25,26,27]. Direct-current cardioversion differs from defibrillation whereby the shock is synchronised to the R wave in the patient's ECG. The patient must be adequately anticoagulated during electrical cardioversion in order to prevent disruption of a pre-existing intra cardiac thrombus which will cause it to embolize to the brain or systemic circulation. The risks of electrical cardioversion include hypotension, bradycardia, pulmonary oedema, systemic embolization, skin burns and ventricular arrhythmias.[28] Risks of emboli range from 0.5% to 3% and is further multiplied in patients who experience recurrence and treated with serial cardioversions.[29,30]

Catheter based ablation techniques were initially developed following Cox's pioneering work with the Maze procedure. These techniques were further influenced by research that demonstrated ectopic foci surrounding pulmonary veins. Isolation of the pulmonary veins remains the cornerstone of most AF catheter ablation procedures. Following heparinization, a percutaneous catheter placed into the femoral vein is advanced to the right atrium. The left atrium is accessed via an interatrial septal puncture. Lesions are created around the pulmonary veins using cryoenergy or radio-frequency energy. These techniques have shown a higher success in treating patients with paroxysmal AF compared to those with enlarged left atrium and persistent or permanent AF.[31,32] Complications of catheter ablation include cardiac tamponade, atrioesophageal fistula and stroke[33]

5. Surgical treatment

Surgery is indicated in patients undergoing elective cardiac surgery that have symptomatic AF or those with asymptomatic AF with low operative risk.[34] It is advised that patients with persistent or permanent AF scheduled for elective cardiac surgery should be considered for concomitant ablation procedure that may increase both short-term and long-term freedom from AF, in addition to lowering the risk of thromboembolism and improving long term survival and cardiac function[35]. Surgery for lone AF may be considered in certain circumstances where patients have failed to respond to catheter ablation or in whom catheter ablation is contraindicated such as a mural thrombus. Patients that develop tachycardia-induced cardiomyopathy will also benefit from surgery. It results in atrial or ventricular dysfunction as a result of increased heart rates in an otherwise structurally normal heart.[36] If left untreated it can lead to heart failure and is reversible if sinus rhythm is restored.[37] In addition patients in whom anticoagulation is contraindicated may also be suitable candidates that may benefit from surgical intervention following failure of catheter based ablation. Patients that continue to experience thromboembolic events despite adequate anticoagulation may also benefit from surgery.[38]

Several procedures were developed in the 1980s aimed at finding a cure to atrial fibrillation. Hoewever, most of these procedures were subsequently abandoned due to their inability to address all three of the detrimental sequelae of AF. Early attempts at surgical treatment of AF attempted to isolate and confine AF to a specific region of the atria and thereby stopping it from propagating its effects upon the ventricles. The left atrial isolation procedure developed by Williams and colleagues was successful in confining AF to the left atrium and thus restoring sinus rhythm to the rest of the heart.[39] It also removed two of the 3 detrimental consequences attributed to AF namely, irregular heart rate and compromised haemodynamics. The latter was achieved because restoring sinus rhythm on the right side permitted a normal right-sided cardiac output that was delivered to the left side of the heart. The left ventricle responded to the normal cardiac output on the right side by delivering a normal cardiac output. Since the left atrium continued to fibrillate this procedure did not reduce the risk of thromboembolism. The 'Corridor' procedure was introduced in 1985 that isolated a strip of atrium that contained both the SA node and AV node from the rest of the atria to create a continuous pathway (corridor) directing the impulses from the SA node to the AV node to maintain sinus rhythm. Since parts of the right and left atrial were free to fibrillate it did not eliminate the risk of thromboembolism and nor did it restore atrioventricular synchrony.

Cox and colleagues described a series of experiments that attempted to cure AF in dogs. A single incision across both atria successfully prevented AF and atrial flutter. Further investigations by Cox and colleagues led to the Cox-Maze procedure in 1987.[16,17,40] The procedure itself was based upon a cut and sew technique whereby multiple incisions were made in the atria. This created lines of scar that interrupted the conduction routes of the most common re-entrant circuits, thus preventing AF or atrial flutter by directing the sinus node impulses along a specified route. It was based around the concept of a maze and as a result was called the Cox-Maze procedure. In contrast to the previous surgical techniques, this was the first that addressed all three sequelae of AF and restored sinus rhythm, AV synchrony and thus significantly reducing the risk of thromboembolism and stroke.[41] The original procedure, known as Cox-Maze I was complicated with a high incidence of heart block requiring pacemaker implantation. It also resulted in the late incidence of two problems. Firstly it led to the frequent inability of patients to generate an appropriate sinus tachycardia and secondly left atrial dysfunction. This was modified to the Cox Maze II procedure which despite decreased incidence of conduction system injury was technically difficult. It was therefore modified to the Cox-Maze III procedure that was associated with a higher incidence of sinus rhythm and improved long-term sinus node function and atrial transport function.[40] In this procedure several dead-end "alleyways "create a maze-like pathway and permit the depolarization of all the atrial tissue. The Cox Maze III procedure can be performed both through median sternotomy as well as a partial lower sternotomy. The patient is fully heparinized and the surgeon cannulates the patient for cardiopulmonary bypass after dividing the sternum. Bicaval cannulation is achieved. The right atrial appendage is excised and a series of incisions are made to the right atrium including a cryolesion. The aorta is occluded preparing for the left atrial portions of the operation. Cold blood potassium cardioplegia is administered via retrograde perfusion of the coronary sinus. The left atrium is exposed by an incision posterior to the interatrial groove close to the orifices of the right pulmonary veins. A number of incisions are made across the left atrium and the left atrial appendage is excised at its base. The incisions to the left atrium interatrial septum and right atrium are closed. Despite its complexity, the Cox-Maze III procedure became the gold standard for surgical treatment of AF. It has been performed in hundreds of patients and proven to be highly successful in ablating any form of AF irrespective of whether patients had concomitant heart disease or not.[42,43] Although it adds to cardiopulmonary bypass and cardiac arrest time it does not increase the operative mortality.[44,45]

Sinus rhythm was reported in 97% at late follow-up and it was equally effective in patients with lone AF as those undergoing concomitant cardiac surgery.[44,46] Similar results were reproduced by other institutions across the world.[47,48]Early postoperative AF is common following a maze procedure and usually abates by 3 months.[44,46] In addition to restoring sinus rhythm the maze procedure is associated with additional clinical benefits for the patients. In those with mitral valve disease restoration of sinus rhythm improves survival. Risks for stroke, systemic thromboembolism and anticoagulant-related haemorrhage are also reduced.[41,49]The freedom from late stroke is likely to be from restoration of sinus rhythm as well as excision of the left atrial appendage, an integral part of the maze procedure.[50]

Despite the excellent results of the cut and sew maze procedure, few surgeons adopted the procedure due to its technical difficulty and is almost obsolete today. Advances in the understanding the pathophysiology of AF and newer ablation technologies fostered the development of novel strategies aimed at simplifying the procedure to make it more accessible to the average surgeon without compromising the results.

Use of ablative energy sources has enabled to replace most of Cox III incisions with a variety of energy sources including radiofrequency, cryoablation and high frequency ultrasound. The development of these technologies has rendered a technically difficult and time-consuming operation easy for all cardiac surgeons to perform. Ablation technologies have also helped foster the development of less invasive procedures through a small incision or port. In order to replace the incision in AF surgery, ablation technology must meet several requirements. It must reliably produce transmural lesion either from the epicardial or endocardial surface to ensure bidirectional conduction block. It should also be safe and render AF surgery simpler and less time consuming to perform. It would also be adaptable to minimally invasive approach. Melby and colleagues[51] described procedure that replaced with cut-and-sew lesions with bipolar radiofrequency lines as the Cox-Maze IV. In this technique, the atrial septal lesion was not performed and an independent isolation of the pulmonary veins was made with a connecting lesion. Although bipolar radiofrequency may reliably produce transmural lines and applied minimally invasively for pulmonary veins, it does not permit secure performance of connecting lines in the left atrial isthmus or inside the right atrium.[53,54]

Early follow-up suggests that the Cox-Maze IV procedure is similar in efficacy with 91% of patients having freedom from AF at 6 months.[55] There was no operative mortality and the group had significantly shorter cross clamp time compared to the Cox Maze III group. Cox also suggested another simplified procedure to cure most patients of AF.[56] This involved three essential lesions that include 1.an incision encircling the pulmonary veins, 2.left atrial isthmus and companion coronary sinus lesions and 3.right atrial isthmus lesion. This modified Cox-Maze procedure has been shown to be nearly as effective as the Cox-Maze III.[57]

6. Lesion sets for the surgical treatment of atrial fibrillation

Three general categories of lesion sets exist for the surgical treatment of AF in adults:

- Pulmonary vein isolation
- Left atrial lesion set
- Biatrial lesion set

Pulmonary vein isolation is only an ideal choice for those who have new onset paroxysmal AF Lesions can be created using a variety of different approaches that include beating heart epicardial techniques or on pump endocardial approaches that use energy devices or the cut and sew technique. Pulmonary vein isolation can be achieved through either a single lesion encircling all pulmonary veins or two lesions encompassing the left and right pulmonary veins. Left atrial lesion sets are advised in patients with recent-onset or paroxysmal AF undergoing elective surgery with no justification to open the right atrium. This includes pulmonary vein isolation with the addition of linear lesions extending to the mitral annulus and left atrial appendage that is usually excised or excluded. This is because more than 90% of left atrial thrombi originate from the left atrial appendage in patients with non-rheumatic AF.[58] Biatrial lesion sets are the most effective treatment option for AF[59]. Patients with longstanding or symptomatic AF, young patients or those undergoing right heart surgery would benefit from this procedure[60]

The Cox maze IV procedure is performed with the patient on CPB with bicaval cannulation. Using blunt dissection, the right and left PVs are dissected. If the patient is in AF, they are cardioverted. Pacing thresholds are obtained from all PVs. The bipolar ablation is performed around the cuff of atrial tissue surrounding the right and left pulmonary veins. Pacing is used to confirm block from both the superior and inferior PVs. Following PVI, the right atrial lesions are performed with the heart beating. An incision is created in the right atrial appendage as shown in figure 3. The bipolar device is used to make a right atrial free wall lesion. Following this a vertical right atriotomy is made around 2cm from the free wall ablation that extends from the crista terminalis toward the intra-atrial septum. The incision is then extended superiorly toward the AV groove. Two cryolesions are placed at the tricuspid annulus using cryoprobe. The bipolar clamp is used to create linear ablation lines from the SVC down to the IVC. The SVC ablation is made as laterally as possible to avoid damage to the SA node. The left sided atrial lesions are performed through a standard left atriotomy. This extends superiorly onto the dome of the left atrium and inferiorly around the orifice of the right inferior pulmonary vein. A lesion is made with the bipolar RF device to create a connecting lesion between the left atrial incision inferiorly to the ablation line encircling left inferior pulmonary vein. In atria greater than 5cm in diameter, a second connecting ablation is placed from the superior aspect of the incision into the left superior pulmonary vein. Finally, a bipolar radiofrequency ablation line is performed from the inferior aspect of the left atrial incision across the mitral valve annulus at a point between the circumflex and right coronary artery circulation. A cryolesion is placed at the mitral valve annulus. The left atrial appendage is amputated and a bipolar RF ablation is performed between the amputated left atrial appendage and superior PV. The left atrial appendage is oversewn. The aorta is unclamped and the right atrial incision is closed.

Patients with lone atrial fibrillation can choose between a catheter based approach or a minimally invasive surgical technique. Minimally invasive surgery to treat lone atrial fibrillation also can benefit patients who have a contraindication to warfarin, antiarrhythmic medications, or a history of cerebrovascular events. The procedure involves groin

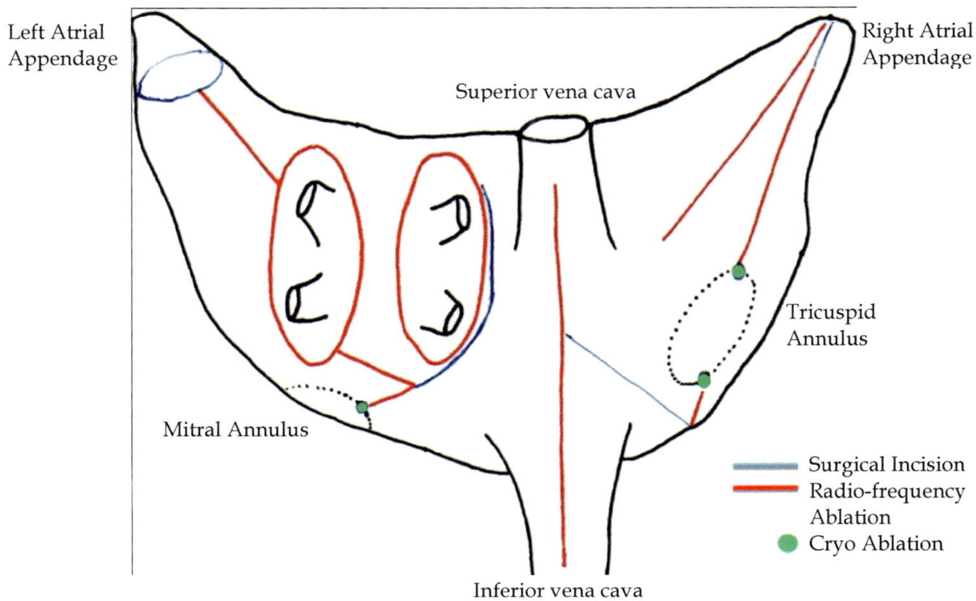

Fig. 3. Cox-Maze IV procedure

cannulation to connect the patient to CPB. The right sided lesions can be completed on a beating heart with or without cardiopulmonary support. After cross clamping the aorta, left sided lesions are created in a similar pattern to the Cox-Maze II procedure, creating a box lesion around all the pulmonary veins with a connecting lesion to the left atrial appendage and to the mitral valve isthmus. The left atrial orifice is closed from the endocardial side. When performed correctly, the results of the minimally invasive approach are excellent.[61]

Minimally invasive surgical techniques have been an area of interest as an alternative to catheter based pulmonary vein isolation. Bilateral thoracotomies or mini sternotomy can be used to isolate the pulmonary veins[62,63]. Its major advantage is that it can be performed in the absence of cardiopulmonary bypass and in many cases left atrial appendage disarticulation can also be offered. However, since AF does not always originate in the pulmonary veins this is not suitable in all patients, particularly those with non-paroxysmal AF.

Surgery for AF reduces medical costs successfully. When performed in conjunction with elective cardiac surgery it is cheaper and more effective than medical or catheter based therapy at a later time and cost effective in patients with a good prognosis[64,65] In summary, surgery for AF has evolved during the previous 2 decades to include several different approaches, lesion sets and energy sources. All patients undergoing concomitant cardiac surgery with AF should undergo surgical treatment for their AF. Ablation technology has simplified the procedure to make it easy for all surgeons to adopt and pave way towards minimal access procedures.

7. References

[1] Feinberg WM, Blackshear JL, Laupacis A, et al. Prevalence, age distribution, and gender of patients with atrial fibrillation. Analysis and implications. Arch Intern Med 1995;155:469-73.

[2] Go AS, Hylek EM, Phillips KA, et al. Prevalence of diagnosed atrial fibrillation in adults: national implications of rhythm management and stroke prevention: the AnTicoagulation and Risk Factors in Atrial Fibrillation (ATRIA) Study. JAMA 2001;285:2370-2375.

[3] Fuster V, Rydén LE, Cannom DS et al; European Heart Rhythm Association; Heart Rhythm Society. ACC/AHA/ESC 2006 guidelines for the management of patients with atrial fibrillation-executive summary. J Am Coll Cardiol 2006;48(4)854-906.

[4] Benjamin EJ, Levy D, Vaziri SM et al. Independent risk factors for atrial fibrillation in a population-based cohort. The Framingham study. JAMA 1994; 271:840-4.

[5] Lloyd-Jones D, Adams R, Carnathon M, et al. Heart disease and stroke statistics-2009 update: a report from the American Heart Association Statistics Committee and Stroke Statistics Subcommittee. Circulation 2009;119:480-486.

[6] Deaton C, Dunbar SB, Moloney M, Sears SF, Ujhelyi MR. Patient experiences with atrial fibrillation and treatment with implantable defibrillation therapy. Heart Lung. 2003:32(5):291-299.

[7] Corley SD, Epstein AE, Di Marco JP, et al. Relationships between sinus rhythm treatment and survival in Atrial Fibrillation Follow-up Investigation of Rhythm Management (AFFIRM) Stduy. Circulation 2004;109:1509-13.

[8] [No authors listed] Adjusted-dose warfarin versus low-intensity fixed-dose warfarin plus aspirin for high-risk patients with atrial fibrillation: Stroke Prevention in Atrial Fibrillation III randomised clinical trial. Lancet 1996;348:633-38.

[9] Copland M, Walker ID, Tait RC; Oral anticoagulation and haemorrhagic complications in an elderly population with atrial fibrillation. Arch Intern Med 2001;161:2125-28.

[10] Di Marco JP, Flaker G, Waldo AL, et al: Factors affecting bleeding risk during anticoagulant therapy in patients with atrial fibrillation: observations from the Atrial Fibrillation Follow-up Investigation of Rhythm Management (AFFIRM) Study. Am Heart J 2005;149(4):650-56.

[11] Hart RG, Halperin JL. Atrial fibrillation and thromboembolism: a decade of progress in stroke prevention. Ann Intern Med 1994;154:1449-57.

[12] Maintenance of sinus rhythm in patients with atrial fibrillation: AN AFFIRM substudy of the first antiarrhytmic drug. J Am Coll Cardiol 2003;42:20-29.

[13] Waldo AL. Management of atrial fibrillation. The need for AFFIRM-ative action. AFFIRM investigators. Am J Cardiol 1999;84:698-700.

[14] Calkins H, Brugada J, Packer DL et al. HRS/EHRA/ECAS expert consensus statement on catheter and surgical ablation of atrial fibrillation: recommendations for personnel, policy , procedures and follow-up. A report of the Heart Rhythm Society (HRS) Task Force on catheter and surgical ablation of atrial fibrillation. Heart Rhythm 2007;4:816-61.

[15] Fuster V, Ryden LE, Cannom DS, Crijns HJ et al: ACC/AHA/ESC 2006 guidelines for the management of patients with atrial fibrillation. Circulation. 2006;114:e257-e354.

[16] Cox JL, Canavan TE, Schussler RB et al. The Surgical treatment of atrial fibrillation II. Intraoperative electrophysiologic mapping and description of the

electrophysiologic basis of atrial flutter and atrial fibrillation. J Thorac Cardiovasc Surg 1991;101:406-26.
[17] Cox JL, Schuessler RB, D'Agostino HJ, et al. The Surgical treatment of atrial fibrillation III Development of a definitive surgical procedure. J Thorac Cardiovasc Surg 1991;101:569-83.
[18] Damiano RJ, Voeller RK. Surgical and minimally invasive ablation for atrial fibrillation. Curr Treat Options Cardiovasc Med 2006;8:371-76.
[19] Haissaguerre M, Jais P, Shah DC, et al. Spontaneous initiation of atrial fibrillation by ectopic beats originating in the pulmonary veins. N Engl J Med 1998;339:659-66.
[20] Narayan S, Cain M, Smith J. Atrial fibrillation. Lancet 1997;350:943-950.
[21] Allessie MA. Atrial fibrillation-induced electrical remodelling in humans :what is the next step ? Cardiovasc Res 1999 ;44 :10-12.
[22] Allessie MA, Penelope AB, Camm AJ. Pathophysiology and prevention of atrial fibrillation. Circulation 2001;103:769-777.
[23] Zipes DP. Electrophysiological remodelling of the heart owing to rate. Circulation 1997;95:1745-48.
[24] Cox JL. Surgical management of atrial fibrillation. Medscape Cardiol. 2005;9(1) http://www.medscape.com/viewarticle/503894 Accessed 28/2/2011.
[25] Synchronised direct-current cardovioversion is an electrical shock administered to the patient in an attempt to restore normal sinus rhythm. Electrical cardioversion was first described in 1962 by Lown et al (Lown B, Neuman J, Amarasingham R, Berkovitz BV: Comparison of alternating current with direct current electroshock across the closed chest. Am J Cardiol 1962;10:223) and its success rates in restoring sinus rhythm ranges from 80-95% depending on the population studied.
[26] Pritchett EL: Management of atrial fibrillation N Engl J Med 1992;326:1264-71.
[27] Dalzell GW, Anderson J, Adgey AA: Factors determining success and energy requirements for cardioversion of atrial fibrillation. Q J Med 1990;76:903-13.
[28] Donahue, Timothy P, Conti, Beth J. Atrial fibrillation: rate control versus maintenance of sinus rhythm. Curr Opin Cardiol 2001;16:46-53.
[29] The steering and publications committees of the acute study. Design of a clinical trial for the assessment of cardioversion using transesophageal echocardiography (The Acute Multicenter Study). Am J Cardiol 1998;81:877-83.
[30] Laupacis A, Albers G, Dalen J, et al. Antithrombotic treatment in atrial fibrillation. Chest 1998;114:579S-589S.
[31] Katritsis D, Merchant FM, Mela T, Singh JP et al. Catheter ablation of atrial fibrillation the search for substrate-driven end points J Am Coll Cardiol. 2010; 55:2293-98.
[32] Del Negro AA. Identifying the AF patient for the primary care physician: When should a patient be referred? Medscape Cardiol. 2005;9(1).
http://www.medscape.com/viewarticle/507147. Accessed 15 Feb 2011.
[33] Cappato, R. et al. Prevalence and causes of fatal outcome in catheter ablation of atrial fibrillation. J Am Coll Cardiol. 2009; 53; 1798–1803.
[34] Fuster V, Ryden LE, Asinger RW, et al. ACC/AHA/ESC guidelines for the management of patients with atrial fibrillation: excecutive summary a report of the American College of Cardiology/American Heart Association Task Force on Practice Guidelines and the European Society of Cardiology Committee for Practice Guidelines and Policy Conferences (Committee to develop guidelines for the

management of patients with atrial fibrillation) developed in collaboration with the North American Society of Pacing and Electrophysiology. Circulation 2001;104:2118-50.

[35] Ad N, Cheng DCH, Martin J, et al. Surgical ablation for atrial fibrillation in cardiac surgery: a consensus statement of the International Society of Minimally Invasive Cardiothoracic Surgery (ISMICS) 2009. Innovations Phila Pa 2010;5:74-83.

[36] Khasnis A, Jongnarangsin K, Abela G et al. Tachycardia-induced cardiomyopathy: A review of literature. Pacing Clin Electrophysiol 2005;28:710-21.

[37] Umana E, Solares CA, Alpert MA. Tachycardia-induced cardiomyopathy. Am J Med 2003;114:51-55.

[38] Bleeding during antithrombotic therapy in patients with atrial fibrillation. The Stroke Prevention in Atrial Fibrillation Investigators. Arch Intern Med 1996;156:409-416.

[39] Williams JM, Ungerleider RM, Lofland GK, et al. Left atrial isolation: New technique for the treatment of supraventricular arrhythmias. J Thorac Cardiovasc Surg 1980;80:373.

[40] Cox JL. The surgical treatment of atrial fibrillation. IV. Surgical technique. J Thorac Cardiovasc Surg 1991;101:584-92.

[41] Cox JL, Ad N, Palazzo T. Impact of the Maze procedure on the stroke rate in patients with atrial fibrillation. J Thorac Cardiovasc Surg 1999;118:833-40.

[42] Cox JL, Schuessler RB, Boineau JP. The development of the Maze procedure for the treatment of atrial fibrillation. Semin Thorac Cardiovasc Surg 2999;12:2-14.

[43] Schaff HV, Dearani JA, Daly RC, et al. Cox-Maze procedure for atrial fibrillation: Mayo Clinic experience. Semin Thorac Cardiovasc Surg 2000;12:30-37.

[44] Prasad SM, Maniar HS, Camillo CJ, et al. The Cox maze III procedure for atrial fibrillation: long-term efficacy in patients undergoing lone versus concomitant procedures. J Thorac Cardiovasc Surg 2003;126:1822-28.

[45] Gillinov AM, Sirak JH, Blackstone EH. The Cox maze procedure in mitral valve disease: predictors of recurrent atrial fibrillation. J Thorac Cardiothorac Surg 2005;130:1653-60.

[46] Cox JL, Ad N, Palazzo T et al. Current status of the Maze procedure for the treatment of atrial fibrillation. Semin Thorac Cardiovasc Surg 2000;12:25-29.

[47] Raanani E, Albage A, David TE et al. The efficacy of the Cox/Maze procedure combined with mitral valve surgery: A matched control study. Eur J Cardiothorac Surg 2001;19:438-442.

[48] McCarthy PM, Gillinov AM, Castle L et al. The Cox-Maze procedure: The Cleveland Clinic experience. Semin Thorac Cardiovasc Surg 2000;12:25-29.

[49] Bando K, Kobayashi J, Kosakia Y. Impact of Cox maze procedure on outcome in patients with atrial fibrillation and mitral valve disease. J Thorac Cardiovasc Surg 2002;124:575-83.

[50] Saltman AE, Gillinov AM. Surgical approaches for atrial fibrillation. Cardiol Clin 2009;27:179-188.

[51] Melby SJ, Zierer A, Bailey MS et al. A new era in the surgical treatment of atrial fibrillation: the impact of ablation technology and lesion set on procedural efficacy. Ann Surg 2006;244:583-92.

[52] Lee AM, Melby SJ, Damiano RJ Jr. The surgical treatment of atrial fibrillation. Surg Clin N Am 2009;89:1001-20.

[53] Shen J, Bailey MS, Damiano RJ. The surgical treatment of atrial fibrillation. Heart Rhythm 2009;6:S45-S50.
[54] Beyer E, Lee R, Lam, BK. Point:Minimally invasive bipolar radiofrequency ablation of lone atrial fibrillation: early multicentre results. J Thorac Cardiovasc Surg 2009;137:521-26).
[55] Gaynor SL, Diodato MD, Prasad SM, et al. A prospective single-center clinical trial of a modified Cox Maze procedure with bipolar radiofrequency ablation. J Thorac Cardiovasc Surg 2004;128:535-42.
[56] Cox JL. Surgical treatment of atrial fibrillation: a review. Eurospace 2004;5(Suppl 1)S20-29.
[57] Cui YQ, Sun LB, Li Y, et al. Intraoperative modified Cox mini-Maze procedure for long-standing persistent atrial fibrillation. Ann Thorac Surg 2008;85:1283-89.
[58] Blacshear JL, Odell JA. Appendage obliteration to reduce stroke in cardiac surgical patients with atrial fibrillation. Ann Thorac Surg 1996;61:755-59.
[59] Damiano RJ Jr, Voeller RK. Biatrial lesion sets. J Interv Card Electrophysiolo 2007;20:95-99.
[60] McCarthy PM, Kruse J, Shalli S, et al. Where does atrial fibrillation surgery fail? Implications for increasing effectiveness of ablation. J Thorac Cardiovasc Surg 2010;139:860-67.
[61] Cox JL Minimally invasive Maze procedure. [abstract]. Circulation 1999; 100: (suppl): I, 778.
[62] Ninet J, Roques X, Seitelberger R, Deville C, Pomar JL, Robin J et al. Surgical ablation of atrial fibrillation with off-pump, epicardial, high-intensity focused ultrasound: results of a multicenter trial. J Thorac Cardiovasc Surg. 2005;130:803-809.
[63] Wolf RK, Schneeberger EW, Osterday R, Miller D, Merrill W, Flege JB Jr, Gillinov AM. Video-assisted bilateral pulmonary vein isolation and left atrial appendage exclusion for atrial fibrillation. J Thorac Cardiovasc Surg. 2005;130:797-802.
[64] Lamotte M, Annemans L, Bridgewater B, Kendall S, Siebert M. A health economic evaluation of concomitant surgical ablation for atrial fibrillation. Eur J Cardiothorac Surg 2007;32:702-710.
[65] Quenneville SP, Xie X, Brophy JM. The cost-effectiveness of Maze procedures using ablation techniques at the time of mitral valve surgery. Int J Technol Assess Health Care 2009;25:485-96.

12

Post-Cardiac Surgery Fungal Endocarditis

Parisa Badiee
Professor Alborzi Clinical Microbiology Research Center,
Shiraz University of Medical Sciences, Shiraz,
Iran

1. Introduction

Infective endocarditis (IE) is a threatening disease associated with a high risk of morbidity and mortality. The most etiologic agents are the bacteria followed by fungi. Fungal Endocarditis (FE) is an uncommon occurrence and the most severe form of IE, however, its rate has increased in recent decades. The first report of FE after a mitral valve replacement was in 1964 (1) but there have been many cases reported in recent years indicating the importance of such infections (2-4). Fungal endocarditis accounts for 1.3% to 6% of all IE cases (5-8). Ranges between 1.7 to 3.8 per 100,000 person-years have been reported in different studies for mean annual incidence (5, 9). Increase in the number of cases of fungemia and FE has been seen during the last 2 decades (10, 11). Men are more at risk of infections than women (7, 12, 13), and younger persons (third to fourth decades of life) are in more risk factor. The incidence of FE varies based on the criteria and methods of diagnosis (5) and population under survey; in liver transplants (14) the incidence of FE after transplantation was 1.7%. The mortality rate was 72% (15) but is still high (about 50%) despite the treatments (7). In an international multicenter prospective cohort study that included 33 cases of *Candida* endocarditis treated between 2000 and 2005, the mortality rate was 30 % (16), and in post-surgical invasive aspergillosis (17) and *Aspergillus* endocarditis the rate was too high (100%) even with combined medical and surgical therapy (2).

Fungi are important causes of prosthetic valve endocarditis, responsible for 1%–10% of these infections (18). Also, there are reports that fungi are responsible for 9.6% of the early cases of prosthetic valve endocarditis (60 days after the insertion of prosthesis) and for 4.3% of late cases (>60 days after the insertion of prosthesis) (19, 20). The incidence of FE in culture-documented cases has been reported to range from 12% to 20% (21) or to 37.5% (22).

Many fungal species cause FE, of which the most important are *Candida albicans* 60%-67% and filamentous *Aspergillus* spp. 20–30% (ratio rate 2/1) (7, 15, 23), In addition, non-*albicans* species of *Candida, Torulopsis glabrata, Candida tropicalis,* and other filamentus fungi like *Aspergillus* spp., *Curvularia genuculata, Hormondendrum dermatitidis, Mucoracae, Scopulariopsis* spp., *Trichosporon spp. and Blastoschizomyces capitatus* have been reported in the literature (10, 15, 22, 24, 25). In some studies, the most common etiologic agent was different, as in Rubinstein E et al. *Candida parapsilosis* accounts for half of the culture-documented patients, whereas *C. albicans* and *Candida stellatoidea* account for 12%-15% only (21). *Pneumocystis jiroveci* caused fungal infection in 9% to 11% of all heart transplant recipients in the past, with a mortality rate of 11% to 38% (26) but with use of prophylaxis, the rate of this infection has decreased.

The source of infection can be internal or external, the former usually with *Candida* spp. This organism is the normal flora of the patient's body and causes contamination during the surgery, and is recognized as the catheter-related blood stream infection (27). However, conidia of the external agents could contaminate the tissues during the surgery or post operative contamination by environmental isolates present in high counts (17).
Time of presenting of infection is different and maybe during the first 2 weeks in hospital period to months after heart surgery at home, and in some cases 12 years later (15). Diagnosis should be prompt because the time interval between the first symptom and hospital admission in some cases is long and may be one year (15). Early diagnosis could be helpful for the patients' survival. The onset of symptoms is usually about 2 weeks or less from the initiating bacteremia.
Anatomical cardiac condition diseases (cardiac abnormality), intravenous drug abusers and open heart cardiac surgery are the top risk factors for the infections. There are many risk factors for progressive FE, including the use of multiple immunosuppressive drugs such as azathioprine, corticosteroids, cyclosporine A, and cyclophosphamide (12, 13, 15). Malignancy, exposure to multiple broad-spectrum antibiotics, prolonged use of intravenous catheters (28), use of high glucose concentrations intravenous catheters especially in premature neonates (29), rheumatic heart disease (22), previous bacterial endocarditis, prior surgery, prolonged intravenous hyper alimentation, pacemaker implantation, and reconstructive cardiovascular surgery are other risk factors (15,30-32). In some cases no predisposing factor has been identified (7, 33)
The mechanism of endocarditis includes high turbulent blood flow due to cardiac abnormality or other risk factors (e.g., particulate material in the repeated injections of drugs in IV drug abusers) which disrupt the surface of endocardia and endothelium. The response of the body is repairing the damaged tissue with platelet-fibrin meshwork which is sticky and proper site for infection. After temporary bacteremia, it sticks to this meshwork and proliferation of organism causes the infection that invades the cardiac valves.
Infective endocarditis is classified into definite, probable, and possible according to Pelletier and Petersdorf (34). Other classifications include definite, probable, possible and rejected by von Reyn (35) and definitive, possible and rejected by Duke criteria (36) (Table 1). Briefly, proven FE is defined as the isolation of fungi from the normally sterile sites, the blood or heart biopsy or vegetation, by culture and/or the evidence of fungal invasion of tissue by histopathological methods. Probable FE is defined as when the culture is negative for the infective agents, and clinical conditions of the respective patients are not recovered despite the administration of standard antibacterial therapy. Role of echocardiography, definition of rejected IE and major and minor clinical criteria were added to the previous definition in 1994 (37). According to Duke criteria, the diagnosis of definitive IE requires the presence of either two major criteria, one major and three minor criteria, or five minor criteria.

2. Clinical manifestations

The clinical manifestations of acute or sub-acute IE are related to the underlying pathophysiology of embolization, bacteremia/ candidemia, immunologic response, and valvulitis (30). Common clinical features are changing heart murmur, fever, and major peripheral emboli (common in fungal endocarditis) (10, 33). Some cases presented with the systemic symptoms associated with bacteremia include fever, tachycardia, septic shock; and the general symptoms and signs of cardiac involvement including chest pain, arrhythmias,

Pelletier and Petersdorf criteria (34)	
Definite IE	-Histologic evidence of vegetation on tissue from surgery or autopsy
Probable IE	- Positive blood cultures with known underlying valvular heart disease and evidence of emboli to viscera or skin - OR fever >38°C with negative blood cultures in individuals, embolic phenomena and new regurgitant valvular heart murmurs
Possible IE	- Positive blood cultures with known underlying heart disease - Embolic phenomena; or negative blood cultures with fever, known underlying valvular heart disease, and embolic episodes.
Property	- Many patients with clinical features of infective endocarditis did not meet the above criteria due to lack of sensitivity.
von Reyn criteria (35)	
Definite	- Histologic evidence from surgery or autopsy - Positive bacteriology evidence of valvular vegetation or peripheral embolus (staining or culture).
Probable	-Persistently positive blood cultures plus one of the following: New regurgitant murmur and predisposing heart disease, vascular phenomena, negative or intermittently positive blood cultures, plus three of the following: new regurgitant murmur, fever, vascular phenomena - petechiae, Roth spots, Osler's nodes, Janeway lesions, splinter hemorrhages, aseptic meningitis, conjunctival hemorrhages, glomerulonephritis, or central nervous system, pulmonary, coronary or peripheral emboli.
possible	-Persistently positive blood cultures plus one of the following: predisposing heart disease - definite valvular or congenital heart disease, or a cardiac prosthesis (excluding permanent pacemakers) , vascular phenomena -Negative or intermittently positive blood cultures with all three of the following: fever, predisposing heart disease, vascular phenomena. -Only for viridans streptococcal endocarditis: fever with at least two positive blood cultures without an extra cardiac source
Rejected	-Endocarditis unlikely, alternative diagnosis generally apparent or endocarditis likely, empiric antibiotic therapy warranted - Culture negative diagnosed clinically as endocarditis, but excluded by postmortem
property	- Lacked prospective validation, but improved the specificity of the classification system, a large proportion of cases being classified as probable or possible (most patients do not require valve surgery).

Duke criteria (36)	
Major clinical criteria	- Persistently positive blood cultures for organisms, new or partial dehiscence of a prosthetic valve or an abscess in the tissues surrounding a heart valve, presented of vegetation or other typical findings of endocarditis in echocardiography; new regurgitate murmur, serological or culture evidence of infection with Coxiella burnetii.
Minor clinical criteria	- Positive blood cultures that do not meet the strict definitions of a major criterion, fever, predisposing valvular condition[a] - OR intravenous drug abuse, elevated erythrocyte sedimentation rate and C-reactive protein hematuria and splenomegaly.
Definitive	- Pathological criterion: vegetation or intracardiac abscess, confirmed by histology showing active endocarditis, positive Gram stain results or cultures of specimens obtained from surgery or autopsy - Clinical criteria: 2 major criteria OR 1 major and 3 minor criteria OR 5 minor criteria
Possible IE	- 1 major criterion and 1 minor criterion OR 3 minor criteria
Rejected IE	- Firm alternate diagnosis for manifestations of endocarditis - Resolution of manifestations of endocarditis, or no pathologic evidence of infective endocarditis at surgery or autopsy after antibiotic therapy for four days or less - Does not meet criteria for possible infective endocarditis, as above

[a] Prosthetic heart valve or a valve lesion that leads to significant regurgitation or turbulence of blood flow; Vascular phenomenon like emboli to the brain or organs, hemorrhages in the mucous membranes around the eyes; Immunologic phenomenon include lesions such as Roth's spots or "Osler's nodes and glomerulonephritis.

Table 1. Definition of three criteria for the diagnosis of infective endocarditis

edema, dyspnea, murmur on examination, cardiac failure, and persistent sepsis would also present. Other symptoms include abdominal pain, malaise, weight loss, night sweats, arthritis, finger clubbing, cough, hemoptysis, sudden death, coagulopathy, jaundice, nausea, hypotension, and renal failure. *Candida spp.* is the most etiologic agent of FE; therefore, patients can present endophthalmitis, meningitis, osteomyelitis and other complications of candidemia. The more specific cutaneous or mucocutaneous lesions of IE include Osler's nodes, Roth spots (rare), and Janeway lesions are more specific signs but less common and not diagnostic . Petechiae and splinter hemorrhages (nonblanching, linear reddish-brown lesions found under the nail bed) are not specific but are common skin manifestations. They may be present on the extremities of skin, or on mucous membranes. Other organs may be involved due to embolic events such as splenic or renal infarcts, or immune reactions like arthritis and glomerulonephritis, or spread by the blood passing to other organs like soft tissues, vertebral osteomyelitis, and the brain causing meningitis and/or encephalitis.

3. Diagnosis of fungal endocarditis

The diagnosis of IE is based upon high index of suspicion, careful history and physical examination, echocardiographic or histopathological findings, laboratory results, and chest radiography. Gold standard tests for the detection of documented infections are the isolation of fungi from the blood, heart biopsy or vegetation by culture and the presence of tissue invasion by histopathology. Isolation of fungi from blood samples is difficult due to non-growth of fungal etiologic agents in blood culture. The rate of culture positive of *Candida* spp. in the blood is about 50% of the documented cases and positive blood culture for *Aspergillus* is rare (38-40). Fungi are cleared rapidly, due to large size, in the blood by the host's reticuloendothelial system; therefore, the blood culture results are negative in many suspicious patients. The use of lysis-centrifugation system (41), or Bactec blood culture (42), may help the isolation of fungal agents but none is recommend as a standard method. Heart tissue is the best sample for the isolation of fungal agents. As resistance to the antifungal agents has been reported in many studies (43-45), in case of positive culture, sensitivity test of the isolated fungi to antifungal agents can contribute to the best management of infections.

Another definitive microbiologic diagnosis depends upon the evidence of fungal tissue invasion with histopathologic investigation. The samples (tissue valve or emboli) are stained with specific stains like Gomori methenamine silver or Periodic acid-Schiff. With histopathology examination, morphological differentiation between *Aspergillus* spp. and other fungi is not completely available.

Given the frequent negative blood cultures, and difficulty in obtaining the material from the surgical sites in the operating rooms, echocardiography, either transthoracic echocardiography (TTE) or transesophageal echocardiography (TEE), are used as the diagnosis tools with the sensitivity of about 77% (15) for the evaluation of FE and the presence of vegetation, based on the major diagnostic Duke criterion. Echocardiography can also detect intra cardiac abscess, new or progressive valvular regurgitation, the size and location of vegetation. The size of vegetation may be small, medium, or large and anatomic site of the vegetation may be aortic valve, on tricuspid, mitral or endocardium, or on the previous aortic valvular surgery.

Transesophageal echocardiography should be considered as the standard diagnostic procedure for IE (46). This method is able to evaluate the prosthetic valves, intracardiac complications, inadequate TTE, fungemia or bacteremia, and has superior sensitivity (47), compared to TTE, but significantly more invasive and expensive than it. Transthoracic echocardiography is the first line procedure for the detection of FE especially in native valve and prosthetic valve vegetations, and local extension of infection. The sensitivity of TTE in infants and younger children is about 80 percent (48, 49), therefore, the negative result of it cannot definitively rule out FE and examination should be repeated in respective patients. If there is a high clinical suspicion for FE and the TTE is negative, we should turn to TEE. Once treatment is completed, repeated evaluation may be necessary to establish a new baseline of valvular and myocardial functions for the patient. Unfortunately, both TTE and TEE may yield false negative results if the vegetations are small, or large size of the vegetation suspected as a mural thrombus, vegetation is attached to the mural endocardium and if embolization of the vegetation has occurred.

Chest radiography and echocardiography are not useful in the diagnosis of IE; x-ray may present the septic pulmonary emboli (Minor Duke's Criteria) and echocardiography may show evidence of some complications.

Over the last several decades, non-culture laboratory methods have been directed at the development for the diagnosis of systemic fungal infections such as FE. Serological diagnostic methods can serve as the non-invasive methods for detecting the circulating fungal antigens, fungal metabolites, or antibody in the blood (50, 51). The major limitation of these methods is unavailability to detect some fungi like *Mucor* spp.

Galactomannan (GM) is a more promising circulating fungal antigen used to detect fungal infections especially invasive aspergillosis, but it is an exoantigen released from the tip of mycelium of many fungi spp. during growth (52), therefore, cross-reactivity has been described with other fungi (53-55). False negative reactivity without any known reason (56) and false positive reactivity with use of some drugs and foods have been reported (57-61). Sensitivity range of GM test, for the diagnosis of documented invasive aspergillosis cases was reported to be between 50.0% (62) and 90.6% (63). There are limited studies using this method for the diagnosis of FE. In one study, GM test to establish the diagnosis of invasive aspergillosis was only positive (≥1 ng/mL) in 2/7 patients with endocarditis and mediastinitis(17) and four out of nine cases in another study (33). To diagnose systemic candidiasis, enolase (64), phospholipase and proteinase enzymes (65), *Candida* mannan antigen (66, 67), and β-D-glucan (68-71) have been detected in some studies. However, there are a few reports on the use of such antigens in patients with FE.

Antibody assays can be helpful for some species of fungi which are not the normal flora but there are problems with both specificity and sensitivity when *Candida spp.* is responsible for infections, since it is a part of the body normal flora. Immunosuppressed hosts may be unable to produce strong antibodies; therefore, the sensitivity of the assay in this high-risk population is decreased.

The current focus of non-culture methods is on the development of a polymerase chain reaction (PCR) assay for the detection of fungal infections (72, 73). Panfungal PCR with universal primers (74), nested PCR (75, 76) and real-time PCR (77, 78) can serve as sensitive and quantitative methods to detect fungal DNA in the human blood specimens (74, 79). The sensitivity and specificity of nested PCR for invasive aspergillosis in the blood are 92.8% and 94%, respectively (55). Although these methods have not been standardized and are not widely used, limited studies indicate a good sensitivity for FE diagnosis and close to blood cultures (33, 80). Using the molecular methods with reduced PCR steps like real time- PCR, the result can be released within 6 hours (81). Due to the inhibitory factors in human blood samples, PCR may yield false negative (82) and for the abundant conidia of fungi in the environment, false positive may also be seen, which is rare and limited. The significance of PCR tests is their ability to detect fungal infections in early stages (83).

Other nonspecific laboratory outcomes include: a normochromic normocytic anemia, elevated erythrocyte sedimentation rate and C-reactive protein indicative of inflammation, elevated rheumatoid factor titers (minor Duke criteria), hematuria and proteinuria (minor Duke criteria).

Totally, in patients suspicious to FE, microscopy examination and culture of tissue materials obtained from heart surgery, with antifungal susceptibility test on the isolated fungi are the best methods for the diagnosis and management of FE. In patients with suspected FE in early stage of infection, use of nonaggressive method (i.e., serologic or molecular) is recommended. Combination of serological and microbiological tests is more useful if we are to avoid over-treatment.

4. Treatment

The high mortality rate, difficulty in sterilizing large fungal vegetation or abscesses, and the risk of embolization associated with medical therapy alone (84) are the reasons for the recommendation of combined surgical and medical treatment in patients with FE for better prognosis (7, 8, 85). It is also the suggestion of the 2009 Infectious Diseases Society of America guidelines for the treatment of native and prosthetic valve *Candida* endocarditis (86). However, there are some reports of *Candida* endocarditis in which medical treatment alone proved successful (85, 87-89) with either caspofungin alone or in combination with flucytosine or fluconazole (87-90). The higher dose of antifungal agents than normal dose is recommended for treatment (86). In critically ill patients for whom surgical resection cannot be done, antifungal therapy is recommended for months and even life-long. In combination therapy a minimum of 6 weeks medication after surgery is advocated (91), but the treatment should be continued till signs and symptoms of the infection disappear and radiographic abnormalities are stabilized, and life-long prophylactic therapy is recommended. Relapses are common either with medical or combined therapy (37, 92, 93) and may appear early or late; mean 25 months (92). Due to high relapse rates, patients should receive life-long therapy (92, 93) and careful follow-up is also essential for successful therapy.

Treatment of FE in immunocompromised patients needs to take into account the underlying disease of patients and the intervention of antifungal agents with the patient's condition. For example, use of amphotericin B deoxycholate, in patients with renal insufficiency or those who are on multiple nephrotoxic drugs is not suggested and for fewer adverse effects, lipid formulations of amphotericin B are recommended (94). Many studies have reported the resistance of some fungi to this antifungal agent (44, 45, 95), therefore, to limit the use of amphotericin B, current treatment options including azole due to its broad antifungal activity, and echinocandins as a new class of antifungal drugs, are recommended (96).

In transplant recipients and HIV patients, use of triazoles which have interaction with human P450 cytochromes (97), can block the metabolism of certain anti-HIV drugs and also some drugs such as cyclosporine, statins, and benzodiazepines (98). Therefore, close monitoring of drug levels needs to be calibrated with the dose of immunosuppressive drugs (99, 100). Physicians should prescribe triazole agents in consultation with a pharmacist because inhibitory activities among triazoles are different and fluconazole is of less active inhibition of P450 than other azole agents such as itraconazole, voriconazole, and posaconazole. In patients receiving these antifungals, monitoring of drug levels in respective sera is suggested (96).

Echinocandins; caspofungin, micafungin, and anidulafungin; are new antifungal agents which damage the fungal cell walls by inhibiting the b-(1, 3)-glucan synthesis. Drug–drug interactions between echinocandins such as caspofungin are observed with tacrolimus and cyclosporine, certain anti-HIV drugs and rifampin (96). Use of caspofungin in patients with impaired liver function and those receiving cyclosporine should be carefully considered, because of the common side effects of this agent including increased liver enzymes, pruritus, facial swelling, headache and nausea. They have fungicidal activity against *Candida* biofilm (101) and most isolates of *Candida* species including *C. glabrata in* vitro and in vivo with benign toxicity profile (102).

If the patients are not responsive to their initial mono-antifungal therapy regimen, the use of the combination antifungal regimen is recommended that include an echinocandins with voriconazole or liposomal amphotericin B. Combination therapy by amphotericin B and a triazole is not suggested in the literature (103). The function of combination antifungal therapy is controversial due to probable increase in side effects and toxicity level (104, 105).

5. Prevention

Fungal endocarditis may be caused by endogenous or exogenous fungi. The prevention of FE could be through adopting two strategies; one is general and useful for all infections like hand-washing, personal hygiene, and indwelling central venous catheters care, and the other is especially for fungal infections. Practical ways to achieve this goal is use of non-drug or drug prevention (prophylaxis). Avoiding opportunistic endogenous agents like *Candida* spp. which colonize in the human body sites is difficult. The best strategy for the management of *Candida* endocarditis is the evaluation of colonization pre-surgery to determine the susceptibility pattern of the isolated organisms, which may cause infection after surgery and enhance the success of management of systemic or endocarditis candidiasis. Care of central venous catheters is important for reducing candidemia and *Candida* endocarditis; and the removal of all existing central venous catheters for the reduction of morbidity and mortality (106-108) is helpful. However, in patients with obligate central venous access, new sites should be obtained (109, 110).

Fungal spores are abundant in the environment, and unfiltered air, dust, and contaminated materials are full of fungal conidia (111, 112). In many cases, fungal infections may occur during the surgery, via contaminated air, surgical site or equipment with conidia. To prevent the contamination, use of high-efficiency particulate air filters for air sterility (113), and sterile equipment in the operation room are recommended.

Antifungal prophylaxis could be used to avoid the development of fungal infections in high risk patients (114), based on the susceptibility patterns of the etiologic agents in each region. Empiric therapy (antifungal treatment of febrile patients at risk for infections) was first introduced to prevent invasive fungal infections in the 1980s in patients with undiagnosed fevers, particularly invasive candidiasis (115). To prevent the relapse in patients with history of fungal infections who have received complete antifungal therapy, clinicians can turn to secondary prophylaxis.

6. Conclusion

Fungal endocarditis is one of the most serious manifestations of invasive fungal infections. The first line of prevention is decreasing fungal conidia transition during surgery in operating rooms by using high-efficiency particulate air filters and sterile equipment. Early diagnosis and immediate appropriate antifungal therapy are critical for the survival of the respective patients. For high quality care of the patients, echocardiography with non-cultural methods such as GM assay and PCR which can detect infection in early stages should be performed. In patients with suspected FE and positive test results, it is recommended that they receive antifungal agents pre-operation and also the clinical management be continued once the documented diagnosis is made based on the sample obtained in the operation room. As high relapses are common, treatment should be followed by careful review of the clinical, mycological (serum GM level and DNA load) and echocardiography sign and symptoms of the infections.

7. Acknowledgement

Our deep gratitude to Hassan Khajehei, PhD, for his valuable copy editing of the chapter.

8. References

[1] Newman WH, Cordell AR. *Aspergillus* endocarditis after open-heart surgery.report of a case and review of the literature. J Thorac Cardiovasc Surg 1964;48:652-60.

[2] El-Hamamsy I, Du¨ rrleman N, et al. Cluster of Cases of *Aspergillus* Endocarditis After Cardiac Surgery. Ann Thorac Surg 2004;77:2184–6.

[3] Vaideeswara P, Mishra P, et al. Infective endocarditis of the Dacron patch-a report of 13 cases at autopsy. Cardiovascular Pathology 2010;32 (3):1-8.

[4] Ryu KM, Seo PW, et al. Surgical Treatment of Native Valve *Aspergillus* Endocarditis and fungemic vascular complications. J Korean Med Sci 2009; (1): 170-2.

[5] Bayer AS, Scheld M. Endocarditis and intravascular infections.In: Mandell GL, Bennett JE, Dolin R, eds.Mandell, Douglas and Bennett's principles and practice of infectious diseases.Philadelphia, PA: Churchill Livingstone, 2000; 857–902.

[6] Karchmer AW. Infections on prosthetic valves and intravasculardevices.In: Mandell GL, Bennett JE, Dolin R, eds. Mandell, Douglas and Bennett's principles and practice of infectious diseases.Philadelphia, PA: Churchill Livingstone 2000; 903–17.

[7] Pierrotti LC, Baddour LM. Fungal Endocarditis, 1995–2000 Chest. 2002; 122(1):302-10.

[8] Tunkel AR, Kaye D. Endocarditis with negative blood cultures. N Engl J Med 1992;326(18):1215-17.

[9] Moreillon P, Que YA. Infective endocarditis. Lancet 2004;10;363(9403):139-49.

[10] Rubinstein E, Lang R. Fungal endocarditis. Eur Heart J 1995;16:84-9.

[11] Fernandez-Guerrero M, Verdejo C, et al. Hospital acquired infective endocarditis not associated with cardiac surgery: an emerging problem. Clin Infect Dis 1995; 20:16–23.

[12] Woods GL, Wood RP, et al. *Aspergillus* endocarditis in patients without prior cardiovascular surgery: report of a case in a liver transplant recipient and review. Rev Infect Dis 1989;11:263–72.

[13] Barst RJ, Prince AS, et al. *Aspergillus* endocarditis in children: case report and review of the literature. Pediatrics 1981;68:73–8.

[14] Paterson DL, Domingues EA, et al. Infective endocarditis in solid organ transplant recipients. Clin Infect Dis 1998: 26: 689-94.

[15] Ellis ME, Al-Abdely H, et al. Fungal endocarditis: evidence in the world literature, 1965-1995.Clin Infect Dis 2001; 32:50-62.

[16] Baddley JW, Benjamin DK, et al. *Candida* infective endocarditis. Eur J Clin Microbiol Infect Dis 2008; 27:519-29.

[17] Jensen J, Guinea J, et al. Post-surgical invasive aspergillosis: an uncommon and under-appreciated entity. J Infect 2010;60(2):162-7.

[18] Giamarellou H. Nosocomial cardiac infections. J Hosp Infect 2002; 50: 91–105.

[19] Gordon SM, Keys TF. Bloodstream infections in patients with prosthetic cardiac valves. Semin Thorac Cardiovasc Surg 1995;7:2–6.

[20] Watanakunakorn C. Prosthetic valve infective endocarditis. Prog Cardiovasc Dis 1979;22:181-92.

[21] Rubinstein E, Noriega ER, et al. Fungal endocarditis: analysis of 24 cases and review of the literature. Medicine 1975;54(4):331-4.

[22] Challa S, Prayaga AK, et al. Fungal endocarditis: An autopsy study. Asian Cardiovasc Thorac Ann 2004;12(2):95-8.

[23] Hauser M, Hess J, et al. Treatment of *Candida albicans* endocarditis: case report and a review. Infection 2003;31(2):125-7.

[24] Jain D, Oberoi JK, et al. *Scopulariopsis brevicaulis* infection of prosthetic valve resembling aspergilloma on histopathology. Cardiovasc Pathol. 2010. (Article in Press)
[25] Kumar P, Muranjan MN, et al. *Candida tropicalis* endocarditis: Treatment in a resource-poor setting. Ann Pediatr Cardiol 2010;3(2):174-7.
[26] Dummer JS. *Pneumocystis carinii* infections in transplant recipients. Semin Respir Infect 1990;5(1):50-7.
[27] Mermel LA, Farr BM, et al. Guidelines for the management of intravascular catheter-related infections. Clin Infect Dis 2001; 32: 1249-72.
[28] Raad I, Hanna H, et al. Intravascular catheter-related infections: advances in diagnosis, prevention, and management. Lancet Infect Dis 2007;7: 645-57.
[29] Levy I, Shalit I, et al. *Candida* endocarditis in neonates: report of five cases and review of the literature. Mycoses 2006; 49:43-8.
[30] Pierotti LC, Baddour LM. Fungal endocarditis, 1995–2000. Chest 2002;122:302–10.
[31] Sohail MR, Uslan DZ, et al. Infective endocarditis complicating permanent pacemaker and implantable cardioverter-defibrillator infection. Mayo Clin Proc. 2008;83(1):46-53.
[32] Cacoub P, Leprince P, et al. Pacemaker infective endocarditis. Am J Cardiol 1998;82:480–4.
[33] McCormack J, Pollard J. *Aspergillus* endocarditis 2003-2009. Med Mycol. 2011;49(1):S30-4.
[34] Pelletier LL, Petersdorf RG. Infective endocarditis: A review of 125 cases from the University of Washington Hospitals, 1963-1972. Medicine 1977;56:287-314.
[35] von Reyn, CF, Levy, BS, et al. Infective endocarditis: An analysis based on strict case definitions. Ann Intern Med 1981;94:505-18.
[36] Durack DT, Lukes AS, et al. New criteria for diagnosis of infective endocarditis: utilization of specific echocardiographic findings. Am J Med 1994; 96:200–09
[37] Melgar GR, Nasser RM, et al. Fungal prosthetic valve endocarditis in 16 patients. An 11-year experience in a tertiary care hospital. Medicine 1997; 76:94-103.
[38] Kahn FW, Jones JM, et al. The role of bronchoalveolar lavage in the diagnosis of invasive pulmonary *Aspergillus*. Am J Clin Pathol 1986;86(4):518-23.
[39] Thaler M, Pastakia B, et al. Hepatic candidiasis in cancer patients: the evolving picture of the syndrome. Ann Intern Med 1988;108(1):88-100.
[40] Goodrich JM, Reed EC, et al. Clinical features and analysis of risk factors for invasive candidal infection after marrow transplantation. J Infect Dis 1991;164(4): 731-40.
[41] Sinha K, Tendolkar U, et al. Comparison of conventional broth blood culture technique and manual lysis centrifugation technique for detection of fungemia. Indian J Medical Microb 2009;27(1):79-80.
[42] Horvath LL, Duane R, et al. Detection of simulated candidemia by the BACTEC 9240 System with Plus Aerobic/F and Anaerobic/F blood culture bottles. J Clin Microb 2003;41:4714–17.
[43] Bodey GP, Mardani M, et al. The epidemiology of *Candida glabrata* and *Candida albicans* fungemia in immunocompromised patients with cancer. Am J Med 2002;112:380 - 85.
[44] Badiee P, Alborzi A, et al. Molecular identification and in-vitro susceptibility of *Candida albicans* and *Candida dubliniensis* isolated from immunocompromised patients. Iranian Red Crescent Medicine Journal 2009;11(4):391-97.
[45] Badiee P, Alborzi A, et al. Susceptibility of *Candida* species isolated from immunocompromised patients to antifungal agents. EMHJ 2011;17(5):425-30.
[46] Karabinos IK, Kokladi M, et al. Fungal endocarditis of the superior vena cava: The Role of Transesophageal Echocardiography. Hellenic J Cardiol 2010; 51: 538-39.

[47] Mylonakis E, Calderwood SB. Infective endocarditis in adults.N Engl J Med 2001;345:1318-30.

[48] Ferrieri P, Gewitz MH, et al. Unique features of infective endocarditis in childhood. Circulation 2002;105:2115-26.

[49] Kavey RE, Frank DM, et al. Two-dimensional echocardiographic assessment of infective endocarditis in children. Am J Dis Child 1983;137:851-6.

[50] Morelle W, Bernard M, et al. Galactomannoproteins of *Aspergillus fumigatus*. Eukaryot Cell 2005;4: 1308-16.

[51] Roger TR, Haynes KA, et al. Value of antigen detection in predicting invasive pulmonary aspergillosis. Lancet 1990;336:1210-13.

[52] Stynen D, Sarfati J, et al. Rat monoclonal antibodies against *Aspergillus* galactomannan. Infect Immun 1992;60:2237-45.

[53] Kappe R, Schulze-Berge A. New cause for false positive results with the Pastorex *Aspergillus* antigen latex agglutination test. J Clin Microbiol 1993;31: 2489–90.

[54] Ikuta K, Shibata N, et al. NMR study of the galactomannans of *Trichophyton mentagrophytes* and *Trichophyton rubrum*. Biochem J 1997;323:297-305.

[55] Swanink CM, Meis JF, et al. Specificity of a sandwich enzyme-linked immunosorbent assay for detecting *Aspergillus* galactomannan. J Clin Microbiol 1997;35:257–60.

[56] Verweij PE, Weemaes CM, et al. Failure to detect circulating *Aspergillus* markers in a patient with chronic granulomatous disease and invasive aspergillosis. J Clin Microbiol 2000;38:3900–1.

[57] Gangneux JP, Lavarde D, et al. Transient *Aspergillus* antigenaemia: think of milk. Lancet 2002;359:1251.

[58] Adam O, Aupe´rin A, et al. Treatment with piperacillin-tazobactam and false-positive *Aspergillus* galactomannan antigen test results for patients with hematological malignancies. Clin Infect Dis 2004;38:917-20.

[59] Mattei D, Rapezzi D, et al. A false-positive *Aspergillus* galactomannan enzyme-linked immunosorbent assay results in vivo during amoxicillin-clavulanic acid treatment. J Clin Microbiol 2004;42:5362-63.

[60] Singh N, Obman A, et al. Reactivity of Platelia *Aspergillus* galactomannan antigen with piperacillin-tazobactam: clinical implications based on achievable concentrations in serum. Antimicrob Agents Chemother 2004;48:1989-92.

[61] Hashiguchi K, Niki Y, et al. Cyclophosphamide induces false positive results in detection of *Aspergillus* antigen in urine. Chest 1994;105:975-6.

[62] Pinel C, Fricker-Hidalgo H, et al. Detection of circulating *Aspergillus fumigatus* galactomannan: value and limits of the Platelia test for diagnosing invasive aspergillosis. J Clin Microbiol 2003;41:2184-86.

[63] Sulahian A, Boutboul F, et al. Value of antigen detection using an enzyme immunoassay in the diagnosis and prediction of invasive aspergillosis in two adult and pediatric hematology units during a 4-year prospective study. Cancer 2001;91: 311-18.

[64] Walsh TJ, Hathorn JW, et al. Detection of circulating *Candida* enolase by immunoassayin patients with cancer and invasive candidiasis. N Engl J Med 1991; 324:1026-31.

[65] Mohan das V, Ballal M. Proteinase and phospholipase activity as virulence factors in *Candida* species isolated from blood. Rev Iberoam Micol 2008;25:208-10.

[66] Sendid B, Poirot JL, et al. Combined detection of mannanaemia and anti-mannan antibodies as a strategy for the diagnosis of systemic infection caused by pathogenic *Candida* species. J Med Microbiol 2002;51:433-42.

[67] Bar W, Hecker H. Diagnosis of systemic *Candida* infections in patients of the intensive care unit. Significance of serum antigens and antibodies. Mycoses 2002; 45:22-28.
[68] Odabasi Z, Mattiuzzi G, et al. Beta-D-glucan as a diagnostic adjunct for invasive fungal infections: validation, cutoff development, and performance in patients with acute myelogenous leukemia and myelodysplastic syndrome. Clin Infect Dis 2004;39:199–205.
[69] Ostrosky-Zeichner L, Alexander BD, et al. Multicenter clinical evaluation of the 1,3-β-D-glucan assay as an aid to diagnosis of fungal infections in humans. Clin Infect Dis 2005;41:654–59.
[70] Smith PB, Benjamin DK, et al. Quantification of 1, 3-β-D-glucan levels in children: preliminary data for diagnostic use of the 1, 3-β-D-glucan assays in a pediatric setting. Clin Vaccine Immunol 2007;14:924–5.
[71] Petraitiene R, Petraitis V, et al. Cerebrospinal fluid and plasma 1, 3-β-D-glucan as surrogate markers for detection and monitoring of therapeutic response in experimental hematogenous *Candida* meningoencephalitis. Antimicrob Agents Chemo 2008;52 (11);4121–29.
[72] Badiee P, Kordbacheh P, et al. Early detection of systemic candidiasis in the whole blood of patients with hematological malignancies. Jpn Infec Dis 2009,62: 1-5.
[73] Badiee P, Alborzi A, et al. Comparative Study of gram stain, potassium hydroxide smear, culture and Nested PCR in the diagnosis of fungal keratitis. Ophthalmic Res 2010; 44:251–6.
[74] Badiee P, Alborzi A, et al. Invasive fungal infection in renal transplant recipients demonstrated by panfungal polymerase chain reaction. Exp Clin Transplant 2007; 5(1):624-9.
[75] Badiee P, Alborzi A, et al. Determining the incidence of aspergillosis after liver transplant. Exp Clinl Transplant 2010; 3:220-3.
[76] Yamakami Y, Hashimoto A, et al. PCR detection of DNA specific for Aspergillus species in serum of patients with invasive aspergillosis. J Clin Microbiol.1996; 34(10):2464-68.
[77] Badiee P, Alborzi A. Detection of *Aspergillus* species in bone marrow transplant patients. J Infect Dev Ctries, 2010;4(8),511-6.
[78] Badiee P, Alborzi A, et al. Early diagnosis of systemic candidiasis in bone marrow transplant recipients. Exp Clin Transplant 2010;2:98-103.
[79] Van Burik JA, Myerson D, et al. Panfungal PCR assay for detection of fungal infection in human blood specimens. J Clin Microbiol 1998:36:1169–75.
[80] Badiee P, Alborzi A, et al. Molecular diagnosis of *Aspergillus* endocarditis after cardiac surgery. J Med Microbiol 2009;58(2):192-5.
[81] Loeffler J, Henke N, et al. Quantification of fungal DNA by using fluorescence resonance energy transfer and the light cycler system. J Clin Microbiol 2000;38: 586–90.
[82] Hebart H, Loeffler J, et al. Early detection of *Aspergillus* infection after allogeneic stem cell transplantation by polymerase chain reaction screening. J Infect Dis 2000;181:1713–19.
[83] Badiee P, Kordbacheh P, et al. Study on invasive fungal infections in immune-compromised patients to present a suitable early diagnostic procedure. Intern J Infect Dis 2009;13:97 – 102.
[84] Utley JR, Mills J, et al. The role of valve replacement in the treatment of fungal endocarditis. J Thorac Cardiovasc Surg 1975; 69:255–8.

[85] Jiménez-Expósito MJ, Torres G, Baraldés A, et al. Native valve endocarditis due to *Candida glabrata* treated without valvular replacement: a potential role for caspofungin in the induction and maintenance treatment. Clin Infect Dis 2004; 39:e70.
[86] Pappas PG, Kauffman CA, et al. Clinical practice guidelines for the management of candidiasis: 2009 update by the Infectious Diseases Society of America. Clin Infect Dis 2009; 48:503-35.
[87] Nguyen MH, Nguyen ML, et al. *Candida* prosthetic valve endocarditis: prospective study of six cases and review of the literature. Clin Infect Dis 1996; 22:262-7.
[88] Melamed R, Leibovitz E, et al. Successful non-surgical treatment of *Candida tropicalis* endocarditis with liposomal amphotericin-B (AmBisome). Scand J Infect Dis 2000; 32:86-9.
[89] Rajendram R, Alp NJ, et al. *Candida* prosthetic valve endocarditis cured by caspofungin therapy without valve replacement. Clin Infect Dis 2005; 40:e72.
[90] Talarmin JP, Boutoille D, et al. *Candida* endocarditis: role of new antifungal agents. Mycoses 2009; 52:60-6.
[91] Gumbo T, Taege AJ, et al. *Aspergillus* valve endocarditis in patients without prior cardiac surgery. Medicine 2000;79:261–8.
[92] Muehrcke DD, Lytle BW, et al. Surgical and long-term antifungal therapy for fungal prosthetic valve endocarditis. Ann Thorac Surg 1995; 60:538-43.
[93] Gilbert HM, Peters ED, et al. Successful treatment of fungal prosthetic valve endocarditis: case report and review. Clin Infect Dis 1996; 22:348-54.
[94] Fortún, J; Martín-Dávila, P; et al. Prevention of invasive fungal infections in liver transplant recipients: the role of prophylaxis with lipid formulations of amphotericin B in high-risk patients. Antimicrob Agents Chemother 2003;52: 813–9.
[95] Badiee P, Alborzi A, et al. Distributions and Antifungal Susceptibility of *Candida* Species from Mucosal Sites in HIV Positive Patients. AIM 2010;13 (4): 282-7.
[96] Limper AH, Knox KS, et al. An official american thoracic society statement: treatment of fungal infections in adult pulmonary and critical care patients. Am J Respir Crit Care Med 2011;183(1):96-128.
[97] Nivoix Y, Ubeaud-Sequier G, et al. Drug interactions of triazole antifungal agents in multimorbid patients and implications for patient care. Curr Drug Metab 2009;10:395–409.
[98] Willems L, van der Geest R, et al. Itraconazole oral solution and intravenous formulations: a review of pharmacokinetics and pharmacodynamics. J Clin Pharm Ther 2001;26:159–169.
[99] Venkataramanan R, Zang S, et al. Voriconazole inhibition of the metabolism of tacrolimus in a liver transplant recipient and in liver microsomes. Antimicrob Agents Chemother 2002; 46:3091–93.
[100] Safdar N, Slattery WR, et al. Predictors and outcomes of candiduria in renal transplant recipients. Clin Infect Dis 2005;40:1413-21.
[101] Kuhn DM, George T, et al. Antifungal susceptibility of *Candida* biofilms: unique efficacy of amphotericin B lipid formulations and echinocandins. Antimicrob Agents Chemother 2002;46:1773–80.
[102] Mora-Duarte J, Betts R, et al. Comparison of caspofungin and amphotericin B for invasive candidiasis. N Engl J Med 2002;347: 2020–9.

[103] J Petraitis V, Petraitiene R, et al. Triazole-polyene antagonism in experimental invasive pulmonary aspergillosis: in vitro and in vivo correlation. J Infect Dis 2006; 194:1008-18.
[104] Viscoli C. Combination therapy for invasive aspergillosis. Clin Infect Dis 2004;39:803-5.
[105] Vazquez JA. Clinical practice: combination antifungal therapy for mold infections: much ado about nothing? Clin Infect Dis 2008;46:1889-901.
[106] Nguyen MH; Peacock JE; et al. Therapeutic approaches in patients with candidemia: evaluation in a multicenter, prospective, observational study. Arch Intern Med 1995;155: 2429–35.
[107] Luzzati R, Amalfitano G, et al. Nosocomial candidemia in non-neutropenic patients at an Italian tertiary care hospital. Eur J Clin Microbiol Infect Dis 2000; 19:602–7.
[108] Rex JH, Bennett JE, et al. Intravascular catheter exchange and duration of candidemia: Niaid Mycoses Study Group and the Candidemia Study Group. Clin Infect Dis 1995;21:994–6.
[109] Nucci, M; Anaissie, E. Should vascular catheters be removed from all patients with candidemia? An evidence-based review. Clin Infect Dis 2002;34:591–99.
[110] Walsh TJ, Rex JH. All catheter-related candidemia is not the same: assessment of the balance the risks and benefits of removal of vascular catheters. Clin Infect Dis 2002;34:600-2.
[111] Sullivan KM, Dykewicz CA, et al. Preventing opportunistic infections after hematopoietic stem cell transplantation: The Centers for Disease Control and Prevention, Infectious Diseases Society of America, and American Society for Blood and Marrow Transplantation practice guidelines and beyond. Hematology 2001;1:392-421.
[112] Partridge-Hinckley K, Liddell GM, et al. Infection control measures to prevent invasive mould diseases in hematopoietic stem cell transplant recipients. Mycopathol;168:329-37.
[113] Infection Control Guidelines Control and Prevention of Aspergillosis. 2002 Pages 1-10 Last revised August 2007.
[114] Saha DC, Goldman DL, et al. Serologic evidence for reactivation of cryptococcosis in solid-organ transplant recipients. Clin Vaccine Immunol 2007;14:1550–4.
[115] Marr KA. Empirical antifungal therapy-new options, new tradeoffs. N Engl J Med 2002; 346:278-80.

13

Sterna Wound Complications Following Cardiac Surgery

Zane B. Atkins[1] and Walter G. Wolfe[2]
[1]*Department of Surgery Durham Veterans Affairs Medical Center Durham, NC*
[2]*Department of Surgery Duke University Medical Center Durham, NC*
USA

1. Introduction

Median sternotomy is a commonly performed incision with distinct advantages for exposure of mediastinal and pulmonary hilar structures [1]. However, a well-defined incidence of wound complications is associated with sternotomy, which are costly and potentially lethal in cases of deep sternal wound infection (DSWI) or mediastinitis [2-13]. Not only is DSWI associated with significant perioperative mortality, but historically even successfully treated DSWI is associated with reduced mid- and long-term survival compared with matched cardiac surgical patients without this dreaded postoperative complication [7-12].

In the past 10 years, we have accumulated extensive experience with managing DSWI as a referral center for these difficult problems. We and others have formalized a protocol for managing mediastinal infection utilizing negative pressure wound therapy which allows sternal salvage and improved outcomes in the majority of cases of DSWI [14-16]. This report describes our protocol for managing mediastinitis and presents our results for the past 18 years.

2. Background

Median sternotomy was originally introduced by Milton in 1897 and was performed infrequently for various conditions of the mediastinum until cardiac surgery as a field blossomed in the 1950s [17]. Shumacker first suggested median sternotomy as the procedure of choice for approaches to the heart and great vessels [18] since it avoided the significant pain and other complications, primarily pulmonary- or pleural-based, of the bilateral anterior thoracotomy ("clamshell") incision, which was most frequently used up to that point. However, not until Julian and colleagues demonstrated discrete advantages of the median sternotomy incision for cardiac surgery, particularly improved surgical efficiency, excellent exposure the heart, great vessels, and pulmonary hila, and reduced pulmonary trauma, was a convincing argument for median sternotomy as the incision of choice for cardiac surgical procedures put forth [19 Table 1]. The utility of this incision, the ease and speed of performance, and the common nature of surgically-treated cardiovascular and

STRUCTURE	STERNOTOMY	RIGHT THORACOTOMY	LEFT THORACOTOMY
RIGHT ATRIUM	+++	++	0
RIGHT VENTRICLE	+++	+	+
LEFT ATRIUM	+++	+	+
LEFT VENTRICLE	++	0	+++
SVC	+++	++	0
IVC	+++	++	0
ASC AORTA/root	+++	+	+
RIGHT SCA	++	++	0
INNOMINATE	+++	++	0
LEFT SCA	+	0	+++
DESC AORTA	0	0	+++
Main PA	+++	0	++
RIGHT PA	++	+++	0
LEFT PA	++	0	+++
PROX TRACHEA	++	+	+
ESOPHAGUS	0	+++	++
HEMIDIAPHRAGM	++	+	+
MAIN STEM BRONCHI	0	+++	++

Table 1. Comparison of exposure of various intrathoracic anatomic structures through median sternotomy, right thoracotomy, or left thoracotomy. (+++ denotes excellent, reliable exposure; 0 denotes no reliable exposure)

thoracic diseases in multiple populations approached through this incision are factors which combine to make median sternotomy the most commonly performed osteotomy worldwide [20]. Recently, several alternatives to median sternotomy have been promoted, including thoracoscopic and robotic approaches to cardiac and thoracic procedures [21, 22]. These approaches are possible as a result of high fidelity instrumentation and video platforms but are limited by steep learning curves and expense. Therefore, for most hospital systems performing cardiac surgical procedures, median sternotomy remains the mainstay incision.

3. Definition and classification

There is still no universally accepted method for treatment of DSWI or other sternal wound complication. One possible explanation for this is that until relatively recently, thorough classification schemes providing specific criteria for assignment as deep sternal infection, mediastinitis, superficial infection, or sterile sternal dehiscence were lacking. However, it is important to distinguish between these individual entities since each demands a different management strategy. Furthermore, results of reported series which include a variety of wound complications will differ from those that report a homogenous population. For example, sternal wound infections that are limited to the superficial soft tissues obviously demand less aggressive intervention for treatment and will generally respond more readily to treatment than deep sternal infection with higher likelihood for success. Therefore, when comparing different treatment modalities for sternal wound infection, it is important to be clear about the extent of infection, since heterogeneity could skew reported results.

Two prominent classification schemes have been proposed and are in use. Mediastinal dehiscence or the more chronic form, sternal nonunion, is defined as sternal wound disruption without any evidence for infection either clinically or pathologically [23, 24]. These entities will not be discussed in any detail. In contrast, mediastinitis, as characterized by the U.S. Centers for Disease Control and Prevention (CDC), is an infection of the mediastinum diagnosed by isolation of pathogenic organisms from the mediastinal fluid or tissue especially when there is obvious evidence of infection at the time of sternal exploration [25]. Alternatively, a combination of clinical features including chest pain, sternal drainage with bony instability, fevers, radiographic findings such as widened mediastinum, and bacterial isolation may also warrant a diagnosis of mediastinitis. Obviously, from the surgical perspective, these definitions are somewhat lacking since either superficial infections, confined to the soft tissues, or deep infections, involving the bone and/or retrosternal space could produce bacteremia and clinical signs of severe infection [23].

Fortunately, more descriptive classification schemes have been introduced and provide more specific insight into the pathologic involvement of the sternal tissues and the clinical consequences and course [23, 26, 27]. For example, the classification scheme introduced by El Oakley and Wright is based on the time at which the patient presents with mediatiastinitis relative to the initial surgical procedure [23]. Schulman et al have advocated a similar classification system [27]. In addition, the El Oakley description also accounts for relevant risk factors underlying the clinical scenario and whether or not previous attempts to treat the sternal wound infection have been made and failed [Table 2]. Therefore, five distinct categories of infection are described, each with important treatment implications. For example, the subtypes I and II appear to respond well to primary sternal closure with mediatinal irrigation, while subtypes III-V appear to require more aggressive sternal debridement and repair techniques [23].

Classification	Description of Infection
Type 1	Mediastinitis within 2 weeks of operation without risk factors
Type 2	Mediastinitis between 2 and 6 weeks of operation without risk factors
Type 3a	Type 1 with one or more risk factors
Type 3b	Type 2 with one or more risk factors
Type 4a	Type 1, 2, or 3 after one failed therapy
Type 4b	Type 1, 2, or 3 after more than one failed therapy
Type 5	Mediastinitis presenting 6 weeks or more after operation

Table 2. Classification scheme of mediastinitis introduced by El Oakley and Wright based on the time at which the patient presents with mediatiastinitis relative to the initial surgical procedure (modified from El Oakley and Wright [23]).

The classification by Jones et al differs from that of El Oakley and Wright in that it is more descriptive anatomically and physiologically [26, TABLE 3]. Three different "types" of sternal infection are described, encompassing both superficial and deep infections, and based on the degree of underlying tissue involvement with infection. We have preferred the use of this classification system as it is simpler to use since it based strictly on features observed or encountered at the time of initial sternal exploration. In addition, Type 3b is physiologically meaningful since it denotes the patient who is systemically ill from the sternal wound process. In our own institutional experience of 222 adult cardiac surgical patients treated for postoperative DSWI, approximately 50% of patients exhibited septicemia (Jones 3b) upon initial presentation [14].

Class	Depth of Involvement	Description
1a	Superficial	Skin/subcutaneous tissue dehiscence
1b	Superficial	Exposed deep fascia, sutures intact
2a	Deep	Exposed bone, stable wired sternotomy
2b	Deep	Exposed bone, unstable wired sternotomy
3a	Deep	Exposed necrotic or fractured bone, unstable, heart exposed
3b	Deep	Types 2 or 3 with septicemia

Table 3. Mediastinal wound classification system modified from Jones et al [26]. Although anatomic involvement by infection in distinguished, the presence of septicemia is the most important feature clinically.

4. Risk factors and pathophysiology

Multiple different etiologies for development of DSWI have been invoked over time. For example, most infections were traditionally thought to arise as a result of breaks in proper surgical technique, prompting strict guidelines for sterile surgical technique. In addition, secondary involvement the mediastinum from remote sites such as leg incisions or the pulmonary tree has also been suggested as a mechanism for DSWI. The "endogenous pathway," seeding of the mediastinum from other host sources, does appear to be important in the development of *S. aureus* mediastinitis. To illustrate, Jakob et al showed that nasal carriage of *S. aureus* was an independent predictor of sternal infection postoperatively [28], while others have demonstrated that application of mupirocin to the nares of *S. aureus* colonized individuals can help reduce postoperative infection [29]. More recently, other factors have been recognized as important contributors to cardiac surgical site infections. For instance, the appropriate timing of perioperative antibiotics and strict perioperative glucose control are both associated with reduced surgical wound infectious complications [30, 31].

Several different patient-related factors have been repeatedly implicated in the development of DSWI, most consistently obesity and diabetes mellitus [5, 6, 32, TABLE 4]. Eklund et al and others have observed that increasing severity of obesity elevates the risk for surgical site infection in a step-wise fashion [6, 13, 33]. Furthermore, when obesity is described in terms of percentage body fat, the relationship between obesity and surgical site infection is nearly linear and appears more accurate than use of body mass index as a descriptor of obesity [34]. Potential explanations for relationship between obesity and DSWI include technical problems

Study	# Patients	Identified Risk Factors
Milano CA, et al. Circulation 1995 [9]	6,459	Obesity, NYHA class, redo surgery, CPB duration
Toumpoulis IK, et al. Chest 2005 [55]	3,760	Diabetes, preoperative hemodynamic instability, renal failure, bilateral IMA, sepsis and/or endocarditis
Immer FF, et al. Ann Thorac Surg 2005 [94]	5,690	Obesity, diabetes mellitus, COPD, bilateral IMA
Fowler G, et al. Circulation 2005 [13]	300,000	Obesity (BMI of 30-40 kg/m^2), diabetes, previous MI, urgent operative status, hypertension
Prabhakar G, et al. Ann Thorac Surg 2002 [32]	559,004	Obesity
Sjorgren J, et al. Ann Thorac Surg 2005 [90]	4,826	Diabetes, obesity, reduced EF, renal failure, multi-vessel CAD
Olsen MA, et al. J Thorac Cardiovasc Surg 2002 [10]	1,980	Obesity (BMI>30 kg/m^2), diabetes, > 4 units RBC transfusion, IABP, current smoking
Cayci C,et al. Ann Plast Surg 2008 [52]	7,978	Obesity (BMI>30 kg/m^2), diabetes, urgent operation, recent smoking; h/o CVA, total HLOS, sepsis/endocarditis postop
Risnes I, et al. Ann Thorac Surg 2010 [12]	18,352	COPD, obesity (BMI > 30 kg/m^2), blood transfusion, advanced age, male sex, diabetes

Table 4. Compiled analyses for underlying risk factors associated with sternal wound infection. Obesity and diabetes mellitus are consistently shown to be independent predictors of poststernotomy mediastinitis.

during surgery owing to the patient's size, increased bleeding, increased deadspace in the wound, and ineffective or inadequate dosing of perioperative antibiotics [6, 9].

Although multiple mechanisms for sternal wound complications are proposed, it is widely accepted that reduced sternal perfusion, often by virtue of internal mammary artery (IMA) harvesting for use as a vascular conduit in coronary artery revascularization, is one of the most important causes of sternal nonhealing and infection [1-6, 8, 26], especially when both IMAs are harvested for bypass graft surgery [5]. Therefore, more cases of DSWI appear to occur after coronary artery bypass grafting or after combined procedures that include coronary artery surgery [7, 35]. Other viable explanations for DSWI etiology include poor bone stock from osteoporosis, malnutrition, and other factors; poorly performed sternotomy leading to sternal fractures and/or costosternal disassociation; and other patient related factors including peripheral vascular disease and lung disease [8, 36]. Several other factors have been implicated in the development of DSWI but may not be manifest in the context of a retrospective review or randomized trial because the numbers are too low. For example, it is generally accepted that postoperative steroids or chronic immunosuppression increases risk for DSWI, but this has been difficult to demonstrate in even large database reviews [13, 37]. Finally, Risnes et al have demonstrated in a review of over 18,000 consecutive patients undergoing coronary artery surgery in Norway, the major preventable risk factor associated with the development of DSWI was the amount of blood product transfusion perioperatively [12].

Several risk analyses are available to estimate the individual patient's propensity for developing DSWI. For example, using Society of Thoracic Surgery National Cardiac Database information, Fowler et al created a model to estimate the risk for systemic infection after coronary artery bypass surgery using patient characteristics available preoperatively [13]. The Fowler model also provides for inclusion of important intraoperative details known to influence postoperative infection including the need for intra-aortic balloon counterpulsation and prolonged cardiopulmonary bypass times [13]. Although the model devised by Fowler et al was based on various cases of major infection after coronary artery surgery, including DSWI, the authors did validate the model as predictive of infection in a test population from the STS Database, and the model was also recently validated in a different cohort of patients from the UK as being predictive of DSWI [38]. The EuroSCORE system also has been shown to predict infection and associated mortality with acceptable discrimination [39].

5. Incidence

Despite advancements in most aspects of perioperative care, rates of sternal wound complications, including mediastinitis, following adult cardiac surgery have varied little over the past 30 years [2-6], although incremental reduction in single center rates of DSWI have been noted and attributed to adjunctive measures such as strict perioperative glucose control [40]. As noted previously, rates of DSWI vary with regard to the specific definition used to describe the pathology encountered and the patient population studied. In general, reported rates of DSWI are relatively low, ranging from 0.25% to 3.6 % [2-9, 38, 39, 41, 42]. However, the incidence of superficial sternal infection excedes that of deep sternal infection by as many as three times [10, 41, 43], and Francel has stated that as many as 70% of patients with poststernotomy infection will have superficial tissue involvement [44].

6. Diagnosis

Depending on the virulent nature of the sternal wound infection, patients typically present within 30 days of cardiac surgery. The most common symptoms include sternal wound drainage, sternal instability, fever, and malaise. In many cases, a high index of suspicion is required to establish the diagnosis, especially when classic signs and symptoms are absent. In addition, it is often difficult to distinguish on physical examination the difference between deep sternal wound infection (infection present beneath the sternum) and superficial sternal infection. Therefore, early wound opening and inspection with appropriate sampling of tissue for bacteriologic assessment is strongly encouraged when sufficient clinical suspicion exists.

One of the most reliable signs of DSWI is sternal instability, which frequently implies a deeper problem than can be appreciated at the superficial level [44]. While sternal instability can be tested on physical examination, we have often noted that the patient themselves will typically report sternal clicking with inspiration, cough, or various other physical maneuvers, so this information should be thoughtfully considered if DSWI diagnosis is being entertained.

The use of various radiographic examinations is often encouraged when evaluating for DSWI, and, in fact, is included as part of the CDC guidelines for defining mediastinitis [25]. Formerly, PA and lateral chest radiograph was the investigative procedure of choice, where details such as a "sternal stripe" indicated present of air between the two sternal halves. The lateral displacement of one or more sternal wires, secondary to tearing of the wire through one side of the sternum, has been a frequently noted finding in the case of poststernotomy infection [37]. More recently, chest computed tomography has been suggested as the procedure of choice for assessing sternal wound infection when a diagnosis cannot be established by clinical examination alone [45, 46]. Mediastial fluid collections, free gas bubbles, soft tissue swelling, pleural effusions, sternal dehiscence, and subcutaneous fluid collections have been the predominant CT findings in cases of DSWI [47], but these features appear to be more specific and sensitive for DSWI presenting more than 3 weeks after surgery [48].

7. Morbidity and mortality

Mediastinal infection negatively impacts early, mid-term, and long-term survival after adult heart surgery [2, 7-12]. While it is intuitive that clinically serious DSWI reduces 30-day and/or in-hospital survival relative to similar patients not suffering this complications, the effect of DSWI on long-term survival is especially insulting since many patients referred for heart surgery expect to gain a survival advantage compared with other treatment options for their underlying heart disease [49].

Prior to the development of modern protocols for DSWI management, which include thorough sternal debridement and use of vascularized flaps to repair the mediastinal defect resulting from debridement, early mortality from DSWI exceeded 50% [50]. In the "modern era," reported rates of in-hospital or 30-day DSWI mortality for range from 7% to over 30% [11,14, 35, 42, 51, 52]. In our own recent experience, early mortality for DSWI is approximately 16% [14]. Therefore, despite many advancements in intensive care medicine, DSWI continues to be a deadly complication. Death in the early period is typicaly the result of sepsis or other infectious complications including multiorgan failure [12]. Morisaki et al. recently demonstrated methicillin-resistent *S. aureus* infection to be an independent risk factor for in-hospital mortality in their cohort of poststernotomy DSWI patients [53].

Patients surviving infectious complications and the acute insult of DSWI exhibit reduced mid-term survival compared with controls. For example, one-year mortality for DSWI following CABG is significantly increased compared with similar patients who did not develop DSWI [2, 8, 10]. Milano et al and Braxton et al both demonstrated a doubling of mid-term mortality among patients with DSWI after CABG compared with controls [9, 54]. Karra et al examined predictors of one-year mortality after treatment for DSWI and found that delay in closing the mediastinal defect; age over 65 years; need for ICU care prior to sternal debridement; and methicillin-resistent *S. aureus* infections were each independently associated with mortality [7].

Long-term survival has consistently been demonstrated to suffer in patients with a history of poststernotomy DSWI [5, 8, 9, 12, 35, 52, 54-56, Figure 1]. For example, Filsoufi et al reviewed nearly 5,800 adult heart surgery patients at a single institution over 8 years and found DSWI to be associated with significantly reduced 5-year survival compared with patients who did not develop DSWI [35]. Similarly, Risnes et al reviewed their experience of over 18,000 cardiac surgical patients with a mean follow-up of over 10 years. Long-term survival for patients whose course was complicated by DSWI was <50% compared with >70% for patients without DSWI, and DSWI was independently associated with reduced long-term survival after cardiac surgery [HR 1.59; 95% CI 1.16 - 2.70, $p = 0.003$] [12]. Similar data have been also been reported by Toumpoulis et al. [55].

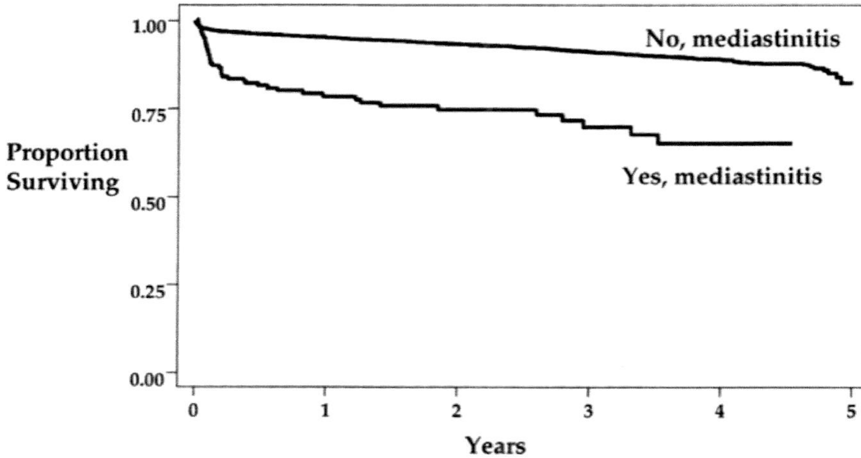

Fig. 1. From Braxton et al with permission [8], patients suffering mediastinal infection after coronary artery bypass grafting have worse overall long-term survival compared with similar patients not experiencing the complication.

It is unclear as to the specific reasons for worse long-term survival after DSWI is successfully treated, but cardiac-related deaths or progression of cardiovascular disease appears to be a common cause of death for those with DSWI [8, 12]. In addition, Chu et al recently reported that patients with peripheral vascular disease had worse outcomes long-term after coronary artery surgery [57]. We recently evaluated long-term survival in a cohort of 222 adult cardiac surgical patients treated at Duke University Hospital for poststernotomy mediastinitis. Using multivariable regression analysis and at a mean follow-up of 5.5 years, the following variables were noted to be independently associated with survival: heart failure [Hazard ratio (HR) 1.58, $p = 0.029$]; sepsis [HR 2.38, $p < 0.001$]; peripheral vascular disease [HR 2.06, $p = 0.001$], age > 65 years [HR 1.61, $p = 0.037$]; and take back for bleeding [HR 2.96; $p = 0.007$] (unpublished data).

Not only does DSWI lead to increased mortality among post-surgical patients, it is also closely associated with other types of postoperative complications. For example, in a recent review of morbidity following coronary surgery from the Virginia Cardiac Surgery Quality Initiative, DSWI was the not only the most expensive complication, but it was also associated with a longer length of hospital stay, by more than two full weeks, than any other single postoperative complication, including perioperative stroke and renal failure [4]. Other reports have corroborated the impact of DSWI on overall hospital length of stay [2, 6, 52]. Speir et al also demonstrated that DSWI was the most likely form of postoperative morbidity to be associated with other complications such as prolonged ventilation, bleeding, renal failure, and atrial fibrillation [4]. DSWI has also been associated with increased rates of stroke, need for inotropic or mechanical cardiac support, and perioperative myocardial infarction, renal failure, and prolonged mechanical ventilation [12, 51].

8. Microbiology

Numerous bacterial pathogens may contribute to DSWI, but the most commonly isolated organisms are *Staphylococcus*, either coagulase-negative *Staphylococcus* (CNS) or *S. aureus*

[58]. In our own recently described experience, methicillin-sensitive and methicillin-resistent *S. aureus* each accounted for 35% of wound isolates, while CNS was present in 12%, and gram negative organisms were found in 18% [14]. It is noteworthy that our protocols for preoperative preparation of the cardiac surgical patient do not routinely incorporate mupirocin treatment. Additionally, many patients included in our cohort of patients treated for DSWI underwent primary cardiac surgery at referring facilities. Therefore, specific details in these patients predisposing to a certain pathogen were often lacking. Risk factors for the development of methicillin-resistent *S. aureus* poststernotomy mediastinitis include previous hospitalization and takeback for bleeding after the original cardiac surgical procedure [59]. Gardlund et al have attributed the development of *S. aureus* infection to the development of bacteremia [60], which is corroborated by our own data in which 50% of patients treated for DSWI had evidence of bacteremia or septicemia (Jones classification 3b) at the time of clinical presentation with DSWI [14]. Finally, it has been demonstrated that methicillin-resistent strains of *S. aureus* are more virulent and deadly than methicillin-sensitive strains, and, in fact, methicillin resistance was the only independent predictor of early mortality in one analysis [61].

In contrast, *S. epidermidis* often presents with a rather indolent course, often not manifesting clinically until 3 weeks or more postoperatively [62]. CNS is frequently isolated in cases of sternal instability or nonunion, which may itself arise from obesity or acute or chronic pulmonary disease [60]. CNS has recently been noted to of increasing incidence and has been reported to be present in roughly 50% of sternal infections in some series [6, 11, 60].

Gram negative organisms contribute less commonly to the pathogenesis of DSWI. Gram-negative infections of the mediastinum classically arise in the setting of other postoperative infectious complications such pneumonia, urinary tract infections, intra-abdominal infections, or other nosocomial infections [58, 60]. Mekontso-Dessap et al reviewed their experience with DSWI after cardiac surgery and found that Enterococcus species were the most common isolates in early cases of DSWI (<14 days), which likely arise from translocation of these bacteria from other sources in the host [63]. In contrast, *Staphylococcus* species, often CNS, were the most common isolates in cases presenting more remotely from the original surgery [63].

9. Cost of DSWI

One of the most impactful consequences of DSWI is the costs incurred in its management, in part due to the multiple associated conditions that frequently complicate the clinical picture of these sick patients [4, 12]. The average hospital costs for patients treated for DSWI is approximately 2.5 to 3 times that of similarly matched patients who enjoy an uncomplicated postoperative course [23, 64, 65]. As noted, increased costs are primarily attributed to associated comorbid conditions that arise during the treatment of mediastinitis, increased length of hospital stays, including frequent need for ICU services, and the need for multiple surgical procedures when using traditional approaches to DSWI [4, 23]. For example, Hollenbeak et al found that patients with DSWI remained hospitalized an average of 3 weeks longer than noninfected patients after coronary artery surgery [2]. Interestingly, in the same study it was noted that DSWI patients who ultimately expired incurred nearly $61,000 US dollars more in costs than other DSWI patients who ultimately survived, presumably secondary to the multiple comorbidities associated with clinically aggressive mediastinitis [2]. Using more recently acquired information, Speir et al found that mediastinitis was the single

most costly complication in Virginia after coronary artery surgery, raising the cost of care by over $62,000 US dollars, or more than 240% increase, on average, [4].
Therefore, it is apparent that treatment of these critically ill patients is extremely expensive to the hospital system, even if the complication is uncommonly encountered. As a result, and based on increased scrutiny of various hospital-associated conditions, the US Center for Medicare and Medicaid Services no longer reimburses for hospital costs incurred in treatment of DSWI following coronary artery bypass surgery [66]. Interestingly, however, it appears that use of negative pressure therapy in the treatment of DSWI contains associated costs. For example, Mokhtari et al reported the use of VAC therapy to be cost effective and efficacious in eradicating mediastinal infection [65]. In our own experience, patients treated with negative pressure therapy for DSWI had costs that were $150,000 US dollars less than the average Medicare charges for treatment required for DSWI ($152,00 vs. $ 300,000) [67].

10. Treatment of DSWI

Upon establishing the diagnosis of sternal wound infection, the immediate goal of treatment is complete eradication of infection followed by stabilization of the sternum and chest wall. Multiple strategies for managing mediastinitis have been proposed and range from open mediastinal packing to debridement with closure over drains, to placement of vascularized tissue flaps. In addition, negative pressure therapy (NPT) has been used to aide in the treatment of mediastinal infection, as first reported in 1999 [68]. Several initial series described the use of NPT for treating mediastinitis and outlined potential benefits of this approach to controlling mediastinal infection [15, 16, 45, 69, 70]. However, a consensus as to best treatment for mediastinal infection has yet to be established. For example, Schimmer et al recently surveyed 79 cardiac surgery programs in Germany to query DSWI management strategies [71]. They found that approximately 1/3 of the centers preferentially used NPT for controlling mediastinal contamination, while another 1/3 use closed chest irrigation, and another 1/3 combine management approaches [71]. Other groups continue to advocate more aggressive surgical therapy in addressing infected sternal wounds [7, 72].
Initially, the primary treatment for DSWI was open packing followed by secondary closure [73]. This method was labor intensive, cumbersome, and was characterized by significant rates of recurrent infection and other complications [58]. Shortly thereafter, Schumaker and Mandelbaum proposed early closure over drains [74], which allowed continual irrigation of the infected mediastinum [73, 74]. Although this approach represented an improvement relative to open packing procedure, the latter procedure was still associated with failure rates of at least 25% [73].
Omental flap repair of the infected mediastinum was originally reported in 1976 by Lee [75] and has been shown to have distinct advantages over continuous antiobiotic irrigation through drains [76] and over muscle flaps for sternal wound defect repair [9, 14]. This is thought to occur by obliterating dead space, a mechanism that can also be credited to muscle flap repair of the open mediastinum [26]. However, the omentum may have angiogenic and immunologic properties that stimulate more complete sternal defect healing [58]. Other advantages of using the greater omentum to flap the sternal defect include superior malleability and excellent blood flow. As originally described, traditional omental flap repair of the mediastinum involves a laparotomy to mobilize and place the graft through the anterior portion of the diaphragm [Figure 2]. More recently, harvesting the

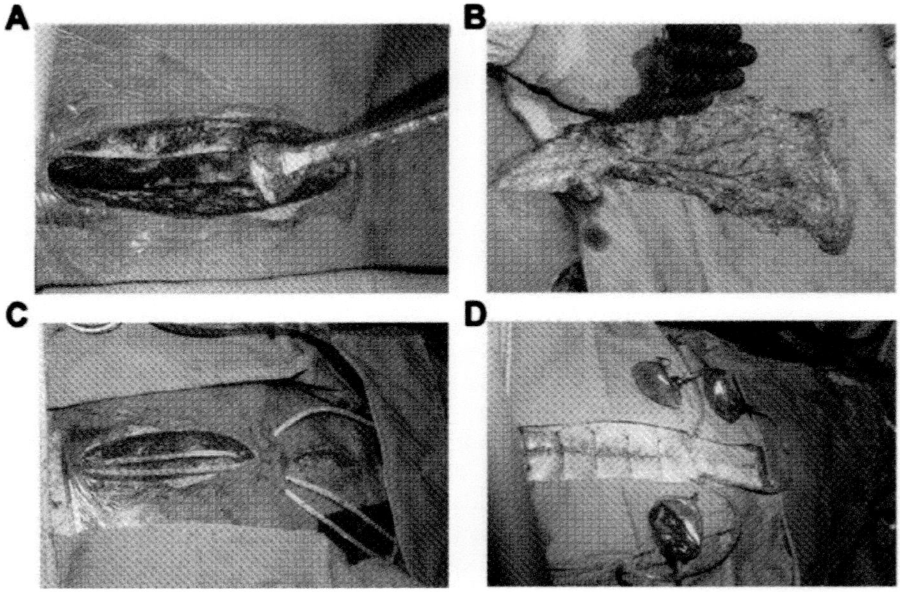

Fig. 2. Preparation of the omental flap graft for transfer to the mediastinum from Milano et al with permission [80]. After preparation of the mediastinum [A], a laparotomy is performed and the greater omental graft is prepared by mobilizing it from the transverse colon [B]. Once the graft is tunneled through an anterior diaphragm incision, it is secured in the mediastinum to fill the defect. Care is taken to avoid twisting or kinking the omental graft as it is delivered from the abdomen into the mediastinum [C]. The mediastinum is then closed over drains with retention sutures. The drains are placed to bulb suction [D].

omental pedicle using a laparoscopic approach may have advantages over open abdominal procedures and has been utilized successfully [77].

Jurkiewicz et al first reported on the successful use of muscle flaps in DSWI in 1980 [78], while the Emory groups' experience with muscle flap repair of the infected mediastinum refined approaches and clarified advantages of these techniques [26]. As with omental flap repair, discrete advantages of complete mediastinal repair with vascularized muscle flaps were demonstrated as compared with closed chest irrigation [26, 79]. Milano et al compared omental and pectoralis muscle flap repairs for the infected mediastinum and found that procedural details, early complications, and hospital length of stay were all improved with omental flap repair [80]. Omental flap repair also trended towards improved survival and reduced chronic pain when compared with pectoralis flap procedures [80]. In fact, significant long-term complications can be associated with muscle flap repair of the mediastinum including paresthesias, sternal instability, truncal weakness, and prolonged pain syndromes [9, 26, 81, 82]. Reporting on the long term results of muscle flap coverage of the mediastinum, Ringelman noted persistent pain in over 50% of patients, numbness and paresthesias in 44%, sternal instability in over 40%, and shoulder weakness in 1/3 of patients [82]. It is worth noting, however, that unfavorable outcomes with open packing and/or mediastinal irrigation prompted recommendations for aggressive mediastinal debridement including radical sternectomy

[78, 83]. While effective in removing devitalized and infected tissue, the resulting sternal defect required large-volume vascularized tissue such as muscle flaps or large omental flaps to obliterate deadspace. As a result, many of the negative long-term consequences often experienced and attributed to muscle flap repair may actually have originated with radical sternal debridement. After the introduction of NPT management of mediastinal sepsis/infection, radical sternal debridement has been de-emphasized [14, 16, 83, 84]. Stated differently, the use of NPT to treat the infected mediastinum helps to avoid radical sternal debridement and likely avoids chronic syndromes previously seen and perhaps erroneously attributed to treatment methods.

Obdeijn et al introduced the use of negative pressure therapy (NPT) for treatment of the infected mediastinum after median sternotomy [68]. The introduction of vacuum-assisted closure (VAC®) technology [Kinetic Concepts Inc. USA San Antonio, TX], based on the application of negative or subatmospheric pressure to the wound, has improved management of DSWI, as demonstrated by several groups including our own, and is now considered a cornerstone in the management of these complex clinical scenarios [14, 15, 70, 73]. Negative pressure therapy appears to induce effective proliferation of the effectors of wound healing [85] removes wound exudates, improves regional blood flow [86], and reduces accumulation of inflammatory mediators such that earlier and more complete wound healing results [70]. Laboratory studies also show that NPT induces early wound healing through microdeformations within the wound, stimulating cell division, proliferation, and angiogenesis [73, 87]. One distinct advantage of the mechanisms of NPT is more thorough eradication of infection, stimulation of vigorous wound granulation, and the subsequent promotion of safe and effective sternal closure either primarily or with rigid osteosynthesis [11, 14, 88]. Wound treatment with NPT appears to be significantly lower rates of recurrent wound complications such as reinfection, seromas, or hematomas [14, 89, 90]. However, there is a recognized tendency for recurrent infection when MRSA is the inciting organism or with prolonged mechanical ventilation [91].

Clinically, NPT has been associated with significantly lower mortality rates in the acute management of mediastinitis [11, 89]. For instance, Petzina et al recently compared 118 patients with poststernotomy DSWI and demonstrated that patients treated with NPT had better survival and less sternal re-infection compared with patients in whom NPT was not used [89]. In addition, as may have been expected, shorter hospital stays were noted within the NPT group. Baillot et al reported similar results by, while documenting a reduction in acute DSWI mortality from 14.1% to less than 5% when NPT was incorporated into treatment regimens [11]. Finally, De Feo et al evaluated 157 patients with poststernotomy DSWI at a single institution over 15 years. Patients in whom NPT was incorporated in the treatment regimen had reduced early mortality rates and, reduced reinfection rates, and slightly reduced overall hospital stays [92].

As noted previously, long term mortality among patients with DSWI has been historically poor compared with similar patients not suffering the complication, but recent evidence suggests this may be changing. The first evidence for this phenomenon was reported by Sjogren et al, who compared 46 patients with poststernotomy mediastinitis managed with NPT with a matched cohort of cardiac surgical patients not experiencing postoperative mediastinitis [93]. Actuarial and adjusted 5-year survival was not different between groups, demonstrating for the first time that long-term results of heart surgery were not negatively impacted by DSWI [Figure 3].

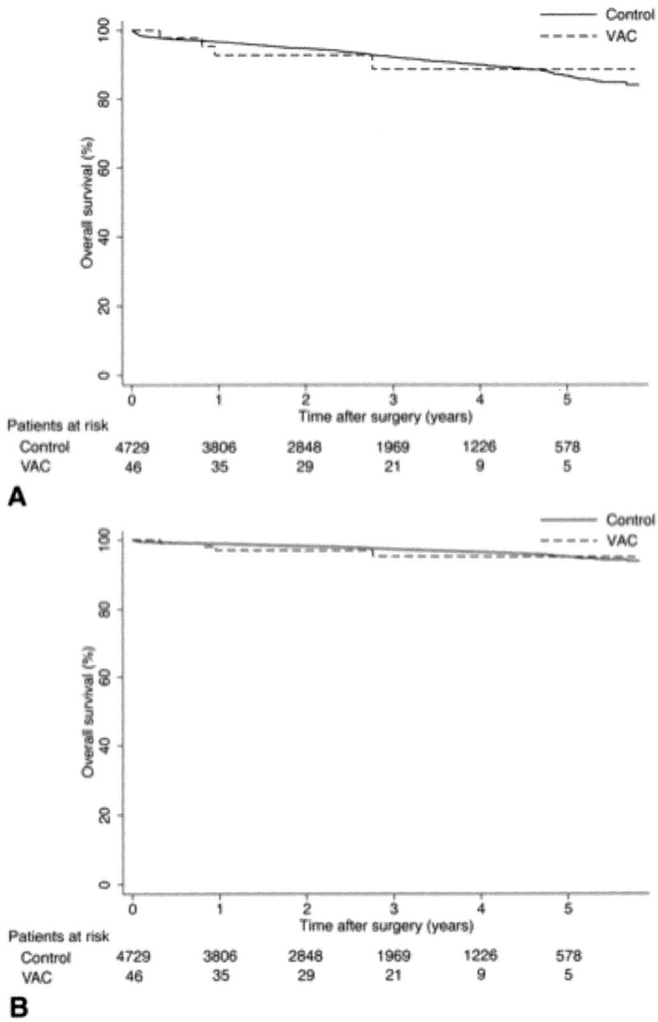

Fig. 3. Actuarial (panel A) and adjusted (panel B) survival curves for patients with poststernotomy mediastinitis treated with vacuum-assisted closure (VAC) as compared to control subjects who did not experience mediastinitis after heart surgery. No difference in long-term survival was demonstrated between the groups. From Sjogren et al [93], with permission.

Another study from the UK demonstrated that midterm survival for patients with postoperative mediastinitis was similar to patients not suffering the complication [51]. Similar results have been reported by Cayci et al from Columbia University, who found that DSWI was associated with increased early mortality but long-term survival was not different from controls. Furthermore, DSWI was not an independent predictor of mortality in their single-center experience [52]. It is unclear as to why this may be the case, but it is notable that NPT was used in over 80% of patients with mediastinitis as a means for clearing infection, and nearly 50% of patients in their cohort were managed with vac therapy alone or vac + secondary sternal closure. In our own series, we found that use of NPT for controlling mediastinal infection was an independent predictor of survival on multivariable analysis [unpublished data], and that patients managed with NPT had significantly improved long term survival compared with patients not treated with NPT [Figure 4].

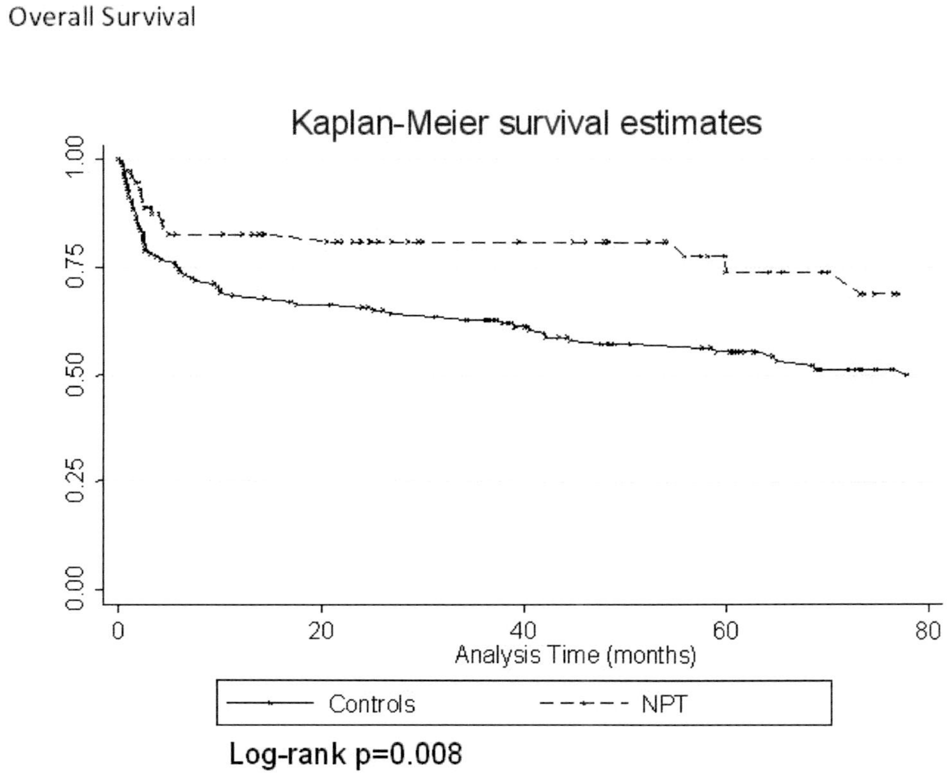

Fig. 4. Kaplan Meier survival curves for patients with poststernotomy mediastinitis treated with negative pressure therapy (NPT) or by traditional means for controlling mediastinal infection (controls). Patients treated with NPT had significantly improved long-term survival by log rank analysis.

11. Suggested treatment algorithms for DSWI

While accumulating extensive experience with DSWI management as a referral center for these difficult problems. We and others have formalized protocols for managing mediastinal infection utilizing NPT which allows sternal salvage and improved outcomes in the majority of cases of DSWI [14-16, Figure 5].

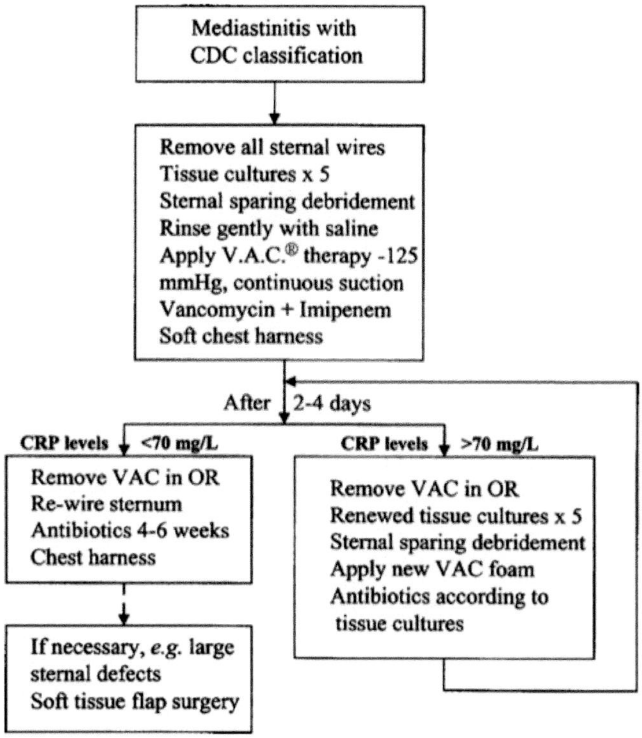

Fig. 5. Suggested algorithm for management of mediastinal infection after cardiac surgery via median sternotomy, with permission from Sjogren et al [15]. Emphasis is placed on gentle sternal debridement, negative pressure therapy to the mediastinum, and closure based on monitored serum C-reactive protein levels.

As noted previously, successful treatment of DSWI begins with recognition of signs and symptoms of sternal infection, which may occasionally be subtle. Sternal wound exploration to ensure a prompt and accurate diagnosis is warranted when signs of mediastinitis are present. This approach also helps to distinguish between superficial and deep sternal infections. At the time of initial sternal exploration, tissues and fluid should be obtained for bacteriologic analysis. Targeted antibiotic therapy for 4-6 weeks duration is prescribed and is determined by the culture results [14, 15]. If the infectious process extends beneath the facial layer, all sternal hardware should be removed. The sternum itself is then gently debrided of grossly devitalized tissue, but wide excision of the sternum is not necessary and may be injurious and counterproductive. Limited sternal debridement is now preferred and good results have been seen with this approach [14, 16, 83, 93, 94]. Negative pressure therapy is then instituted on the opened incision after limited sternal debridement. The polyurethane foam is subsequently changed in the operating room or at the bedside every 2-3 days. During this time, assessment as to the state of the sternum is made to determine if mediastinal flap repair is required or if secondary sternal closure is possible. Our general approach for determining when the sternum can reliably be reapproximated is based on the state of the sternum after several days of NPT. Wound characteristics precluding secondary sternal reapproximation include multiple transverse sternal fractures, poor bone stock, costosternal separation, or the requirement for such extensive sternal debridement that reapproximation of the sternal halves is not feasible. Gustafsson en et al have advocated use of serum C-reactive protein levels to guide wound closure timing [95, Figure 6]. C-reactive protein levels less than 70 mg/L corresponded with successful sternal reapproximation [95]. Successes have also been reported with sternal plating as a treatment for the fractured sternum [11, 96], but our approach has been conservative in this regard since any residual infectious process could contaminate the implanted hardware [91].

Numerous clinical advantages for DSWI management protocols incorporating NPT have been observed, many centered upon the sternal stabilization achieved when vacuum-assisted clousure is engaged [70]. The sternal stability afforded by NPT improves pain compared with open packing or other approaches for addressing the infected mediastinum [88]. In addition, the stabilized sternum yields several pulmonary benefits, the first of which is the ability to successfully separate from mechanical ventilation. This promotes earlier and more effective patient mobilization and prevents the patient from being confined to bed, where other complications common to DSWI therapy are often incurred [70]. Negative pressure therapy also improves ventilation and overall pulmonary function and leads to more effective chest physiotherapy [70, 97]. Importantly, no deleterious hemodynamic effects of NPT have been documented although this has been speculated [70].

12. Complications of treating mediastinitis

It has been estimated that approximately 15% of patients develop recurrent infection [98]. In the experience of Bapat et al, this has included recurrent infection with the same organism associated with the original sternal infection [99], and we speculate that if the polyurethane foam required for NPT is not adequately inserted with each dressing change, small, isolated spaces may arise within the wound that can become superinfected. We recently reported rates of recurrent wound complications associated with various mediastinal flap coverages. For example, muscle flap repair of the treated mediastinum, consisting predominantly of pectoralis muscle flaps, was associated with increased rates of recurrent wound complications such as hematoma, seromas, and recurrent infection [14]. Conversely, use of NPT prior to definitive repair of the sternal wound defect was associated with increased rates of successful secondary sternal closure without the need for any flap transfer, and with shortened length of hospital stay after definitive repair. Excellent results have been reported elsewhere when NPT is incorporated into management protocols for DSWI [65].

Petzina et al recently reported a 7.2% rate of "major complications" associated with NPT for DSWI in a cohort of 69 patients. Most complications were bleeding-related [100]. On the other hand, cardiac function and hemodynamics appear to be stable during NPT to the open mediastinal wound [101, 102].

When NPT is used, caution should be exercised with regard to the length of therapy. In our own experience, prolonged use of NPT leads to a "frozen" mediastinum, making subsequent closure by vascularized flaps or other technique difficult to perform and places the cardiac structures at risk for injury during subsequent sternal repair. Others have noted the similar difficultiess [99]. In such cases, continued application of NPT to closure by secondary intent may be the best therapeutic option rather than to place the mediastinal structures at risk for injury during attempted flap repair.

13. Can mediastinitis be prevented?

Loop has stated: "prevention and better treatment of sternal wound complications must be a major goal in assuring the highest quality of cardiovascular care…[5]. Although most efforts towards DSWI have focused on the treatment of DSWI, several methods to reduce rates of mediastinitis have been proposed and validated recently. As a result, efforts to prevent mediastinal infection may already be working. For instance, investigators from Boston recently reported on their experience with DSWI between 1992 and 2006, separating analysis into early and late time periods. They noted that DSWI had decreased from 1.57% to 0.88% over the last 5 years of their analysis and attributed the positive findings to adoption of strict glucose control algorithms [40]. Tight glycemic control appears to be effective in significantly reducing rates of DSWI. [30, 103]. In addition, Lazar et al demonstrated improved coronary surgery outcomes with a strategy for strict glucose control (125 - 200 mg/dL) using glucose-insulin-potassium solution, including reduced ischemic events and improved rates of wound infection in a cohort of diabetic patients undergoing CABG [31].

Antimicrobial therapy has also positively impacted rates of DSWI. Most notably, appropriate timing and selection of preoperative antibiotics has been associated with reduced rates of sugical site infection [6, 104]. Furthermore, use of nasal mupirocin in patients undergoing cardiac surgery via median sternotomy eradicates 95 - 100% of *S. aureus* for up to one year postoperatively [105], and sternal wound infections are also reduced by nearly 2/3 in some series with the use of mupirocin in patients colonized with *S. aureus* [106, 107].

Technical details of the median sternotomy incision and closure almost certainly impact the likelihood for DSWI postoperatively. Baskett et al have argued that assiduously following technical details and proper surgical and aseptic techniques can also dramatically reduce rates of poststernotomy infection [42]. They emphasize the importance of accurate reapproximation of the sternal halves and caution against the use of bone wax to gain sternal hemostasis [42]. Since sternal instability is often evoked as one mechanism contributing to the development of sternal infection, evaluation of the most effective sternal closure methods has been undertaken. For example, Schimmer et al compared standard closure techniques by transsternal or peristernal wiring with techniques using additional lateral wire reinforcement in the method described by Robicsek in a cohort of 815 high-risk patients [108]. There were no differences observed in the rates of sternal dehiscence or superficial or deep sternal wound infections, but they did show that more sternal wires placed for closure was associated with significantly reduced rates of DSWI [108]. Others have emphasized that rigid sternal closure techniques are preferred, particularly in those considered at high risk for sternal wound complications such as dehiscence and infection. These techniques are widely used in most surgical practices that incorporate osteotomy incisions. In fact, cardiac surgery is now the only discipline not routinely repairing osteotomies with rigid plating techniques [109]. Lee et al recently reported their experience with titanium plate fixation of the sternum in 750 patients at high risk for sternal wound complications, noting 97.6% freedom from sternal infection or dehiscence [110]. Levin et al have also introduced another form of rigid sternal closure as an alterntive to wire circlage and highlighted advantages to this approach [111]. Although rigid sternal closure techniques have not been compared prospectively with wire circlage, cadaveric studies have shown rigid plate fixation techniques to be superior to wire circlage by providing increased stiffness to the wound closure and less lateral displacement of the sternal halves [112].

Other suggested techniques for reducing the incidence of DSWI include ensuring true midline sternotomy as this is thought to preserve periosteal blood flow and limits transverse sternal fractures which contribute to sternal nonunionn and instability [42, 44]. Since sternal ischemia is thought to play an important role in most cases of DSWI, limiting the length of internal mammary artery harvested for use as a coronary artery bypass conduit or avoiding its use altogether in prohibitively high risk patients may help to reduce DSWI [44]. Harvesting the internal mammary artery as a skeletonized conduit is also preferable to harvesting the graft as a pedicle since this preserves more peristernal blood flow [113]. Finally, sternal foreign bodies that may impede bony union, especially bone wax, should be avoided [42, 44]. In contrast, vancomycin paste or gentamicin-soaked absorbable sponges applied to the sternum upon closure have been shown to reduce rates of sternal bacterial contamination [114, 115]. However a more recent randomized controlled trial evaluating the impact of gentamicin-soaked collagen sponge on poststernotomy wound infection did not show an advantage of this approach over controls [116].

Based on the aforementioned successes with NPT in the treatment of documented DSWI we and others have recently evaluated the application of NPT to clean, closed incisions as a method to prevent complications in high-risk wounds [117, 118]. We initially applied this form of "well wound therapy" in a cohort of 57 adult cardiac surgery patients known to be at increased risk for DSWI based on a validated risk stratification model [13]. No cases of superficial or deep sternal wound infections were noted although the group had an estimated 6% risk for DSWI [118]. This form of NPT was noted to be easy to apply, well-tolerated by the patients, and was also judged to be cost-effective when utilized in patients with increased demonstrated risk for DSWI [117]. Since the time of the original report, we have used this novel wound treatment system in over 200 high risk patients and continue to observe reduce rates of sternal wound complications (unpublished data). However, residual problems have been encountered with gross technical errors including off-center sternal incisions, sternal fractures, and costo-sternal separation.

The mechanisms underlying such positive clinical findings are not well understood, but based on well described mechanisms of vacuum-assisted therapy in open incisions, it is hypothesized that applying NPT to the closed incision also favorably affects wound perfusion. Therefore, we assessed peristernal perfusion after median sternotomy and under various degrees of reduced native sternal perfusion as a result of mammary artery harvesting using laser Doppler flowmetry, demonstrating that after median sternotomy and IMA harvesting, peristernal perfusion is significantly reduced and recovers little in the first 4 postoperative days [119]. However, NPT applied to the closed incision increases peristernal perfusion compared with controls regardless of the status of the ipsilateral IMA, providing a rare piece of physiologic evidence for the efficacy of NPT and supports use of NPT as a form of "well wound therapy," particularly in patients at high-risk for sternotomy complications [119] These findings are clinically important and relevant, implying that NPT can augment peristernal soft tissue perfusion made relatively ischemic by IMA harvesting. Although this study does not address bony perfusion, per se, Fokin et al proposed that substrate diffusion through peristernal tissues may be an important mechanism to maintain perfusion in sternal wounds rendered ischemic by mammary artery harvesting until collateral blood supply to the sternum is well-established [120, 121]. If so, NPT may indeed augment sternal and/or periosteal perfusion via improved peristernal "diffusion" through improved soft tissue perfusion.

14. Conclusions

Deep sternal wound infections remain dreaded and deadly complications associated with cardiac surgery. However, incremental improvements have been made recently with regard to lowering rates of observed infections due to a variety of measures. In addition, it appears that management of DSWI with negative pressure therapy alleviates the impact of this condition on short- and long-term survival. Further investigation is needed to determine the potential impact of negative pressure therapy on closed incisions as a novel method to prevent sternal wound complications.

15. References

[1] Durrleman N, Massard G. Sternotomy. Multimedia Manual Cardio Thorac doi:10.1510/mmcts.2006.001875.

[2] Hollenbeak CS, Murphy DM, Koenig S, Woodward RS, Dunagan WC, Fraser VJ. The clinical and economic impact of deep chest surgical site infections following coronary artery bypass graft surgery. Chest 2000; 118: 397-402.

[3] Taylor GJ, Mikell FL, Moses HW, et al. Determinants of hospital charges for coronary artery bypass surgery: the economic consequences of postoperative complications. Am J Cardiol 1990; 65: 309-13.

[4] Speir AM, Kasirajan V, Barnett SD, Fonner E, Jr. Additive costs of postoperative complications for isolated coronary artery bypass grafting patients in Virginia. Ann Thorac Surg 2009; 88: 40-6.

[5] Loop FD, Lytle BW, Cosgrove DM, et al. Maxwell Chamberlain memorial paper. Sternal wound complications after isolated coronary artery bypass grafting: early and late mortality, morbidity, and cost of care. Ann Thorac Surg 1990; 49: 179-87.

[6] Eklund AM, Lyytikainen O, Klemets P, et al. Mediastinitis after more than 10,000 cardiac surgical procedures. Ann Thorac Surg 2006; 82: 1784-9.

[7] Karra R, McDermott L, Connelly S, Smith P, Sexton DJ, Kaye KS. Risk factors for 1-year mortality after postoperative mediastinitis. J Thorac Cardiovasc Surg 2006; 132: 537-43.

[8] Braxton JH, Marrin CAS, McGrath PD, Ross CS, Morton JR, Norotsky M, Charlesworth DC, Lahey SJ, Clough RA, O'Connor GT. Mediastinitis and long-term survival after coronary artery bypass graft surgery. Ann Thorac Surg 2000; 70: 2004-7.

[9] Milano CA, Kesler K, Archibald N, Sexton DJ, Jones RH. Mediastinitis after coronary artery bypass graft surgery. Risk factors and long-term survival. Circulation 1995; 92: 2245-51.

[10] Olsen MA, Lock-Buckley P, Hopkins D, Polish LB, Sundt TM, Fraser VJ. The risk factors for deep and superficial chest surgical-site infections after coronary artery bypass graft surgery are different. J Thorac Cardiovasc Surg 2002; 124: 136-45.

[11] Baillot R, Cloutier D, Montalin L, et al. Impact of deep sternal wound infection management with vacuum-assisted closure therapy followed by sternal osteosynthesis: a 15-year review of 23,499 sternotomies. Eur J Cardiothorac Surg 2010; 37: 880-7.

[12] Risnes I, Abdelnoor M, Almdahl SM, Svennevig JL. Mediastinitis after coronary artery bypass grafting risk factors and long-term survival. Ann Thorac Surg 2010; 89: 1502-10.

[13] Fowler VG Jr, O'Brien SM, Muhlbaier LH, Corey GR, Ferguson TB, Peterson ED. Clinical predictors of major infections after cardiac surgery. Circulation 2005; 112 [Suppl 1]: I-358-65.

[14] Atkins BZ, Onaitis MO, Hutcheson KA, Kaye K, Petersen RP, Wolfe WG. Does method of sternal repair influence long-term outcome of postoperative mediastinitis? Am J Surg 2011. In Press.

[15] Sjogren J, Malmsjo M, Gustafsson R, Ingemansson R. Poststernotomy mediastinitis: a review of conventional srugical treatments, vacuum-assisted closure therapy and presentation of the Lund University Hospital mediastinitis algorithm. Eur J Cardiothorac Surg 2006; 30: 898-905.

[16] Domkowski PW, Smith ML, Gonyon DL Jr, et al. Evaluation of vacuum-assisted closure in the treatment of post-sternotomy mediastinitis. J Thorac Cardiovasc Surg 2003; 126: 386-90.

[17] Milton H. Mediastinal surgery. Lancet 1897; 1: 872-5.

[18] Shumacker HB, Jr, Lurie PR. Pulmonary valvulotomy: description of a new approach about diagnostic characteristics of pulmonic valvular stenosis. J Thorac Surg 1953: 25: 173-86.

[19] Julian OC, Lopez-Belio M, Dye WS, Javid H, Grove WJ. The median sternal incision in intracardiac surgery with extracorporeal circulation: a general evaluation of its use in heart surgery. Surgery 1957; 42: 753-61.

[20] Raman J, Straus D, Song DH. Rigid plate fixation of the sternum. Ann Thorac Surg 2007; 84: 1056-8.

[21] McGinn JT Jr, Usman S, Lapierre H, Pothula VR, Mesana TG, Ruel M. Minimally invasive coronary artery bypass grafting: dual-center experience in 450 consecutive patients. Circulation 2009; 120: S78-84.

[22] de Canniere D, Wimmer-Greinecker G, Cichon R, et al. Feasibility, safety, and efficacy of totally endoscopic coronary artery bypass grafting: multicenter European experience. J Thorac Cardiovasc Surg 2007; 134: 710-6.

[23] El Oakley RM, Wright JE. Postoperative mediastinitis: classification and management. Ann Thorac Surg 1996; 61: 1030-6.

[24] Olbrecht VA, Barreiro CJ, Bonde PN, et al. Clinical outcomes of noninfectious sternal dehiscence after median sternotomy. Ann Thorac Surg 2006; 82: 902-7.

[25] Horan TC, Andrus M, Dudeck MA. CDC/NHSN surveillance definition of health care-associated infection and criteria for specific types of infections in the acute care setting. Am J Infect Control 2008; 36: 309-32.

[26] Jones G, Jurkiewicz MJ, Bostwick, et al. Management of the infected median sternotomy wound with muscle flaps. Ann Surg 1997; 225: 766-78.

[27] Schulman NH, Subramanian V. Sternal wound reconstruction: 252 consecutive cases. The Lenox Hill experience. Plast Reconstr Surg 2004; 114: 44-8.

[28] Jakob HJ, Borneff-Lipp M, Bach A, et al. The endogenous pathway is a major route for deep sternal wound infection. Eur J Cardiothorac Surg 2000; 17: 154-60.

[29] Kluytmans JA, Mouton JW, VandenBergh MF, et al. Reduction of surgical-site infections in cardiothoracic surgery by elimination of nasal carriage of Staphylococcus aureus. Infect Control Hosp Epidemiol 1996; 17: 780-5.

[30] Furnary AP, Gao G, Grunkemeier GL, et al. Continuous insulin infusion reduces mortality in patients with diabetes undergoing coronary artery bypass grafting. J Thorac Cardiovasc Surg 2003; 125: 1007-21.
[31] Lazar HL, Chipkin SR, Fitzgerald CA, Bao Y, Cabral H, Apstein CS. Tight glycemic control in diabetic coronary artery bypass graft patients improves perioperative outcomes and decreases recurrent ischemic events. Circulation 2004; 109: 1497-502.
[32] Prabhakar G, Haan CK, Peterson ED, Coombs LP, Cruzzavala JL, Murray CF. The risks of moderate and extreme obesity for coronary artery bypass grafting outcomes: a study from the Society of Thoracic Surgeons' database. Ann Thorac Surg 2002; 74: 1125-31.
[33] Eagle KA, Guyton RA, Davidoff R, et al. ACC/AHA 2004 guideline update for coronary artery bypass graft surgery: a report of the American College of Cardiology/American Heart Association Task Force on Practice Guidelines (Committee to Update the 1999 Guidelines for Coronary Artery Bypass Graft Surgery.) American College of Cardiology Web Site. Available at http://www.acc.org/clinical/guidelines/cabg/cabg.pdf
[34] Waisbren E, Rosen H, Bader AM, Lipsitz SR, Rogers SO, Eriksson E. Percent body fat and prediction of surgical site infection. J Am Coll Surg 2010; 210: 381-9.
[35] Filsoufi, F, Castillo JG, Rahmanian PB, et al. Epidemiology of deep sternal wound infection in cardiac surgery. J Cardiothorac Vasc Anesth 2009; 23: 488-94.
[36] Pevni D, Uretzky G, Mohr A, et al. Routine use of bilateral skeletonized internal thoracic artery grafting: long-term results. Circulation 2008; 118: 705-12.
[37] Graeber GM, McClelland WT. Current concepts in the management and reconstruction of the dehisced median sternotomy. Semin Thorac Cardiovasc Surg 2004; 16: 92-107.
[38] Ariyaratnam P, Bland M, Loubani M. Risk factors and mortality associated with deep sternal wound infections following coronary bypass surgery with or without concomitant procedures in a UK population: a basis for a new risk mode? Interact Cardiovasc Thorac Surg 2010; 11: 543-6.
[39] Paul M, Raz A, Leibovici L, Madar H, Holinger R, Rubinovitch B. Sternal wound infection after coronary artery bypass graft surgery: validation of existing risk scores. J Thorac Cardiovasc Surg 2007; 133: 397-403.
[40] Matros E, Aranki SF, Bayer LR, et al. Reduction in incidence of deep sternal wound infections: random or real? J Thorac Cardiovasc Surg 2010; 139: 680-5.
[41] Ridderstolpe L, Gill H, Granfeldt H, Ahlfeldt H, Rutberg H. Superficial and deep sternal wound complications: incidence, risk factors, and mortality. Eur J CTS 2001; 20: 1168-75.
[42] Baskett RJF, MacDougall CE, Ross DB. Is mediastinitis a preventable complication? A 10-year review. Ann Thorac Surg 1999; 67: 462-5.
[43] Blanchard A, Hurni M, Ruchat P, Stumpe F, Fischer A, Sadeghi H. Incidence of deep and superficial sternal infection after open heart surgery. A ten years retrospective study from 1981 to 1991. Eur J Cardiothorac Surg 1995; 9: 153-7.
[44] Francel TJ. A rational approach to sternal wound complications. Semin Thorac Cardiovasc Surg 2004; 16: 81-91.

[45] Cowan KN, Teague L, Sue SC, Mahoney JL. Vacuum-assisted wound closure of deep sternal infections in high-risk patients after cardiac surgery. Ann Thorac Surg 2005; 80: 2205-12.
[46] Goodman LR, Kay HR, Teplick SK, Mundth ED. Complications of median sternotomy: computed tomographic evaluation. Am J Roentgenol 1983; 141: 225-30.
[47] Yamashiro et al; and Misawa Y, Fuse K, Hasegawa T. Infectious mediastinitis after cardiac operations: computed tomographic findings. Ann Thorac Surg 1998; 65: 622-4.
[48] Yamashiro T, Kamiya H, Murayama S, et al. Infectious mediastinitis after cardiovascular surgery: role of computed tomography. Radiat Med 2008; 26: 343-7.
[49] Hoffman SN, TenBrook JA Jr., Wolf MP, Pauker SG, Salem DN, Wong JB. A meta-analysis of randomized controlled trials comparing coronary artery bypass graft with percutaneous transluminal coronary angioplasty: one-to eight-year outcomes. J Am Coll Cardiol 2003; 41: 1293-304.
[50] Sarr MG, Gott VL, Townsend TR. Mediastinal infection after cardiac surgery. Ann Thorac Surg 1984; 38: 415-23.
[51] Sachithanandan A, Nanjaiah P, Nightingale P, et al. Deep sternal wound infection requiring revision surgery: impact on mid-term survival following cardiac surgery. Eur J Cardiothorac Surg 2008; 33: 673-8.
[52] Cayci C, Russo M, Cheema FH, et al. Risk analysis of deep sternal wound infections and their impact on long-term survival: a propensity analysis. Ann Plast Surg 2008; 61: 294-301.
[53] Morisaki A, Hosono M, Sasaki Y, et al. Evaluation of risk factors for hospital mortality and current treatment for poststernotomy mediastinitis. Gen Thorac Cardiovasc Surg 2011; 59: 261-7.
[54] Braxton JH, Marrin CAS, McGrath, et al. 10-year follow-up of patients with and without mediastinitis. Semin Thorac Cardiovas Surg 2004; 16: 70-6.
[55] Toumpoulis IK, Anagnostopoulos CE, Derose JJ Jr, Swistel DG. The impact of deep sternal wound infection on long-term survival after coronary artery bypass grafting. Chest 2005; 127: 464-71.
[56] Stahle E, Tammelin A, Bergstrom R, Hanbreus A, Nystrom SO, Hansson HE. Sternal wound complications-incidence, microbiology, and risk factors. Eur J Cardiothorac Surg 1997; 11: 1146-53.
[57] Chu D, Bakaeen FG, Wang XL, et al. The impact of peripheral vascular disease on long-term survival after coronary artery bypass graft surgery. Ann Thorac Surg 2008; 86: 1175-80.
[58] Tang GHL, Maganti M, Weisel RD, Borger MA. Prevention and management of deep sternal wound infection. Semin Thorac Cardiovasc Surg 2004; 16: 62-9.
[59] Lin CH, Hsu RB, Chang SC, Lin FY, Chu SH. Poststernotomy mediastinitis due to methicillin-resistent Staphylococcus aureus endemic in a hospital. Clin Infect Dis 2003; 37: 679-84.
[60] Gardlund B, Bitkover C, Vaage J. Postoperative mediastinitis in cardiac surgery-microbiology and pathogenesis. Eur J Cardiothorac Surg 2002; 21: 825-30.
[61] Mekontso-Dessap A, Kirsch M, Brun-Buisson C, Loisance D. Poststernotomy mediastinitis due to Staphylococcus aureus: comparison of methicillin-resistent and methicillin-susceptible cases. Clin Infect Dis 2001; 32: 877-83.

[62] Tegnell A, Aren C, Ohman L. Coagulase-negative staphylococi and sternal infections after cardiac operation. Ann Thorac Surg 2000; 69: 1104-9.

[63] Mekontso Dessap A, Vivier E, Girou E, Brun-Buisson C, Kirsch M. Effect of time to onset on clinical features and prognosis of post-sternotomy mediastinitis. Clin Microbiol Infect 2011; 17: 292-9.

[64] Graf K, Ott E, Vonberg RP, Kuehn C, Haverich A, Chaberny IF. Economic aspects of deep sternal wound infections. Eur J Cardiothorac Surg 2010; 37: 893-6.

[65] Mokhtari A, Sjogren J, Nilsson J, Gustafsson R, Malmsjo M, Ingemansson R. The cost of vacuum-assisted closure therapy in treatment of deep sternal wound infection. Scand Cardiovasc J 2008; 42: 85-9.

[66] Center for Medicare and Medicaid Services; http://www.cms.hhs.gov/HospitalAcqCond/

[67] O'Reilly KB. Medicare's no-pay events: coping with the complications. http://www.ama-assn.org/amednews/2008/07/14/prsa0714.htm

[68] Obdeijn MC, de Lange MY, Lichtendahl DH, et al. Vacuum-assisted closure in the treatment of poststernotomy mediastinitis. Ann Thorac Surg 1999; 68: 2358-60.

[69] Luckraz H, Murphy F, Bryant S, Charman SC, Ritchie AJ. Vacuum-assisted closure as a treatment modality for infections after cardiac surgery. J Thorac Cardiovasc Surg 2003; 125: 301-5.

[70] Malmsjo M, Ingemansson R, Sjogren J. Mechanisms governing the effects of vacuum-assisted closure in cardiac surgery. Plast Reconstr Stur 2007; 120: 1266-75.

[71] Schimmer C, Sommer SP, Bensch M, Elert O, Leyh R. Management of poststernotomy mediastinitis: experience and results of different therapy modalities. Thorac Cardiovasc Surg 2008; 56: 200-4.

[72] Cabbabe EB, Cabbabe SW. Immediate versus delayed one-stage sternal debridement and pectoralis muscle flap reconstruction of deep sternal wound infections. Plast Reconstr Surg 2009; 123: 1490-4.

[73] Orgill DP, Austen WG Jr, Butler CE, et al. Guidelines for treatment of complex chest wounds with negative pressure wound therapy. WOUNDS 2004; Suppl B: 1-23.

[74] Schumaker HB, Mandelbaum I. Continuous antibiotic irrigation in the treatment of infection. Arch Surg 1963: 86; 384-7.

[75] Lee AB, Schimert G, Shaktin S, et al. Total excision of the sternum and thoracic pedicle transposition of the greater omentum; useful stratagems in managing severe mediastinal infection following open heart surgery. Surgery 1976; 80: 433-6.

[76] Kutsal A, Ibrisim E, Catav Z, et al. Mediastinitis after open heart surgery. Analysis of risk factors and management. J Cardiovasc Surg (Torino) 1991; 32: 38-41.

[77] van Wingerden JJ, Coret ME, van Nieuwenhoven CA Totte ER. The laparoscopically harvested omental flap for deep sternal wound infection. Eur J Cardiothorac Surg 2010; 37: 87-92.

[78] Jurkiewicz MJ, Bostwick J, hester TR, et al. Infected median sternotomy wound. Successful treatment by muscle flaps. Ann Surg 1980; 191: 738-44.

[79] Nahai F, Rand RP, Hester TR, et al. Primary treatment of the infected sternotomy wound with muscle flaps: a review of 211 consecutive cases. Plast Reconstr Surg 1989; 84: 434-41.

[80] Milano CA, Georgiade G, Muhlbaier LH, Smith PK, Wolfe WG. Comparison of omental and pectoralis flaps for poststernotomy mediastinitis. Ann Thorac Surg 1999; 67: 377-81.

[81] Yuen JC, Zhou AT, Serafin DT, et al. Long-term sequelae following median sternotomy wound infection and flap reconstruction. Ann Plast Surg 1995; 35: 585-9.

[82] Ringelman PR, Vander KC, Cameron D, Bumgartner WA, Manson PN. Long-term results of flap reconstruction in median sternotomy wound infection. Plast Reconstr Surg 1994; 93: 1208-14.

[83] Gottlieb LJ, Pielet RW, Karp RB, Krieger LM, Smith DJ Jr, Deeb GM. Rigid internal fixation of the sternum in postoperative mediastinitis. Arch Surg 1994; 129: 489-93.

[84] Douville EC, Asaph JW, Dworkin RJ, et al. Sternal preservation: a better way to treat most sternal wound complications after cardiac surgery. Ann Thorac Surg 2004; 78: 1659-64.

[85] Chen SZ, Li J, Li XY, et al. Effects of vacuum-assisted closure on wound mcrocirculation: an experimental study. Asian J Surg 2005; 28: 211-7.

[86] Wackenfors A, Gustafsson R, Sjogren J, et al. Blood flow responses in the peristernal thoracic wall during vacuum-assisted closure therapy. Ann Thorac Surg 2005; 79: 1724-30.

[87] Saxena V, Hwang C-W, Huang S, Eichbaum Q, Ingber D, Orgill DP. Vacuum-assisted closure: microdeformations of wounds and cell proliferation. Plast Reconstr Surg 2004; 114: 1086-96.

[88] Gustafsson RI, Sjogren J, Ingemansson R. Deep sternal wound infection: a sternal-sparing technique with vacuum-assisted closure therapy. Ann Thorac Surg 2003; 76: 2048-53.

[89] Petzina R, Hoffmann J, Navasardyan A, et al. Negative pressure wound theapy for post-sternotomy mediastinitis reduces mortality rate and sternal re-infection rate compared to conventional treatment. Eur J Cardiothorac Surg 2010; 38: 110-3.

[90] Sjogren J, Gustafsson R, Nilsson J, Malmsjo M, Ingemansson R. Clinical outcome after poststernotomy mediastinitis: vacuum-assisted closure versus conventional treatment. Ann Thorac Surg 2005; 79: 2049-55.

[91] Gaudreau G, Costache V, Houde C, et al. Recurrent sternal infection following treatment with negative pressure wound therapy and titanium transverse plate fixation. Eur J Cardiothorac Surg 2010; 37: 888-92.

[92] De Feo M, Della Corte A, Vicchio M, Pirozzi F, Nappi G, Cotrufo M. Is post-sternotomy mediastinitis still devastating after the advent of negative-pressure wound therapy? Tex Heart Inst J 2011; 38: 375-80.

[93] Sjogren J, Nilsson J, Gustafsson R, Malmsjo M, Ingemansson R. The impact of vacuum-assisted closure on long-term survival after post-sternotomy mediastinitis. Ann Thorac Surg 2005; 80: 1270-75.

[94] Immer FF, Durrer Muhlemann KS, Erni D, Gahl B, Carrrel TP. Deep sternal wound infection after cardiac surgery: modality of treatment and outcome. Ann Thorac Surg 2005; 80: 957-61.

[95] Gustafsson R, Johnsson P, Algotsson L, Blomquist S, Ingemansson R. Vacuum-assisted closure therapy guided by C-reactive protein level in patients with deep sternal wound infection. J Thorac Cardiovasc Surg 2002; 123: 895-900.

[96] Voss B, Bauernschmitt R, Will A, et al. Sternal reconstruction with titanium plates in complicated sternal dehiscence. Eur J Cardiothorac Surg 2008; 34: 139-45.

[97] Ramnarine IR, McLean A, Pollock JC. Vacuum-assisted closure in the paediatric patient with post-cardiotomy mediastinitis. Eur J Cardiothorac Surg 2002; 22: 1029-31.

[98] Kaye AE, Kaye AJ, Pahk B, McKenna ML, Low DW. Sternal wound reconstruction: management in different cardiac populations. Ann Plast Surg 2010; 64: 658-66.

[99] Bapat V, El-Muttardi N, Yound C, Venn G, Roxburgh J. Experience with vacuum-assisted closure of sternal wound infections following cardiac surgery and evaluation of chronic complications associated with its use. J Card Surg 2008; 23: 227-33.

[100] Petzina R, Malmsjo M, Stamm C, Hetzer R. Major complications during negative pressure wound therapy in poststernotomy mediastinitis after cardiac surgery. J Thorac Cardiovasc Surg 2010; 140: 1133-6.

[101] Malmsjo M, Lindstedt S, Ingemansson R. Effects on heart pumping function when using foam and gauze for negative pressure wound therapy of sternotomy wounds. J Cardiothorac Surg 2011; 6: 5.

[102] Torbrand C, Ugander M, Engblom H, et al. Changes in cardiac pumping efficiency and intra-thoracic organ volume during negative pressure wound therapy of sternotomy wounds, assessment using magnetic resonance imaging. Int Wound J 2010; 7: 305-11.

[103] Kramer R, Groom R, Weldner D, et al. Glycemic control and reduction of deep sternal wound infection rates. Arch Surg 2008; 143: 451-6.

[104] Bratzler DW, Houck PM for the Surgical Infection Prevention Guidelines Writers Workgroup. Antimicrobial prophylaxis for surgery: an advisory statement from the National Surgical Infection Prevention Project. Clin Infect Dis 2004; 38: 1706-15.

[105] Perl TM, Golub JE. New approaches to reduce *Staphylococcus aureus* nosocomial infection rate: treating aureus nasal carriage. Ann Pharmacother 1998; 32: S7-16.

[106] Cimochowski G, harostock M, Brown R, et al. Intranasal mupirocin reduces sternal wound infection after open heart surgery in diabetics and nondiabetics. Ann Thorac Surg 2001; 71: 1572-9.

[107] Carrier M, Marchand R, Auger P, et al. Methicillin-resistant *Staphylococcus aureus* infection in a cardiac surgical unit. J Thorac Cardiovasc Surg 2002; 123: 40-4.

[108] Schimmer C, Reents W, Berneder S, et al. Prevention of sternal dehiscence and infection in high-risk patients: a prospective randomized multicenter trial. Ann Thorac Surg 2008; 86: 1897-904.

[109] Song DH, Lohman RF, Renucci JD, Jeevanandam V, Raman J. Primary sternal plating in high-risk patients prevents mediastinitis. Eur J Cardiothorac Surg 2004; 26: 367-72.

[110] Lee JC, Raman J, Song DH. Primary sternal closure with titanium plate fixation: plastic surgery effecting a paradigm shift. Plast Reconstr Surg 2010; 125: 1720-4.

[111] Levin LS, Miller AS, Gajjar AH, et al. An innovative approach for sternal closure. Ann Thorac Surg 2010; 89: 1995-9.

[112] Ozaki W, Buchman SR, Iannettoni MD, Frankenburg EP. Biomechanical study of sternal closure using rigid fixation techniques in human cadavers. Ann Thorac Surg 1998; 65: 1660-5.

[113] Kamiya H, Akhyari P, Martens A, Karck M, Haverich A, Lichtenberg A. Sternal microcirculation after skeletonized versus pedicled harvesting of the internal thoracic artery: a randomized study. J Thorac Cardiovasc Surg 2008; 135: 32-7.
[114] Friberg O, Svedjeholm R, Soderquist B, Granfeldt H, Vikerfors T, Kallman J. Local gentamicin reduces sternal wound infections after cardiac surgery: a randomized controlled trial. Ann Thorac Surg 2005; 79: 153-62.
[115] Vander Salm T, Okike O, Pasque M, et al. Reduction of sternal infection by application of topical vancomycin. J Thorac Cardiovasc Surg 1989; 98: 618-22.
[116] Bennett-Guerrero E, Ferguson TB Jr, Lin M, et al. Effect of an implantable gentamicin-collagen sponge on sternal wound infections following cardiac surgery. JAMA 2010; 304: 755-62.
[117] Stannard JP, Atkins BZ, O'Malley D, et al. Use of negative pressure therapy on closed surgical incisions: a case series. Ostomy Wound Manage 2009; 55: 58-66.
[118] Atkins BZ, Wooten MK, Kistler J, Hurley K, Hughes GC, Wolfe WG. Does negative pressure wound therapy have a role in preventing poststernotomy wound complications? Surg Innov 2009; 16: 140-6.
[119] Atkins BZ, Tetterton JK, Petersen RP, Hurley K, Wolfe WG. Laser Doppler flowmetry assessment of peristernal perfusion after cardiac surgery: beneficial effect of negative pressure therapy. Int Wound J 2011; 8: 56-62.
[120] Fokin AA, Robicsek F, Masters TN, Fokin A Jr, Reames MK, Anderson JE, Jr. Sternal nourishment in various conditions of vascularization. Ann Thorac Surg 2005; 79: 1352-7.
[121] Medalion B, Katz MG, Lorberboym M, Bder O, Schachner A, Cohen AJ. Decreased sternal vascularity after internal thoracic artery harvesting resolves with time: an assessment with single photon emission computed tomography. J Thorac Cardiovasc Surg 2002; 123: 508-11.